LEARNING DISABILITY NURSING

Modern Day Practice

LEARNING DISABILITY NURSING

Modern Day Practice

Bob Gates

Professor of Learning Disabilities, University of West London, Institute for Practice, Interdisciplinary Research and Enterprise (INSPIRE); Emeritus Professor, The Centre for Learning Disability Studies, University of Hertfordshire; and Honorary Professor of Learning Disabilities, Hertfordshire Partnership University NHS Foundation Trust, United Kingdom.

Kay Mafuba

University of West London, United Kingdom

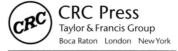

CRC Press
Taylor & Francis Group
Boca Raton   London   New York

CRC Press is an imprint of the
Taylor & Francis Group, an **informa** business

CRC Press
Taylor & Francis Group
6000 Broken Sound Parkway NW, Suite 300
Boca Raton, FL 33487-2742

Printed on acid-free paper
Version Date: 20141103

International Standard Book Number-13: 978-1-4822-1558-8 (Paperback)

Visit the Taylor & Francis Web site at
http://www.taylorandfrancis.com

and the CRC Press Web site at
http://www.crcpress.com

Contents

Preface

In recent years, learning disability nursing has moved from a narrowly defined role, within long-term care, to a much broader role within the National Health Service in the United Kingdom, and beyond. Hence, there is a need for a brand new learning disability textbook that will inform students and practitioners alike of the continued development of modern-day learning disability nursing roles. Roles that span community support specialists, liaison roles between services and agencies, transitional roles, and roles in secure or forensic health settings offer support across the age continuum. Learning disability nursing is a health profession supported and endorsed by many, as unique in its breadth of employment base, and located as it is among the various sectors of the health and social care economies. Uniquely, the content of this book has been benchmapped against current Nursing and Midwifery Councils for the United Kingdom (2010) and An Bord Altranais, Ireland (2005) standards for competence for each chapter. The nomenclature for identifying competences, competencies and indicators uses a numbering system that can be found in Appendices A and B, and these relate to those corresponding competencies and indicators identified at the commencement of each chapter. Also at the commencement of each chapter is a helpful box that identifies the content that the chapter will focus on, along with further reading and resources given at the end of each chapter.

A note at the outset on terminology used in this text, generally speaking, within the United Kingdom, the term *learning disability* is used to describe that group of people who have significant developmental delay resulting in arrested or incomplete achievement of the 'normal' milestones of human development. Other terms are used elsewhere, such as developmental disability and intellectual disability, and in the past, mental retardation and mental handicap were widely used. Notwithstanding the wide variety of terminology, we have chosen to adopt the term *learning disability* throughout this book as we believe it is still the more widely used term in the United Kingdom. Therefore, throughout the text, the term *learning disability* is used; save where certain Acts and/or other technical works require us to use another term for accuracy.

In the first chapter, the nature and manifestation of learning disabilities, along with their relationship to learning disability nursing are explored. The second half of this chapter explores learning disability nursing, and its strong value base, and long relationship in supporting people with learning disabilities, their families and services, and how they can contribute to the health and well-being of people with learning disabilities – making a small but nonetheless valuable contribution in improving the quality of lives for this group of often marginalised and vulnerable group of people.

In Chapter 2, the long and complex history and tradition of how learning disability nurses have supported, and continue to offer support to, people with learning disabilities and their families is further explored, and in more detail.

In Chapter 3, the nature of learning disability throughout the lifespan and its relationship to learning disability nursing are explored. Learning disability is a lifelong condition, and therefore it is not unusual for learning disability nurses to work with, and/or offer support to people with learning disabilities throughout their lifespan, quite literally from the cradle to the grave. Holistic approaches in learning disability nursing seek to promote interventions that adopt a whole person–centred approach are promoted. This means providing nursing that responds to the various dimensions of being, and these typically include attention to the physical, emotional, social, economic and spiritual needs of people. Therefore, this chapter focuses on the knowledge as well as the kinds of practical skills that learning disability nurses will need when working with people with learning disabilities across their lifespan. The role of the learning disability nurse during childhood and adolescence of people with learning disabilities is explored in the context of diagnosis of learning disability, parenting children with learning disabilities, transitioning, psychological and physical changes during adolescence and transition into adulthood. The lifestyle and health needs of adults and older adults with learning disabilities, employment and retirement, personal relationships and parenting needs of adults with learning disabilities are explored. The chapter concludes by exploring end-of-life care needs, decisions and palliative care for people with learning disabilities.

In Chapter 4, the key concepts and policies in public health are included as well as the key policy drivers that are refocusing nursing interventions to be centrally concerned with prevention of ill health. The role of learning disability nursing in helping people with learning disabilities plan for good health and well-being is explored in detail. Learning disability nurses' public health roles, and in particular the importance of health promotion in care planning, health facilitation and health action planning will be addressed, as well as newer roles such as health liaison nursing in primary care and acute settings. These roles are explored in the context of some well-known health issues such as cardiovascular fitness, obesity, epilepsy, mental ill health, sexuality, diets and smoking. It is pointed out that many of these conditions will require learning disability nurses to develop careful and imaginative ways of constructing nursing interventions to improve and/or maintain the health status of people with learning disabilities. This takes us to Chapter 5 where mental ill health in people with learning disabilities is outlined. It is well known that people with learning disabilities are at greater risk of developing mental health problems than is the general population. And because of the high prevalence of mental health problems in this population, there is need to prepare learning disability nurses to promote good mental health and well-being, and/or its maintenance in those who are particularly vulnerable. In this chapter, the nature of, and manifestations of, good mental health, as well as the manifestations of mental ill health, assessment tools used in nursing practice and how to conduct a mental state examination are all explored. A range of approaches to treatments is outlined, as well as the Care Programme Approach. Finally, relevant mental health legislation and assessment of mental capacity, Independent Mental Capacity Advocates (IMCAs), Deprivation of Liberty and safeguarding issues are outlined.

Chapter 6 outlines the nature of and special needs of people with profound learning disabilities and complex needs. It is pointed out that they likely represent one of the most marginalised and potentially vulnerable groups of people in any society. They are at continuing risk from social exclusion, and simultaneously experience poorer health than the rest of the population (Mansell, 2010). Therefore, arguably, the role of the learning disability nurse in supporting, and where necessary providing direct care for this group of people, is particularly relevant because of the high levels of dependence they may have on others throughout their lives. Nursing or directed social care should be regarded as a way of systematically planning and documenting interventions to meet the needs of and to support this group of people in all aspects of their lives. This chapter considers both the direct and the indirect roles of learning disability nurses in supporting and/or caring for this group of people.

Chapter 7 explores the key competencies, skills and the knowledge base required for learning disability nursing in forensic settings. It is pointed out that in learning disability the term *forensic* is usually applied, although not always, to people who have offended and been dealt with by the courts. In relation to those who have not offended, the term *forensic* is still applied to people with learning disabilities who present a significant risk to others, and who may commit an offence and those who have a significant history of self-harm. Learning disability nursing in forensic settings is a highly complex area of practice involving balancing the tensions between offering person-centred and therapeutic care, within a framework of a contemporary rights culture, and the need to manage risk within controlling systems and environments. People with learning disabilities and forensic histories have a diverse range of complex needs and their behaviours constitute a risk, and often result in offending that include arson, sexually inappropriate behaviour, physical aggression, destruction of property and self-harming behaviours. It is pointed out that causation of these behaviours is often extremely complex, with a multifactorial range of other contributory factors that includes dual diagnosis of mental disorder and learning disabilities, the presence of autism or Asperger syndrome, acquired brain injury and psychosocial issues such as dysfunctional family dynamics, abuse and institutionalisation.

In Chapter 8, community learning disability nursing is explored in some detail and depicts its practice as typically working with a wide cross section of people with learning disabilities and agencies. This chapter, therefore, explores current and changing roles of learning disability nurses working in the community. It is pointed out that, depending on local configuration of services, they can often occupy a number of new and exciting roles. Many, for example work as specialist practitioners, and will work on time-limited interventions that can include personal and sexual relationships in people with learning disabilities, challenging behaviours, teaching direct carers, managing groups, dealing with loss and bereavement issues, working in multidisciplinary teams, assessing individuals, supporting clients, working as epilepsy specialists, facilitating self-advocacy groups and helping people access mainstream services. This chapter will serve as a template for good care planning within the context of community learning disability teams and/or where nurses are attached to Local Authorities, NHS Trusts. Current health and social policy, for example, Clinical Commissioning, will inevitably make further demands on the development on everyday practice of learning disability nurses working in the community; seemingly the public health agenda is becoming central to the role of this group of health care workers.

In the penultimate chapter, the support of people with learning disabilities who present with challenging and/or distressed behaviour by learning disability nurses is presented. The chapter promotes the unique contribution that learning disability nursing can provide in promoting holistic support, whilst drawing from a strong value and professional base. It is pointed out that understanding challenging and/or distressed behaviour in people with learning disabilities is problematic, and managing such behaviours has been the subject of much past and recent controversy. This chapter asserts that the management and support of individuals with learning disabilities who present with challenging behaviours are of critical importance to learning disability nurses; this is because the collective professional integrity of this specialist field of nursing can easily be contaminated by the few who choose not to practice within an ethical and legal framework of nursing practice. Crucially, that is why this chapter focuses on the knowledge and practical skills that learning disability nurses will need to meet the needs of people with learning disabilities who present with challenging and/

or distressed behaviours. The final chapter contextualises the current and future roles of learning disability nursing within an arena of ever-changing health and social care political imperatives. This can be seen at policy level both nationally and internationally, and it is articulated that with the ever-growing move towards citizenship, and the importance of human rights, learning disability nursing needs to place itself carefully – both within the family of nursing – and yet simultaneously appeal to a complex landscape of human service organisations and the wider community of learning disability. This chapter briefly reflects on the past, but most importantly looks to the future of the modern learning disability nurse practitioner. It discusses issues affecting learning disability nursing, such as changing professional requirements, policy directions and ever-growing opportunities for learning disability nurses to assert their role in a widening practice arena.

We believe that *Learning Disability Nursing: Modern Day Practice* is destined to become a key nursing textbook – not only for the field of learning disability nursing practice but also more widely used by many professionals and students from a wide range of different professional and academic backgrounds who have an interest in the lives of those with learning disabilities. We earnestly hope that all who read this book find it helpful, and that its use will assist us in helping people with learning disabilities enjoy health and well-being in their lives.

REFERENCES

An Bord Altranais (2005) *Requirements and Standards for Nurse Registration Education Programmes* (3rd Edition). Dublin. An Bord Altranais.

Mansell, J (2010) *Raising Our Sights: Services for Adults with Profound Intellectual and Multiple Disabilities*. Kent. Tizard Centre.

Nursing and Midwifery Council (2010) *Standards for Pre-Registration Nursing Education*. London. NMC.

Authors

Bob Gates, MSc, PGCE (Social Anthropology), BEd (Hons), Dip. Nurs. (Lond), RNMH, RMN, Cert.Ed, RNT, is a professor of learning disabilities, University of West London, Institute for Practice, Interdisciplinary Research and Enterprise (INSPIRE). He is also an emeritus professor, the Centre for Learning Disability Studies, University of Hertfordshire, and an honorary professor of learning disabilities, Hertfordshire Partnership University NHS Foundation Trust. He has a long career of over 42 years in learning disabilities and is known nationally and internationally for his contribution to the field. During his career, he has held numerous positions across the United Kingdom in learning disability services, management and education settings. Recently, he worked at the University of Hertfordshire, where he established the Centre for Learning Disability Studies. He was the founding editor-in-chief of *Journal of Intellectual Disabilities* published by Sage, and he serves on numerous editorial boards of international journals. In January 2014, he was appointed editor-in-chief of the *British Journal of Learning Disabilities*. He is a patron for 'Friendly Bombs', a theatre group for people with learning disabilities based in Slough, and also patron for 'Razed Roof', an inclusive performing arts group based in Harlow. He has an extensive publication record that extends over 150 outputs including peer-reviewed articles, numerous textbooks, chapters, commentaries, commissioned research reports and editorials. His main research interests include advocacy, challenging behaviour, workforce issues, families, people with profound and complex needs, and the education and training of carers. He has been the holder of numerous research grants, and has recently been awarded one by the National Institute for Health Research for undertaking a randomised controlled feasibility trial of the 'Books Beyond Words' intervention to improve the management of epilepsy in people with learning disabilities. He is also currently working with the Department of Health on workforce issues and safer staffing in learning disability services.

Kay Mafuba, PhD, SEDA-PDF, MA, PGCertResearch, FellowHEA, PGCertLTHE, BA, RNT, RNLD, DipHE, is an associate professor of learning disabilities in the College of Nursing, Midwifery and Healthcare at the University of West London, London, United Kingdom. He has an MA in Health and Social Policy and a PhD in Health from the University of West London. His research interests are learning disabilities, public health policy, staffing and professional roles. He has a number of publications in these areas, and has extensive experience in teaching learning disabilities nursing, public health and research methods at both undergraduate and postgraduate levels.

Contributor

We are indebted to Mick Wolverson for his contribution of Chapter 7 to this book.

Michael Wolverson, BA (Hons), BSc (Hons), RNMH, MSc, PGCE, is a lecturer in learning disabilities at York University, United Kingdom. He has been involved with supporting people with a learning disability since 1983. He initially worked as a nursing assistant in a hospital in Sheffield before commencing learning disability nurse training in 1984 and qualifying in 1987. His career in nursing has covered a variety of roles including supporting those with complex needs in specialist units, community nursing, being a challenging behaviour nurse specialist and managing services. His practice roles have been based in Sheffield, Rotherham and Hull. He became involved with teaching at the University of Hull in 1998 before moving to York in 2002.

1

The nature of learning disabilities and their relationship to learning disability nursing

Bob Gates

INTRODUCTION

This chapter explores the nature and various manifestations of learning disabilities, along with their relationship to learning disability nursing. It commences by describing in some detail learning disabilities, along with criteria that are used in determining whether someone has learning disabilities, and this leads to defining what learning disabilities mean. This is sometimes difficult, as the term learning disability means different things to different people—not only in England and the United Kingdom, but also internationally (Gates, 2007). Furthermore, it will be shown that the term learning disability has different meanings between the many health and social care professionals, service agencies and other disciplines involved in supporting people with learning disabilities. Next, the chapter outlines some of the important issues surrounding the incidence and prevalence of learning disabilities. Distinctions will be made between pre-, peri-, and postnatal factors of causation. This is followed by an outline of causation, and some of the more common genetic and chromosomal abnormalities, and their manifestation, and the chapter will identify aspects of co-morbidity, and some of the health challenges that people with learning disabilities may experience because of these particular clinical manifestations. The second half of this chapter will then explore learning disability nursing, its strong value base, and its long relationship in supporting people with learning disabilities and their families. Also explored will be services, and how such services can contribute to the health and well-being of people with learning disabilities, making a small but nonetheless valuable contribution to improving the quality of lives for this often marginalised and vulnerable group of people. The content of this chapter is contextualised within the Nursing and Midwifery Council (NMC) of the United Kingdom (2010) and Ireland's An Bord Altranais (2005) standards for competence.

> **This chapter will focus on the following issues:**
>
> - Understanding learning disabilities: a conceptual minefield
> - Legislative definitions of learning disability
> - Adaptive ability or social (in)competence
> - Defining learning disability
> - Incidence and prevalence of learning disabilities

- Classification of learning disabilities
- Genetic causes of learning disabilities
- Chromosomal abnormalities
- Manifestation of autosomal abnormalities
  - Manifestation of sex-chromosome abnormalities
- Genetic abnormalities
- Autosomal dominant conditions
- Autosomal recessive conditions
- X-linked recessive conditions
- Environmental factors
- Infections
- Diagnosing learning disabilities
- Learning disability nursing
- Case history 1.1: Mohammad

Competences

NMC Competences and Competencies

Domain 1: Professional values - Field standard competence and competencies – 1.1; 2.1; 3.1; 4.1.

Domain 2: Communication and interpersonal skills - Field standard competence and competencies – 1.1; 2.1; 3.1.

Domain 3: Nursing practice and decision making - Field standard competence and competencies – 3.1; 5.1.

Domain 4: Leadership, management and team working - Field standard competence and competencies – 1.1; 1.2; 2.1; 6.1; 6.2.

An Bord Altranais Competences and Indicators

Domain 1: Professional/ethical practice – 1.1.4; 1.1.6; 1.1.8.

Domain 2: Holistic approaches to care and the integration of knowledge – 2.1.1; 2.1.2; 2.1.3; 2.2.1; 2.2.3; 2.4.1; 2.4.2; 3.1.3; 3.2.1; 3.2.2; 5.1.1; 5.1.2; 5.1.3.

UNDERSTANDING LEARNING DISABILITES: A CONCEPTUAL MINEFIELD

In this first section, learning disabilities, as a concept, is explored through a number of different lenses of interpretation. These include intelligence, legislation, social competence, and adaptive behaviour. This leads to an articulation of definitions about what this term means. It has been said that intelligence is an obvious indicator that may be used to judge whether someone has a learning disability (Rittey, 2003). If this is so, then we must ask *'What is intelligence, and how might it be measured?'* Intelligence is concerned with logic, abstract thought, understanding, self-awareness, communication, learning, emotional knowledge, retaining, planning, and problem solving. To a lesser or greater extent, as this chapter will show, these are the things that many, if not most, people with learning disabilities struggle with. Within psychology, the complexity of intelligence is evidenced by numerous schools of thought on the subject (Weinberg, 1989). But one particular way psychology has attempted to measure intelligence is by psychometric assessment through the well-established method of employing intelligence tests, which have now been used widely since the early part of the twentieth century. These tests enable comparison of the intellectual ability of one individual, after completing a range of standardised tests, against a large and representative sample of the general population. Contemporary opinion about their usefulness is divided, with a view that the tests have many limitations. Some alleged limitations include failure to measure creative insight and the more practical side of intelligence, and a criticism that such tests limit people to a fixed time to complete, thus equating intelligence with speed.

Once undertaken and completed, the score attained is converted into a mental age, which is then divided by the chronological age of an individual and multiplied by 100. This process converts the score into a percentile, which is then known as an intelligence quotient (IQ) (see Figure 1.1). The IQ enables us to compare how any individual compares with others of a similar chronological age in the general population.

This has been (and continues to be) used as one of the principal processes for identifying learning disabilities. Given that intelligence is present in the general population, and that it is evenly distributed, it is possible to measure how far an individual moves away from what constitutes a *'normal'* IQ (Figure 1.2). The World Health Organisation (1992) has classified the degrees of learning disability (retardation) according to how far an individual moves away from the normal distribution of IQ for the general population.

$$\frac{\text{Mental age}}{\text{Chronological age}} \times 100 = \text{IQ}$$

Figure 1.1 The intelligence quotient formula.

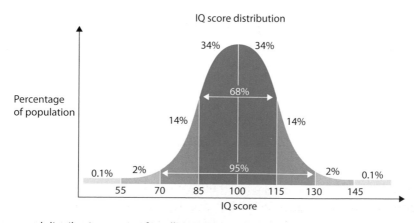

Figure 1.2 The normal distribution curve of intelligence.

Learning Activity 1.1

If an individual consistently scored two standard deviations above the 'norm' of an IQ test, that is, a measured IQ of greater than 130, how might that be explained or described?

Using this system, an individual who consistently scores two standard deviations below the 'norm' of an IQ test, that is, a measured IQ of less than 70, would be defined as having a learning disability. Those with an IQ between 71 and 84 are said to be on the borderline of intellectual functioning, whereas those within the range 50–69 are generally identified as having *mild* learning disabilities (mild mental retardation).

The term *moderate* learning disability (moderate mental retardation) is used when the measured IQ is in the range of 35–49. *Severe* learning disability (severe mental retardation) is reserved for people whose IQ is in the range of 20–34. Finally, the term *profound* learning disability (profound mental retardation) is used to refer to people with complex additional disabilities, for example, sensory, physical or behavioural. This group of people is referred to as those with profound learning disabilities and complex needs (see Chapter 6). Calculating an IQ in such cases can prove extremely difficult, owing to the severity of cognitive impairment and an absence of verbal communication, but there is general agreement that this is <20.

LEGISLATIVE DEFINITIONS OF LEARNING DISABILITY

Legislation, in both the United Kingdom and other countries, has attempted over centuries to use law to define the nature of learning disabilities. Generally speaking, law has done so within the framework of mental health legislation, which may explain (in part) why many people confuse learning disability with mental illness. This unfortunate conflation has resulted in people with learning disabilities being the subject of considerable unnecessary legislation over many centuries. The following brief exploration considers legislation passed during the twentieth century principally in the United Kingdom, focusing in particular upon legislation directly or indirectly related to people with learning disabilities. In 1904, a Royal Commission on the care and control of what was then called the *'feeble-minded'** was established. The commission's report, published in 1908, was known as the Radnor Report. The report was highly influential in informing the subsequent Mental Deficiency Act 1913, which was the first specific piece of legislation by the British government to focus on people with learning disabilities. Up until that point in history, institutions provided care both for those who were *'feeble-minded'* and for those who were *'insane'*.

---

* Throughout the twentieth and twenty-first centuries, terms used in the United Kingdom to describe people with learning disabilities have continued to change. At the beginning the twentieth century, the term feeble-minded was in common use. Also commonly used were mentally defective, idiot, and imbecile, mental and severe mental subnormality, and then mental handicap and severe mental handicap.

> ### Box 1.1   Classifications of the Mental Health Act 1959
>
> **Sub-normality:** A state of arrested or incomplete development of mind, not amounting to severe sub-normality, which includes sub-normality of intelligence, and is of such a nature or degree which requires, or is susceptible to, medical treatment or other special care or training of the patient.
>
> **Severe sub-normality:** A state of arrested or incomplete development of mind that includes sub-normality of intelligence and is of such a nature or degree that the patient is incapable of living an independent life or guarding himself/herself against serious exploitation, or will be so incapable when of an age to do so.
>
> **Psychopathic disorder:** A persistent disorder or disability of mind, whether or not including sub-normality of intelligence, which results in abnormally aggressive or seriously irresponsible conduct on the part of the patient, and requires, or is susceptible to, medical treatment.

The Mental Deficiency Act 1913 embodied two important principles that included the separation of the feeble-minded from their communities, and control, which was overseen by a regulatory body set up under the Act, the Board of Control (Cox, 1996; Thomson, 1996). This Act was to cast a long shadow over the lives of people with learning disabilities for many decades to come. The Act of 1913 defined what we now know as learning disabilities as follows

> **Mental defectiveness means a condition of arrested or incomplete development of mind existing before the age of eighteen years, whether arising from inherent causes or induced by disease or injury.**

Following the Radnor Commission, the Mental Deficiency Act of 1913 reflected the strong eugenics (*'the science of using controlled breeding to increase the occurrence of desirable heritable characteristics in a population'* [Oxford English Dictionary, 2013]) movement of the early twentieth century. So, unsurprisingly, the Act required that *defectives* be identified and subsequently segregated from the rest of society. By 1959, terminology, and, possibly, to some small extent, attitudes had changed. The Mental Health Act 1959 introduced yet more new terms for people with learning disabilities (see those listed in Box 1.1).

The Mental Health Act 1959 required local authorities, for the first time, to make both day service and residential provision for people with a mental sub-normality, and placed a new emphasis on the reintegration of this group of people into the communities to which they belonged. However, although the terminology seems derogatory this Act should be judged in a temporal context, particularly that it followed the implementation of the National Health Service Act 1946. The consequent medicalisation of 'mental sub-normality', following the National Health Service Act, is clearly reflected in the Mental Health Act 1959, and therefore its definitions reflected this. For example, it is noteworthy that a strong emphasis in the definitions was placed on treatment (Box 1.1). In addition, the Act made extensive reference to the 'Responsible Medical Officer'. And

> ### Box 1.2 Classifications of the 1983 Mental Health Act
>
> **Severe mental impairment:** A state of arrested or incomplete development of mind, which includes severe impairment of intelligence and social functioning and is associated with abnormally aggressive or seriously irresponsible conduct of the person concerned.
>
> **Mental impairment:** A state of arrested or incomplete development of mind (not amounting to severe mental impairment), which includes significant impairment of intelligence and social functioning and is associated with abnormally aggressive or seriously irresponsible conduct on the part of the person concerned.

it is at this point in the history of mental health legislation, arguably, that the influence of medicine in defining the nature of learning disabilities exerted its greatest impact. Notwithstanding, due to continued social reform, and continuing pressure from lobby groups, mental health legislation was again reformed in 1983–1984; but on this occasion this Act was to bring about positive outcomes for people with learning disabilities. Thus the Act of 1959 was subsequently replaced with the Mental Health Act 1983; and once again old terminology was changed, and replaced with the terms shown in Box 1.2.

Thus, it can be seen that the nature of these definitions at last excluded the large majority of people with learning disabilities; that is, unless learning disability (mental or severe mental impairment) coexisted with aggressive or seriously irresponsible behaviour, from mental health legislation. The 1983 Act represented a major shift in the perception of people with learning disabilities within mental health legislation. For the first time, this legislation distinguished between and separated the majority of people with learning disabilities from mental health legislation. Finally, in 2007 severe mental impairment and mental impairment were removed from mental health legislation as categories of mental health disorder (see Chapter 7).

ADAPTIVE ABILITY OR SOCIAL (IN)COMPETENCE

Adaptive ability or social competence is the final criterion (or indicator) used to identify learning disabilities that will be outlined in this chapter. It has been suggested that it is helpful to use criteria based on social competence that include the ability of an individual to adapt to the changing demands made by the society in which that individual lives (British Psychological Society, 2000). These abilities are suggested to include

- Conceptual skills: For example, the use of language, the ability to read and write, being able to use currency, understanding how to tell the time, using numbers, and being able to find one's way around a familiar environment.
- Social skills: For example, interpersonal skills, acting in a responsible manner, enjoying a positive self-esteem, avoiding being exploited, being able to solve social problems, and recognising and responding appropriately to social and cultural expectations.

- Everyday living skills: For example, activities of daily living (washing, teeth cleaning, bed making, cooking), occupational skills, looking after yourself to maintain a healthy body, being able to use the bus and train, being able to use your own money, and being able to use a personal computer and other common electronic devices.

Thus, at one level, it may sound relatively straightforward to identify how this criterion might be used to categorise or identify someone with learning disabilities. One might simply identify people who are able to adapt to their environment and demonstrate social competence, and distinguish them from those who do not respond well to changing societal demands. The latter group could then be said to have learning disabilities. Burton (1996) has said

> **Social competence concerns such areas as understanding and following social rules, adjusting social behaviour to the situation, social problem-solving, and understanding others. These are the areas where people typically fail independent living.**

> *(Burton, 1996, p. 40)*

Based on an individual's performance being significantly 'below' what could be considered *normal*, for the general population one might say that some people with learning disabilities are socially incompetent or unable to adapt readily to their environments. However, there are a number of problematic issues to consider in relation to the criterion of social competence and adaptation. Firstly, social incompetence, or an inability of an individual to adapt to his or her environment, can be found in a wide cross-section of people in the population, and not just those with learning disabilities. Consider, for example, people with chronic mental health problems, or those with dementia, as well as those who actively choose to reject societal norms; alternatively, there may be problems of communication and cultural idiosyncrasies. Hearing and vision difficulties could cause social incompetence, and may not necessarily involve learning disabilities. Equally, there is an issue concerning level of expectation, and the notion of the so-called '*self-fulfilling prophecy*'. Let us assume that an individual is identified as having a learning disability, because of poor adaptation, based on some measure of social competence. Problematic is whether this should be interpreted as a learning disability or as poor adaptation as a result of a hospital setting where this individual may have spent his or her formative years. Such a finding is still not beyond the realm of credibility. In the United Kingdom, it is still only relatively recently that the old large learning disability hospitals have begun to close. Tens of thousands of people with learning disabilities had been segregated from society, and consequently led highly devalued lifestyles. Opportunities for the development of social competence were rare in such institutions. There have been numerous studies undertaken on the effects of people who were deprived of 'normal' nurturing environments. For example, Dennis (1973) found that institutionalised children were delayed in basic competencies such as sitting, standing, and walking, and reported that they had no opportunity to practise these skills. He also noted that with the additional lack of stimulation, there was significant delay in language acquisition, social skill development, and emotional expression

> **…as babies they lay on their backs in their cribs throughout the first year and often for much of the second year…. Many objects available to most children did not exist…. There were no building blocks, no sandboxes, no scooters, no tricycles, no climbing apparatus, no swings. There were**

> no pets or other animals of any sort… they had had no opportunities to learn what these objects were. They never saw persons who lived in the outside world, except for rather rare visitors.
>
> *(Dennis, 1973, pp. 22–23)*

In short, the expectations of people in such environments were low; therefore it is reasonable to assume that their ability to develop social competence was reduced. Despite the criticisms presented in this section, the use of social competence and adaptation as a means to identify learning disabilities still remains a globally used criterion.

DEFINING LEARNING DISABILITY

In the United Kingdom, the term *learning disability* is generally used and accepted to mean

> [a] significantly reduced ability to understand new or complex information, to learn new skills (impaired intelligence), with a reduced ability to cope independently (impaired social functioning) and which started before adulthood, with a lasting effect on development.
>
> *(DOH, 2001, p. 14)*

In Ireland, the term *intellectual disability* is used to mean

> …a greater than average difficulty in learning. A person is considered to have an intellectual disability when the following factors are present: general intellectual functioning is significantly below average; significant deficits exist in adaptive skills and the condition is present from childhood (eighteen years or less).
>
> *(Inclusion Ireland, 2013)*

In the United States, the American Association of Intellectual and Developmental Disability recently revised its definition of what was previously known as *'mental retardation'*, which was drawn up in that country in 2002

> Intellectual disability is a disability characterized by significant limitations in both intellectual functioning and in adaptive behaviour, which covers many everyday social and practical skills. This disability originates before the age of 18
>
> *(American Association of Intellectual and Developmental Disability, 2010)*

Finally, the World Health Organisation (1992) still uses the term *mental retardation* to mean

> A condition of arrested or incomplete development of the mind, which is especially characterized by impairment of skills manifested during the developmental period, skills which contribute to the overall level of intelligence, i.e., cognitive, language, motor, and social abilities. Retardation can occur with or without any other mental or physical condition.
>
> *(1992, pp. 225–231)*

INCIDENCE AND PREVALENCE OF LEARNING DISABILITIES

Calculating the incidence of learning disabilities is problematic because there is no way to detect the vast majority of infants who have a learning disability at birth. Therefore, to arrive at any estimate, one must use cumulative incidence, and this has been calculated at the age of 8 as 4.9, and for severe learning disabilities as 4.3 per 100 live births (Emerson et al., 2001).

Nonetheless, generally speaking, it is calculated that 2–3% of the population is likely to have learning disabilities, but it is estimated that a large proportion of this population will never come into contact with a caring agency. Therefore, it is more common to refer to *'administrative prevalence'*, which refers to the number of people provided with some form of service from caring agencies.

Historically, the general consensus has been that the overall administrative prevalence of severe learning disabilities is approximately three to four persons per 1000 of the general population (DH, 2001).

The Department of Health has suggested that mild learning disability is more common; the prevalence has been estimated to be in the region of 20 per 1000 of the general population. In the United Kingdom it has been further calculated that, of the three to four persons per 1000 of the general population with a learning disability, approximately 30% will present with severe or profound learning disabilities. Within this group it is common to find multiple disabilities, including physical or sensory impairments or disabilities, as well as behavioural difficulties.

Emerson et al. (2001), drawing on extensive epidemiological data, have confirmed the estimation of prevalence for severe learning disabilities. They have stated it to be somewhere in the region of three to four persons per 1000 of the general population. The prevalence rate Emerson et al. give for the learning disabled population referred to as having *mild learning disabilities* is much more imprecise. It is estimated that it might be between 25 and 30 people per 1000 of the general population. Based on these estimates, one can be assume that there are some 230,000–350,000 persons with severe learning disabilities, and possibly 580,000–1,750,000 persons with mild learning disabilities in the United Kingdom.

More recently, Emerson et al. (2010) has revised these estimates and calculated that in England 1,198,000 people have learning disabilities. This includes

- 298,000 children (188,000 boys and 110,000 girls) ages 0–17
- 900,000 adults ages 18+ (526,000 men and 374,000 women), of whom 191,000 (21%) are known to learning disability services

There is a slight imbalance in the ratio of males to females in people with both mild and severe learning disabilities, with males having slightly higher prevalence rates. Also, there is some evidence of slightly higher prevalence rates amongst some ethnic groups, and this includes 'Black Groups in the USA and South Asian Groups in the United Kingdom' (Emerson et al., 2001).

CLASSIFICATION OF LEARNING DISABILITIES

A learning disability may be classified in a number of ways. One way is to do so by the nature of its causation. This may fall into two broad main categories: genetic or environmental. Genetic aberrations may originate prior to conception or during the very early stages of the development of the foetus. The second category is defined by the stage of development at which the damage to the child occurred. Environmental causes, on the other hand, include those external factors that can affect the development of a foetus or a child in the preconceptual or pre-, peri- or postnatal periods. Where the cause of the learning disability is unknown, then generally such manifestation is usually described as *idiopathic*.

The following sections will portray some of the clinical features associated with specific conditions or syndromes found within the population of people with learning disabilities. When reading each section, you may wish to reflect upon the type of health care support that may be required in responding to the needs of such individuals and their families.

GENETIC CAUSES OF LEARNING DISABILITIES

Many of our physical features (phenotype) originate from our genetic makeup (genotype). The information required for the development of these characteristics exists in the form of genes passed from parents to their offspring, and are shaped within a complex interaction with the environment. Genes are found located on chromosomes, of which humans have 23 pairs; 22 pairs are known as autosomes and the 23rd pair is known as the sex chromosomes. See Figure 1.3 for an example of a normal karyotype, this is the number and appearance chromosomes, of a male. These are present within the nucleus of every human cell and comprise the genetic material DNA (deoxyribonucleic acid).

It is believed that between 30% and 40% of moderate to severe learning disabilities are caused by changes in the genetic makeup of an individual (Knight et al., 1999). Developments in genetic technology arising from the Human Genome Project have suggested that the percentage may be even higher. A study by Knight et al. (1999) has shown that a number of previously undiagnosed conditions in learning disabilities could be attributed to subtle chromosomal rearrangements. Figure 1.4 presents a simple classification system of the genetic causes of learning disabilities. An example is given for each group, and further examples are provided in the following section of this chapter.

CHROMOSOMAL ABNORMALITIES

This following section provides specific examples of conditions in learning disabilities that result from changes in the structure or number of autosomes and sex chromosomes. Where changes in the structure of the chromosome may occur, this can include the deletion, duplication, translocation, non-disjunction, or inversion of genetic material.

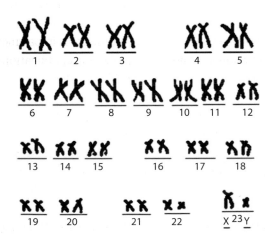

Figure 1.3 Normal karyotytpe of a male.

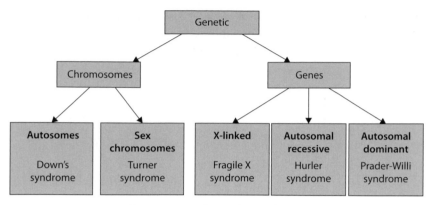

Chromosome and gene abnormalities

Figure 1.4 Simple classification system of the genetic causes of learning disabilities.

MANIFESTATION OF AUTOSOMAL ABNORMALITIES

Down syndrome (Trisomy 21)

Down syndrome was first described by John Langdon Down in 1866, and the condition results from the non-disjunction of chromosome 21 pair during cell division, resulting in an individual having three rather than two of chromosome 21. The incidence rate of this syndrome is between 1 in 650 and 1 in 700 (Mueller and Young, 1998), and the rate becomes higher with an increase in maternal age. Typical characteristics of individuals include short stature, small ears, ear and eye defects, heart defects, and an increased susceptibility to infections, particularly upper-respiratory tract and eye infections. In rare cases, some individuals with Down syndrome may have a mixture of cells that contain either trisomy 21 or the normal number of chromosome 21 and this condition is known as *mosaicism*.

Health challenges include

Management of weight: //www.ndss.org/Resources/Wellness/Nutrition/Recreation-Friendship21/

Congenital heart disease: http://www.ndss.org/Resources/Health-Care/Associated-Conditions/ The-Heart-Down-Syndrome/

Hearing challenges: http://www.sense.org.uk/content/hearing-impairment-and-down-syndrome

Thyroid disorder: http://www.downs-syndrome.org.uk/shop/publications/medical-and-health/ for-families/from-birth-11-years/1075-thyroid-disorder-among-people-with-downs -syndrome.html

Respiratory tract infection: https://www.ndss.org/PageFiles/3185/respiratory_concerns_in_ children_with_down_syndrome_slides.pdf

Eye abnormalities: http://www.seeability.org/eyecare_hub/carersandsupportersinfo/healthy_ eyes/downs_syndrome_and_eye_conditions.aspx

Cri-du-Chat

Cri-du-Chat is a relatively rare condition with an incidence rate of approximately 1 in 37,000 live births. It was first described in 1963 by Lejeune et al. and given this name because affected infants are found to have high-pitched cries similar to those of a cat. Typical characteristics include microcephaly, low-set ears, and wide-spaced eyes. This condition is usually associated with moderate to severe learning disabilities. More often, infants present with feeding problems because of difficulty swallowing and sucking, they may have low birth weight, and they may develop challenging behaviour (Wiedemann et al., 1992; Gilbert, 2000).

Health challenges include

Congenital heart disease: http://pediatrics.aappublications.org/content/117/5/e924.long

Eye abnormalities: http://www.oepf.org/sites/default/files/23_4_SWEENEY.pdf

MANIFESTATION OF SEX-CHROMOSOME ABNORMALITIES

Klinefelter syndrome (XXY)

Klinefelter syndrome, first described by Klinefelter and his associates in 1942, affects only males. It results from the non-disjunction of the XY chromosomes during cell division, resulting in an individual having an extra X chromosome. The incidence rate of this syndrome is between 1 in 500 and 1 in 1000 births. Typical characteristics include a large forehead, ears, and jaw, and, following the onset of puberty, hypogonadism (small testicles) and gynecomastia (enlarged breasts). Psychosocial problems are said to be common. The degree of learning disability is said to be moderate, with a few cases of individuals presenting with profound learning disability (Wiedemann et al., 1992; Gilbert, 2000).

Health challenges include

Management of diabetes: http://care.diabetesjournals.org/content/29/7/1591

Thyroid disorder: http://www.apeg.org.au/Portals/0/Resources/Hormones_and_Me_13_
        Klinefelter_Syndrome.pdf

Testosterone therapy: http://www.klinefelter.org.uk/about_ks.html

Turner syndrome (XO)

Turner syndrome affects only females and results from the loss of one of the two XX chromosomes. Its incidence rate is estimated to be 1 in 2500 births. Typical characteristics include short stature, web-like neck, non-functioning ovaries, and, in some cases, learning disabilities. However, a normal range of intelligence is generally associated with this syndrome (Wiedemann et al., 1992; Gilbert, 2000).

Health challenges include

Management of weight: http://www.nhs.uk/Conditions/Turners-syndrome/Pages/Treatment.aspx

Coarctation of the aorta: http://www.patient.co.uk/health/Coarctation-of-the-Aorta

Hearing challenges: http://www.ncbi.nlm.nih.gov/pubmed/19081146

Thyroid disorder: http://www.nhs.uk/Conditions/Turners-syndrome/Pages/Introduction.aspx

Eye abnormalities: http://www.nhs.uk/Conditions/Turners-syndrome/Pages/Symptoms.aspx

GENETIC ABNORMALITIES

This section provides specific examples of conditions in learning disabilities that result from changes in the structure of the genetic material making up a gene. These changes may include the deletion, duplication, addition, inversion, and substitution of the parts of the DNA. Gene abnormalities are generally categorised by the mode of transmission of the defective gene. You may want to refer to the simple classification system depicted in Figure 1.4. These forms of transmission can be described as autosomal dominant, autosomal recessive, or X-linked, and are all described briefly in the following. Some conditions may also result from the interaction of various genes (polygenic), though these are not described in this book. A further reading section about specific conditions or syndromes found in the population of people with learning disabilities is provided at the end of this chapter.

Autosomal dominant conditions

In the case of autosomal dominant conditions, transmission is reliant upon only one parent being a carrier of the defective gene, and there is a 50% chance of the condition occurring in the offspring (Figure 1.5). The following provides examples of disorders inherited through this process.

Prader–Willi syndrome

Prader–Willi syndrome is a condition that results from deletion of part of the genetic material on the long arm of chromosome 15 and usually originates from the father. The incidence rate is approximately 1 in 15,000 and affects both males and females. Characteristics of this condition include small hands and feet, hypogenitalism (underdeveloped testes), and cryptorchidism (undescended testes) in males. One of the most notable characteristics, however, is hyperphagia (excessive overeating). Without professional help and support, people with this syndrome commonly experience

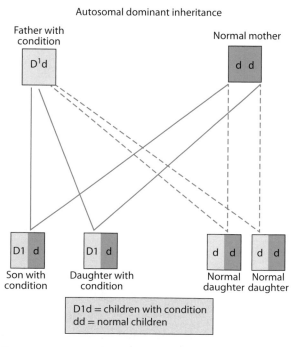

Figure 1.5 Dominant inheritance.

gross obesity and the related conditions of heart disease and diabetes, which may result in premature death (Wiedemann et al., 1992; Gilbert, 2000).

Health challenges include

Management of weight: http://www.pwsa.co.uk/index.php/what-is-pws/131-weight
-management-in-pws

Scoliosis: http://www.ncbi.nlm.nih.gov/pubmed/7215706

Diabetes: http://ghr.nlm.nih.gov/condition/prader-willi-syndrome

Tuberous sclerosis (epiloia)

First described in 1880 and estimated to affect between 1 in 30,000 to 40,000 births, tuberous sclerosis is a condition characterised by growths on the brain and major organs. A butterfly-shaped rash (adenoma sebaceum) will be present on the face. Epilepsy is common in people with this condition. Whereas normal intelligence may be present, 60% of affected people will have some degree of learning disability (Wiedemann et al., 1992; Gilbert, 2000).

Health challenges include

Dental care: http://www.nhs.uk/Conditions/Tuberous-sclerosis/Pages/Treatment.aspx

Epilepsy: http://www.nhs.uk/conditions/tuberous-sclerosis/Pages/Introduction.aspx

Monitoring of lesions in vital organs: http://www.nhsdirect.wales.nhs.uk/encyclopaedia/t/article/
tuberoussclerosis/

Autosomal recessive condition

In the case of autosomal recessive conditions, transmission is reliant on both parents being carriers of the defective gene, and in this case, there is a 25% chance of the condition manifesting in the offspring (Figure 1.6). The following section provides examples of disorders inherited through this process.

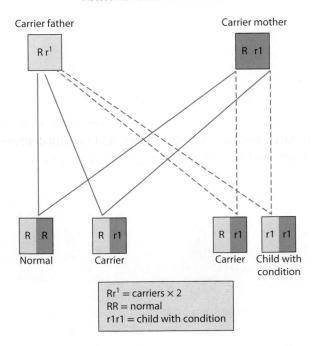

Figure 1.6 Recessive inheritance.

Phenylketonuria

Described by Fölling in 1934, phenylketonuria is a disorder that affects protein metabolism, resulting in raised levels of phenylalanine in the blood. If protein levels are not maintained at a normal level through diet control, they may subsequently become toxic and cause brain damage. This condition is thought to affect 1 in 12,000 live births. The condition is commonly diagnosed using the Newborn blood spot test, which is carried out 6 to 14 days after birth. If left untreated, typical characteristics include lack of pigmentation in the eyes, skin, and hair; hyperactivity; autistic features; epilepsy; and a severe degree of learning disability (Wiedemann et al., 1992; Gilbert, 2000).

Health challenges include

Management of diet: http://www.nhs.uk/Conditions/Phenylketonuria/Pages/Treatment.aspx

Hurler syndrome

One of a number of mucopolysaccharide disorders, Hurler syndrome has an estimated prevalence rate of 1 in 1,50,000 births. It is characterised by the abnormal storage of mucopolysaccharides in connective tissue. Affected individuals are short in stature and described as having thick, coarse facial features and a low nasal bridge. Hirsutism is a common characteristic, as is the presence of heart abnormalities. Affected individuals may also have sight and hearing impairments; death normally occurs during adolescence (Wiedemann et al., 1992; Gilbert, 2000).

Health challenges include

Joint management: http://www.nlm.nih.gov/medlineplus/ency/article/001204.htm

Hearing and sight abnormalities: http://www.patient.co.uk/doctor/retinitis-pigmentosa

Hernias: http://www.patient.co.uk/doctor/Hurler's-Syndrome.htm

Cardiac abnormalities https://www.mpssociety.org/wp-content/uploads/2011/07/Cardiac_
Problems_ 11-05.pdf

X-linked recessive conditions

Fragile X syndrome

Fragile X syndrome occurs more commonly in males than in females, with a prevalence rate of 1 in 4000 and 1 in 8000, respectively. It is believed to be the most common cause of learning disability, next to Down syndrome. The condition arises from the bottom tip of the X chromosome breaking off, making the site fragile, hence its name. Common characteristics include an oversized head, long face, prominent ears, large jaw, language difficulties, and varying degrees of learning disability. Behavioural challenges in affected individuals are also a characteristic of this condition.

Health challenges include

Epilepsy: http://www.cafamily.org.uk/medical-information/conditions/f/fragile-x-syndrome/

Recurrent infections: http://www.fragilex.org/fragile-x-associated-disorders/fragile-x-syndrome/
medical-issues/

ENVIRONMENTAL FACTORS

Environmental factors have an important influence on the physical and intellectual development of individuals. Where an environment contains the positive factors necessary for healthy growth, such as food, warmth, love, safety, and sensory stimulation, normal development should occur. However,

Preconception	Prenatal	Perinatal	Postnatal
Diet, substance abuse, pre-existing medical conditions	Infections (viral/bacterial, e.g., congenital rubella, congenital syphilis), trauma, anoxia, x-rays	Premature birth, asphyxiation, trauma (forceps delivery)	Infection, trauma, toxic agents, nutrition, sensory/ social deprivation, untreated conditions

Figure 1.7 Causation of learning disabilities.

in some cases, certain environmental conditions may hinder the growth and development of an individual, which might result in a learning disability. Environmental factors that may exert influence on development might occur at the preconceptual, prenatal, perinatal, and postnatal periods of human development and typically include, for example, infections, trauma, substance abuse, and social deprivation (Figure 1.7).

Environmental causes of learning disabilities include trauma during the prenatal, perinatal, and postnatal phases, as well as accidental and non-accidental injury during human growth. At the prenatal stage, this could also include the delivery of a baby using forceps or suction. Restriction of the oxygen supply to the foetus during the prenatal and perinatal phases can also result in brain damage. In the latter stage, asphyxiation may occur if the umbilical cord becomes wrapped around the baby's neck for a prolonged period of time.

The consumption of drugs, including alcohol [substance abuse], also accounts for stunted growth and lack of brain development observed in some children. Toxic agents, lead poisoning, strontium poisoning, chemical pollutants, and hard metals, such as mercury and manganese, are also recognised causes of brain damage. In the postnatal phase of development, poor nutrition and a lack of sensory and social stimulation can impair development and result in learning disabilities.

Infections

Other causes of learning disabilities include acquired infections that can result in brain damage at the prenatal, perinatal, and the postnatal stages of development, and encompass rubella (German measles), mumps and chickenpox. In the past syphilis was also a common cause of learning disability, but this is now rare in Western countries. Viral infections may give rise to encephalitis (inflammation of the brain), and the subsequent degree of learning disability can be severe; dehydration occurs rapidly, leading to brain haemorrhage and subsequent brain damage.

Congenital rubella

First described by Gregg in 1941, congenital rubella is a condition characterised by a number of abnormalities that include cataracts, deafness, congenital heart defects, and learning disabilities. Damage occurs when the rubella virus passes across the placenta barrier and attacks the developing nervous tissue in the unborn foetus. In recent years, the prevalence of congenital rubella has declined with the introduction of rigorous immunisation programmes.

DIAGNOSING LEARNING DISABILITIES

This following section explores briefly how one arrives at a diagnosis of learning disability. Most parents are not made aware that their child could have a learning disability before birth. In most instances, only a small number of parents are given advance information, and this will come as a

Research Edwards syndrome, and answer the following questions:
  What causes this syndrome?
  What potential health challenges might this condition present to individuals affected?

result of some form of screening investigation, such as blood tests, ultrasound scans, or diagnostic investigations such as amniocentesis, chorionic villous sampling, or other tests. These are generally undertaken because the parents are perceived as being at high risk. For example, increased maternal age is highly correlated with a diagnosis of Down syndrome in any offspring: age 20, 1:1450; age 29, 1:1050; age 39, 1:110; age 49, 1:25 (Morris et al., 2003). Newer tests being developed, such as the CytoScan Dx Assay, may help identify causation of developmental delay or intellectual disability, and it is believed that this particular test may be superior to karyotyping and chromosomal testing.

However, unless a definite physical abnormality or characteristic signs (as in children with Down syndrome) are present at birth, or a traumatic delivery has taken place, a learning disability is seldom suspected or diagnosed at birth. A diagnosis can vary from the confirmation of the presence of a specific condition (for example, Edwards syndrome) to a much broader diagnosis of global developmental delay, with no particular condition being identified. A learning disability is generally identified during childhood, but sometimes it may not be finally diagnosed until early adolescence.

Generally speaking, children with severe or profound learning disabilities with complex needs are much more likely to be more noticed as having learning disabilities at a younger age than those with mild to moderate learning disabilities. A learning disability is most often diagnosed in early childhood, and usually when a child fails to reach the 'normal' but critical developmental milestones. During this period, parents may have expressed concerns over the nature of their child's progress, and suspected that some kind of a problem exists. When this happens, a regular check should be kept on the child's progress, more frequently than the usual screening checks, and records should be kept. It will be a huge relief to both parents and professionals, after a period of observation, to be able to show that a child is reaching the normal milestones of development. Unless managed sensitively, it may be the case that active family involvement will be damaged in the short term, and possibly for many years, when a learning disability diagnosis is finally confirmed, despite repeated concerns having been raised previously but dismissed or largely ignored. That is why it is important to identify both the nature and extent of learning disabilities, and exclude or include other more specific developmental disorders that are sometimes present. For example, some developmental disorders include autistic spectrum conditions, attention deficit hyperactivity disorder, and dyspraxia. Finally, identifying possible causes of learning disabilities, and the provision of an early diagnosis are important to

- Limit potential feelings of self-blame that some parents may experience
- Reduce possible challenges in the adaptation of parents to their child and hopefully avoid rejection

Other reasons for identifying the presence of a learning disability and forming a diagnosis include a need to

- Understand the possible manifestation and trajectory of an identified condition over time
- Identify a range of therapeutic approaches that may be used to ameliorate the effects of the condition, which will include mobilising and accessing resources (Gates, 2000)
- Establish, in some cases, the degree of risk to other family members of the condition reoccurring in their siblings and offspring through genetic counselling

LEARNING DISABILITY NURSING

Nursing has a long association of supporting or caring for people with learning disabilities. Currently, in the United Kingdom and Ireland, pre-registration undergraduate students of nursing choose to follow one of four fields of practice: children, adults, people with learning disabilities, or people with mental health challenges. These students then qualify in their chosen area of practice at the point of initial registration. Ireland and the United Kingdom are the only countries internationally to follow this approach; other countries provide a generic pre-registration education. Until 2011, all U.K. nurse education programmes were structured so that all students followed the same programme for the first year of their course (the Common Foundation Programme), and then focused on their chosen area for the two-year 'Branch' programme. The three-year programme consisted of 50% of the time being spent in the university and 50% being spent in a range of clinical placements, including schools, residential units, assessment and treatment units, hospitals, and community-based teams.

In Ireland, intellectual disabilities nursing, as it is known there, has undergone a similar trajectory in its professional development to support people with learning disabilities (Doody et al., 2012). In 2002, intellectual disabilities nursing, along with other fields of nursing practice, moved to a four-year undergraduate programme of study. Students of nursing, as do their U.K. counterparts, spend the practice component of the programme in a range of clinical placements that includes hospitals, schools, residential units, assessment and treatment units, day centres, recreation departments, and physiotherapy units, as well as employment settings.

Recently in the United Kingdom, the Nursing and Midwifery Council launched new standards for pre-registration nurse education in 2010 to be met by 2013 (NMC, 2010). All new programmes must now be at the undergraduate level, and students will focus on one of four 'fields of nursing practice'. However, rather than having a one-year common foundation programme, and a two-year branch programme, as was the case in the recent past, generic and field-specific elements are now integrated throughout the programme. The programme must be a minimum of three years in length, with 2300 hours in theoretical instruction and 2300 hours practice learning. The programmes are competency based and require that students demonstrate competence in both generic and field-specific aspects of four domains to qualify as a registered nurse. The four domains are professional values; communication and interpersonal skills; nursing practice and decision making; and leadership, management, and team working.

In Ireland in 2005 the An Bord Altranais published the third edition of its requirements and standards for nurse registration education programmes (An Bord Altranais, 2005). The theoretical and clinical instruction comprises not less than 4600 hours. In Ireland, the academic component comprises no less than one-third of these 4600 hours, or 1533 hours. Time spent in practice comprises not less than one-half of these 4600 hours, or 2300 hours.

Nationally and internationally, the specialisation of learning disability nursing at a pre-registration level for this field of nursing practice has been a subject of much debate over the past three decades. At various points, it has been proposed that there should be a generic pre-registration programme, and that learning disabilities should become a post-registration specialism. However, such a model has not been effective elsewhere, such as in Australia and New Zealand (Barr and Sines, 1996), and its cessation has brought with it many challenges that need to be addressed (Barr and Sines, 1996). Subsequently, within the United Kingdom and Ireland, a specific field has been maintained, and this is further endorsed on an ongoing basis within the educational programmes that universities offer.

The new standards for pre-registration nurse education in the United Kingdom and Ireland also require that education in physical and mental health provided to learning disability nurses must increase; nurses will be further prepared to support people with learning disabilities to develop and maintain better physical and mental health across their lifespan.

Ongoing educational opportunities for all learning disability nurses are essential in the context of changing service configurations and the increasing complexity of client need in this population of people. Learning disability nurses must maintain a wide range of clinical nursing skills that enable them to assess complex needs and plan interventions in a person-centred manner (RCN, 2011). Some have thus decided to further their education by studying post-qualifying courses in diabetes, palliative care, epilepsy, challenging behaviour, and supporting older people, and they use this knowledge to support people with learning disabilities, building on the knowledge and skills obtained in their pre-registration degree programme.

Today the modern practice setting for learning disability nursing is located in a complex landscape of service provision. This includes, for example, residential care homes, independent living homes, supported living arrangements, and people with learning disabilities living in their own homes, as well as family homes. There are also larger, but now much fewer than in the past, service configurations, and a range of very specialist settings, such as treatment and assessment services, challenging behaviour units, and other specialist health or social care settings. There are hospices for children with life-limiting conditions and homes for older people. In addition, learning disability nurses may be found supporting people with learning disabilities in mainstream health and social care settings, such as in general hospitals, in prison services, and in other settings. Therefore, learning disability nurses work with people who have learning disabilities and their families from birth to death, and who may require a range of support throughout their lives that will range from none, or minimal support, to intensive holistic nursing aimed at meeting the multi-dimensional health needs of people with learning disabilities. This is why learning disability nursing is often referred to as the 'purist' form of nursing. Unlike other fields of nursing practice, learning disability nurses do not concentrate on specific manifestations of physical ill health or trauma, nor do they just focus on mental health and well-being or children or child birth. Instead, learning disability nurses offer all-embracing support to those with learning disabilities and their families that is quite literally from the cradle to the grave.

To offer comprehensive nursing interventions that meet the multi-dimensional needs of people with learning disabilities, it is necessary to adopt a structured approach to this field of practice. This typically consists firstly of completion of a comprehensive needs assessment (physical, psychological, social and spiritual, emotional). If a learning disability nurse is required to work with someone who has learning disabilities, or such a person's family, it is necessary to assess such a person's needs and incorporate them into an individual care plan that addresses their desires, wishes, and aspirations. The nurse must work closely with the client's family, with care providers, and with other professionals. Adopting this broad approach may bring very important and essential information to light for assessment. This first stage is followed by the construction of a written care plan that is then implemented and followed by ongoing review and evaluation. It is this structured approach along with partnership working, and a consideration of the multi-dimensionality of people, coupled with person-centred planning, that allows learning disability nursing to lay claim, which is attested by others, that they offer the purist form of nursing (Gates, 2009). In response to social and political influences, learning disability care models, along with that of care planning, have, over the past few years, undergone unprecedented change. Therefore, so has the practice of learning disability nurses (Alaszewski et al., 2001; Gates, 2011; U.K. Chief Nursing Officers, 2012).

During the past century, learning disabilities services were dominated by a medical model of care that emphasised the biological needs of people and the need to *'cure'* physical problems to allow a person to function in society. The majority of people with learning disabilities have now moved out of the old long-stay hospitals, but there remain concerns that the powerful effects of the medical model continue to influence care provided in smaller community-based residences. Klotz (2004) has argued that the use of the medical model has pathologised and objectified people with learning disabilities, leading to them being seen as *'less human'*. Therefore, learning disability nurses need to consider adopting a 'nursing model' to guide their care in practice, to counter this potentially pathologising effect, to ensure that what is offered is holistic and meets the many needs of this client group. It must remembered that the use of any model must hold the person with learning disabilities as central to the care-planning process and that the nurse must be mindful that he or she uses such a model to promote what is best for that patient. A number of nursing models can be adapted and used in a variety of health and social care settings. Some nursing models, such as Orem's (1991) self-care, Roper's (1980) activities of daily living, and Aldridge's (2004) model for practice, are well known, often cited, and used in learning disability nursing. It should be remembered that these models may not be seen as relevant or ideal for all people with learning disabilities, but such models can generally be adapted relatively easily and become ideal frameworks for assessing health and well being as well as more general needs.

Case study 1.1

Mohammad, an 18-year-old man, has very severe learning disabilities. His general practitioner has recently referred Mohammad to his local community team—learning disability (CTLD). He lives at home with his parents, who worry about his future, as he has just finished school, and they are not sure what will happen him. He has to use a wheelchair, he cannot speak, and he seemingly does not understand words. He is unable to look after even his most basic needs. He is prone to chest and urine infections, and he regularly develops pressure sores in the sacral area of his lower back. He needs a great deal of support to provide his basic care, and for others to understand what he is trying to communicate. Sometimes, for example, he cries and bangs the back of his head against the back of his wheelchair. He also needs, and in some ways relies upon, an environment with special equipment. His parents report that he loves to get out and meet new people, who always seem to make him happy.

Learning Activity 1.3

Spend some time reflecting on the case history for Mohammad. What do you think your role might be as his learning disability nurse in assisting to help meet his needs and plans for the future? Structure your answer under two columns—one for direct support and the other for indirect support for Mohammad and his family.

Temporally, learning disability nursing in the United Kingdom and Ireland is located within an ongoing paradigm shift of service ideologies. These ideologies have moved in recent years rapidly from an NHS (UK) dominated or congregated hospital provision (Ireland) of residential services for people with learning disabilities to a complex landscape of private, voluntary, and not-for-profit providers. In the United Kingdom, for example, this has resulted in nearly all NHS campuses being closed (Mair, 2009), bringing with it questions about the need to continue commissioning a specialist learning disability nursing workforce. Regardless of this shift in service ideologies, some people with learning disabilities and their families arguably will always need to be supported by specialist health services, and a specialist learning arguably nursing workforce. This is because the population of people with learning disabilities is increasing, owing to an increased overall life expectancy and survival into adulthood of young people with complex health needs (Parrot et al., 2008).

There is now a growing and irrefutable body of evidence indicating that people with learning disabilities have a profile of health needs that differs from the health needs of the wider population (for example, Mencap, 2007; Mencap, 2012; Michael, 2008; Heslop et al., 2013).

These needs often go unrecognised and unmet, and the health services that those with learning disabilities receive may not be appropriate. Learning disability nurses have an important role to play in addressing such deficits, and this has been articulated by the U.K. Chief Nursing Officers (2012). However, as learning disability nurses' numbers have declined, there is need for urgent attention to workforce planning issues. Many have advocated this, because current evidence points to a potential crisis looming in the learning disability nursing workforce. However, this may not yet be the case for Ireland (Gates, 2011; Glover and Emerson, 2012). Here, and in Chapter 2, it will be shown that learning disability nursing has moved away from a very narrowly defined role, within long-term institutionalised-based care, to a much broader role. The learning disability nursing field of practice spans such areas of practice as community support specialists, liaison nurses between and within services and agencies, and secure or forensic health settings, and these roles offer support across the age continuum (Manthorpe, 2004). And, as the Chief Nursing Officers have said recently

> **We want to ensure that people with learning disabilities of all ages, today and tomorrow, will have access to the expert learning disabilities nursing they need, want and deserve.**
>
> *(U.K. Chief Nursing Officers, 2012, p. 4)*

CONCLUSION

This chapter has portrayed the complexities inherent in our understanding of the nature of learning disabilities. Many textbooks refer to 'people with learning disabilities' as a homogenous group. This is both simplistic and unhelpful, not only for people with learning disabilities, but also for their families and health and social professional carers.

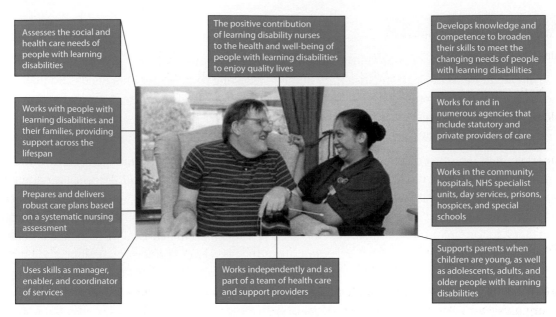

Assesses the social and health care needs of people with learning disabilities

The positive contribution of learning disability nurses to the health and well-being of people with learning disabilities to enjoy quality lives

Develops knowledge and competence to broaden their skills to meet the changing needs of people with learning disabilities

Works with people with learning disabilities and their families, providing support across the lifespan

Works for and in numerous agencies that include statutory and private providers of care

Prepares and delivers robust care plans based on a systematic nursing assessment

Works in the community, hospitals, NHS specialist units, day services, prisons, hospices, and special schools

Uses skills as manager, enabler, and coordinator of services

Works independently and as part of a team of health care and support providers

Supports parents when children are young, as well as adolescents, adults, and older people with learning disabilities

Figure 1.8 Modern-day practice of learning disability nursing.

This chapter has also examined the varying causes and manifestations of common conditions of learning disabilities. It has been demonstrated that changes in the genetic makeup of individuals results in the manifestation of specific syndromes, whereas environmental factors can also cause learning disabilities during the prenatal, perinatal, and postnatal periods. Diagnosing the cause of learning disabilities is important for families to allow them to adapt to, and value, their child for who he or she is, rather than for what he or she might have been. It is also important for health services, as it provides specific information about actual and potential needs of individuals, allowing the mobilisation of appropriate resources when needed. Caution, however, must be exercised, because providing diagnostic labels may reduce an approach of recognising the importance of individuality; a danger with labels is forgetting the importance of the person behind them.

As a health professional, you must ensure that you endeavour to see and value every person and their individual characteristics before any diagnosis, and also to influence the approach others may adopt in the wider health and social care economies. This issue will be further developed in subsequent chapters. Reflect on the information in Figure 1.8, which depicts the complexities of learning disability nurses' role in contemporary practice.

People with learning disabilities share a common humanity with us all. Most people desire love and a sense of connection with others to feel safe, to learn, to lead a meaningful life, to be free from ridicule and harm, and to be healthy and free from poverty. People with learning disabilities are no different in this respect. It is in the spirit of our collective common humanity that this learning disability nursing text is presented. It is our aim that this text will, in some small part, assist learning disability nurses to continue making a strong contribution in bringing about the inclusion of people with learning disabilities into their communities. It is for all learning disability nurses to ensure that either directly through their interventions, or indirectly through directing and leading other health and social care practitioners, equitable health care is provided to all people, regardless of their perceived differences.

REFERENCES

Alaszewski, A., Motherby, E., Gates, B., Ayer, S., and Manthorpe, J. 2001. *Diversity and Change: The Changing Roles and Education of Learning Disability Nurses*. London: English National Board.

Aldridge, J. 2004. Intellectual disability nursing: A model for practice. In: Turnbull, J. (Ed.), *Learning Disability Nursing*. Oxford: Blackwell Publishing.

American Association of Intellectual and Developmental Disability. 2010. *Intellectual Disability: Definition, Classification, and Systems of Supports* (11th ed.). AAIDD: Washington, DC.

An Bord Altranais. 2005. *Requirements and Standards for Nurse Registration Education Programmes* (3rd ed.). Dublin: An Bord Altranis.

Barr, O. and Sines, D. 1996. The development of the generalist nurse within preregistration nurse education in the UK: Some points for consideration. *Nurse Education Today*, 16(4):274–277.

British Psychological Society. 2000. Learning disability: Definitions and contexts. http://www.bps. org.uk/system/files/documents/ppb_learning.pdf (accessed August 19, 2014).

Burton, M. 1996. Intellectual disability: Developing a definition. *Journal of Learning Disabilities for Nursing, Health and Social Care,* 1(1):37–43.

Cox, P. 1996. Girls, deficiency and delinquency. In: Wright, D. and Digby, A. (Eds.), *From Idiocy to Mental Deficiency.* London: Routledge, pp. 184–206.

Dennis, W. 1973. *Children of the Crèche.* New York: Appleton Century - Crofts.

Department of Health 2001 *Valuing People: A New Strategy for Learning Disability for the 21st Century.* CM 5086. London: The Stationery Office.

Doody, O.L., Slevin, E., and Taggart, L. 2012. Intellectual disability nursing: Identifying its development and future. *Journal of Intellectual Disabilities*, 16(1):7–16.

Emerson, E., Hatton, C., Felce, D., and Murphy, G. 2001. *Learning Disabilities: The Fundamental Facts.* London: The Foundation for People with Learning Disabilities.

Emerson, E., Hatton, C., Robertson, J., Roberts, H., Baines, S., and Glover, G. 2010. *People with Learning Disabilities in England 2010.* Lancaster: Improving Health and Lives: Learning Disabilities Observatory.

Gates, B. 2000. Knowing: The importance of diagnosing learning disabilities. *Journal of Intellectual Disabilities*, 4(1):5–6.

Gates, B. 2007. What's in a name? *Journal of Intellectual Disabilities*, 9(1):5–7.

Gates, B. and Barr, O. 2009 (Eds.). *The Oxford Handbook of Intellectual Disability Nursing.* Oxford: Oxford University Press.

Gates, B. 2011. Envisioning a workforce for the 21st Century. *Learning Disability Practice.* 14(1):12–18.

Gilbert, P. 2000. *A–Z of Syndromes and Inherited Disorders.* 3rd ed. Cheltenham: Stanley Thornes.

Glover, G. and Emerson, E. 2012. Patterns of decline in numbers of learning disability nurses employed by the English National Health Service. *Tizard Learning Disability Review,* 4 (17):194–198.

Heslop, P., Blair, P., Fleming, P., Hoghton, M., Marriott, A. et al. 2013. *Confidential Inquiry into premature deaths of people with learning disabilities, final report.* Bristol: Norah Fry Research Centre.

Inclusion Ireland. 2013. *Intellectual Disability Causes and Prevention: Your Questions Answered,* http://www.inclusionireland.ie/sites/default/files/documents/causesandpreventionbooklet.pdf (accessed August 19, 2014).

Klotz, J. 2004. Sociocultural study of intellectual disability: Moving beyond labeling and social constructionist perspectives. *British Journal of Learning Disabilities,* 32: 93–94.

Knight, S.J.L., Regan, R., and Nicod, A. 1999. Subtle chromosomal rearrangements in children with unexplained mental retardation. *The Lancet,* 345(9191):1676–1681.

Lejeune, J., Lafourcade, J., Berger, R., Vialatte, J., Boeswillwald, M., Serineg, P., and Turpin, R. 1963. Trois casde délétion partielle du bras court d'un chromosome 5. *CR Acad. Sci.* (D) 257:3098–3102.

Mair, R. 2009. Trying to get it right with campus closure. *Learning Disability Today,* 9(6):10–11.

Manthorpe, J., Alaszewski, A., Motherby, E., Gates, B., Ayer, S. 2004. Learning disability nursing: A multi-method study of education and practice. *Learning in Health and Social Care,* 3(2):92–101.

Mencap. 2007. *Death by indifference: Following up the* Treat me right! *report.* London: Mencap.

Mencap. 2012. *Death by indifference: 74 deaths and counting – a progress report 5 years on.* London, Mencap.

Mental Deficiency Act 1913. London: HMSO.

Mental Health Act 1959. London: HMSO.

Mental Health Act 1983. London: HMSO.

Mental Health Act 2007. London: HMSO.

Michael, J. 2008. *Healthcare for All: Report of the Independent Inquiry into Access to Healthcare for People with Learning Disabilities.* London: HMSO.

Morris, J.K., Wald, N.J., Mutton, D.E., and Alberman, E. 2003. Comparison of models of maternal age-specific risk for Down syndrome live births. *Prenatal Diagnosis,* 23(3):252–258.

Mueller, R.F. and Young, D. 1998. *Emery's Elements of Medical Genetics.* 10th ed. Edinburgh: Churchill Livingstone.

National Health Service Act 1946. London: HMSO.

Nursing and Midwifery Council. 2010. *Standards for Pre-Registration Nursing Education,* London: NMC.

Orem, D.E. 1991. *Nursing: Concepts of Practice*. St Louis: Mosby.

Oxford English Dictionary. 2013. http://oxforddictionaries.com/definition/english/eugenics?q=eugenics (accessed August 19, 2014).

Parrott, R., Tilley, N., and Wolstenholme, J. 2008. Changes in demography and demand for services from people with complex needs and profound and multiple learning disabilities. *Tizard Learning Disability Review,* 13(3):26–34.

Rittey, C.D. 2003. Learning difficulties: What the neurologist needs to know. *Journal of Neurological Neurosurgery Psychiatry,* 74:130–136.

Roper, N., Logan, W., and Tierney, A. 2002. *The Elements of Nursing*, 4th ed. Edinburgh: Churchill Livingstone.

Royal College of Nursing. 2011. *Learning from the Past—Setting Out the Future: Developing Learning Disability Nursing in the United Kingdom.* London: RCN.

Royal Commission on the Care and Control of the Feeble-Minded (1904–1908). *The Radnor Report.* Cd 4202. London: HMSO.

Thomson, M. 1996. Family, community, and state: The micro-politics of mental deficiency. In: Wright, D. and Digby, A. (Eds.) *From Idiocy to Mental Deficiency.* London: Routledge, pp. 207–230.

U.K. Chief Nursing Officers. 2012. *Strengthening the Commitment: The Report of the UK Modernising Learning Disabilities Nursing Review.* Scottish Government, Edinburgh, pp. 55.

Weinberg, R.A. 1989. Intelligence and IQ: Landmark issues and great debates. *American Psychologist*, 44(2):98–104.

WHO. 1992. *ICD-10 Classification of Mental and Behavioural Disorders. Clinical Descriptions and Diagnostic Guidelines.* Geneva: World Health Organisation.

Wiedemann, H.R., Kunze, J., and Dibbern, H. 1992. *An Atlas of Clinical Syndromes: A Visual Aid to Diagnosis,* 2nd ed. London: Mosby-Wolfe.

FURTHER READING

Department of Health. 2007. *Good Practice in Learning Disability Nursing*. London: Department of Health.

Gates, B. 2006. *Care Planning and Care Delivery in Intellectual Disability Nursing*. London: Blackwell Science.

Grant, G., Ramcharan, P., Flynn, M., and Richardson, M. 2010. *Learning Disability: A Life Cycle Approach*. Berkshire: OU Press.

Northway, R., Hutchinson, C., and Kingdon, A. 2006. *Shaping the Future: A Vision for Learning Disability Nursing*. UK Learning Disability Consultant Nurse Network.

Turnbull, J. 2004. *Learning Disability Nursing*. Oxford: Blackwell Publishing.

USEFUL RESOURCES

BILD: http://www.bild.org.uk/

Contact a Family: http://www.cafamily.org.uk/medical-information/conditions/

Enable Scotland: http://www.enable.org.uk/Pages/Enable_Home.aspx

Foundation for People with Learning Disabilities: http://www.learningdisabilities.org.uk/

Inclusion Ireland: http://www.inclusionireland.ie/

Intellectual Disability Info Web Pages: http://www.intellectualdisability.info/

Mencap: http://www.mencap.org.uk/

Mencap Northern Ireland: http://www.mencap.org.uk/northern-ireland

Mencap Wales: http://www.mencap.org.uk/wales

POLICY

England: Department of Health. 2009. Valuing people now: a new three year strategy for people with learning disabilities. http://www.dwp.gov.uk/docs/dla-reform-andover-and-district-mencap-appendix-3.pdf [archived and as such England has no current, coherent national policy specifically for people with learning disabilities] (accessed March 31, 2014).

Northern Ireland: Department of Health and Social Security. 2005. Equal lives: review of policy and services for people with a learning disability in Northern Ireland. www.dhsspsni.gov.uk /learning-disability-report (accessed March 31, 2014).

Scotland: Scottish Government. 2013. The keys to life: improving quality of life for people with learning disabilities. http://www.scotland.gov.uk/Publications/2013/06/1123 (accessed March 31, 2014).

Wales: Learning Disability Advisory Group. 2001. Fulfilling the promises: report of the learning disability advisory group. http://www.allwalespeople1st.co.uk/fulfillingthepromises.asp (accessed March 31, 2014).

2 History and modern-day practice of learning disability nursing

Kay Mafuba

INTRODUCTION

In this chapter, students of nursing will explore the nature of learning disabilities and their relationship to learning disability nursing. This will be contextualised within the Nursing and Midwifery Council for the United Kingdom (2010) and An Board Altranis (2005) standards for competence.

Learning disability nursing has a long and complex history and a tradition of supporting people with learning disabilities and their families. This chapter addresses the history of learning disability nursing, and its relationship with changing social policy in the 1930s, 1950s, 1960s, 1980s, and 1990s through to the present day. Some of this history has been blighted by scandal, isolated instances of abuse, and poor practice.

This chapter will demonstrate how learning disability nursing has moved from a narrowly defined role, within long-term care, to a much broader role within the National Health Service in the United Kingdom and beyond. So whereas this text is primarily aimed at a U.K. readership, social policy and governance differences will be explored briefly. Modern-day learning disability nursing roles span community support specialists, liaison roles between services and agencies, and roles in secure or forensic health settings, and these roles offer support across the age continuum.

It is known that people with learning disabilities carry a disproportionate health burden when compared with people in the general population (Emerson et al., 2011). Whereas people with learning disabilities have largely moved away from long-term residential care provided by the National Health Service, some still require specialist support from a specialist National Health Service provision, as well as a specialist National Health Service learning disability nursing workforce. And all people with learning disabilities, regardless of these specialist services and staff, will need to access the wider National Health Service. When they do access the wider National Health Service, people with learning disabilities are entitled to receive care and support from a workforce that will treat them as equal citizens.

There is a known and acknowledged history of inequity in mainstream health services for people with learning disabilities, and this is not acceptable (Disability Rights Commission, 2006; Mencap, 2007, 2012; Michael Report, 2008; Parliamentary and Health Ombudsmen, 2009). Given all of this, there remains a crucial role for learning disability nurses to assist in addressing these inequities as well as contributing to the lives of people with learning disabilities across the lifespan in a range of services and agencies. References will be made to the Nursing and Midwifery Council (NMC, 2010) and An Bord Alranais (An Board Altranais, 2005) standards for competence.

This chapter will focus on the following issues:

- What is learning disability nursing?
- Origins of learning disability nursing in the United Kingdom
- From 'mental deficiency nursing' to 'mental handicap' nursing in the United Kingdom
- From mental handicap nursing to learning disability nursing
- Strengthening the commitment
- History of intellectual disability nursing in Ireland
- Modern-day drivers for learning disability nursing practice in the United Kingdom
  - Health needs
- Policy
- Modern-day professional requirements of learning disability nurses
- Current services in the United Kingdom
- Wider learning disability nursing roles
- Select specialist learning disability nursing roles
  - Specialist assessment and treatment roles
  - Public health roles
  - Non-medical prescribing
- Future learning disability nursing roles

Competences

NMC Competences and Competencies

Domain 1: Professional values - Field standard for competence and competencies – 1.1; 2.1; 3.1; 4.1.

Domain 2: Communication and interpersonal skills - Field standard for competence and competencies – 1.1; 2.1; 4.1.

Domain 3: Nursing practice and decision-making - Field standard for competence and competencies – 1.1; 3.1; 5.1; 8.1.

An Bord Altranais Competences and Indicators

Domain 1: Professional/ethical practice – 1.1.5; 1.1.6; 1.1.8.

Domain 3: Interpersonal relationships – 3.1.2; 3.1.3; 3.2.1; 3.2.2.

WHAT IS LEARNING DISABILITY NURSING?

In the United Kingdom, learning disability nursing is defined as follows:

Learning disability nursing is a person-centred profession with the primary aim of supporting the well-being and social inclusion of people with learning disabilities through improving or maintaining physical and mental health

(DH 2007, p. 10)

Learning disability nurses work with people who have learning disabilities and who require a wide range of health and social care needs to be met, along with their families, and with their carers. Learning disability nurses work in a wide range of settings. They provide generalist and specialist nursing and health care. Such nurses require a wide range of generic nursing skills (for example, nursing assessment and care planning), and specialist skills (for example, behavioural and psychological assessments) (see Figure 2.1 and Box 2.1).

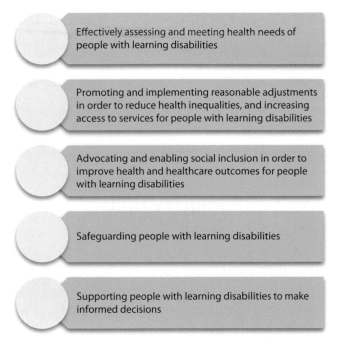

Effectively assessing and meeting health needs of people with learning disabilities

Promoting and implementing reasonable adjustments in order to reduce health inequalities, and increasing access to services for people with learning disabilities

Advocating and enabling social inclusion in order to improve health and healthcare outcomes for people with learning disabilities

Safeguarding people with learning disabilities

Supporting people with learning disabilities to make informed decisions

Figure 2.1 Key roles of learning disability nurses in the United Kingdom. (From DH et al., *Strengthening the Commitment: The Report of the UK Modernising Learning Disability Nursing Review,* Edinburgh: The Scottish Government, 2012.)

Box 2.1 *Key roles of learning disability nurses in Ireland (An Bord Altranais, 2013)*

Developing life skills and social skills for people with learning disabilities in order for people with learning disabilities to live independently in the community.

Working as part of a multi-disciplinary team and making referrals to them. This team may include, for example, professionals such as doctors, speech therapists, schoolteachers, and physiotherapists.

(continued)

Advocating, particularly for people with learning disabilities and communication difficulties.

Enhancing the quality of life for people with learning disabilities.

Providing support for families and carers of people with learning disabilities.

Providing health promotion and health education to people with learning disabilities, their families, carers, and the wider community.

Counseling.

Case management.

Budgeting.

Staff education and training.

Planning activities (i.e., social events and holidays).

Promotion of choice and independence.

Learning Activity 2.1: The roles of learning disability nurses

Having explored the roles of learning disability nurses above, consider the following:

Reflect on your own experience and identify other roles learning disability nurses could be involved in.

ORIGINS OF LEARNING DISABILITY NURSING IN THE UNITED KINGDOM

It could be argued that the introduction of asylums in the early part of the nineteenth century to accommodate the *'feeble-minded, imbeciles, or idiots'* with lifelong institutional care laid the foundations of learning disability nursing as we know it today. The purpose of this institutional care was aimed primarily at preventing sexual relations that were presumed to produce more people with mental deficiency. The fear that these people, deemed to be mentally deficient, would 'infect' the rest of the population led to the beginning of the eugenics movement in the 1860s. The eugenics movement came to an end only after World War II, during which Nazi Germany used eugenics theory to justify the horrors of the Holocaust.

The Mental Deficiency Act 1913 provided a distinct legal identity for people with learning disabilities. The operational segregation of service provision for people with learning disabilities provided for in the Act has had a long and lasting effect on the provision of nursing care. Under the Act, service provision for people with learning disabilities was based in large asylums under the remit of psychiatry. According to Mitchell (2004), before the introduction of the Mental Deficiency Act of 1913, training for the nurses working in mental deficiency institutions was developed and provided by the Royal Medico-Psychological Association. This training was designed for the nurses who were working in mental institutions of the time. According to Sines (2000), the training was flexible and was adapted to meet the needs of each institution.

FROM 'MENTAL DEFICIENCY NURSING' TO 'MENTAL HANDICAP' NURSING IN THE UNITED KINGDOM

The legal identity of people with *'mental deficiency'* (people with learning disabilities, as they were known then) introduced by the Mental Deficiency Act 1913 resulted in the development of a distinct qualification for mental deficiency nurses (as learning disability nurses were then known) by the Royal Medico-Psychological Association. According to Mitchell (2004), there were four distinct training courses for learning disability nurses (bedside nursing, occupational therapy, crafts training, and industrial therapy) designed to meet the individual needs of institutions. Following the Nurses Registration Act of 1919, the General Nursing Council created a separate Mental Nurses Supplementary Register for learning disability nurses. However, like mental health nurses, the majority of learning disability nurses continued to register with the Royal Medico-Psychological Association rather than the General Nursing Council (GNC) until after World War II. According to Dingwall et al. (1988), this was because the Royal Medico-Psychological Association examination was cheaper. In addition, medical superintendents supported the Royal Medico-Psychological Association examination. The inception of the National Health Service (NHS) in 1948 incorporated most learning disability institutions, and their training into the NHS. In the early 1950s the GNC took over training for nurses working in the NHS, and that included the training of mental health nurses and learning disability nurses. The incorporation of both mental health institutions and learning disability institutions contributed to the medicalisation of mental heath nurses and learning disability nurses. Despite this, literature demonstrates that there was a long history of debate as to whether learning disability nurses should be called nurses at all (Herringham, 1926; General Nursing Council, 1926).

The debate about the position of learning disability nursing within the nursing regulatory framework has existed since the Nurses Registration Act 1919. In the 1970s two reports were published suggesting that mental handicap nurses, as learning disability nurses were then known, should not be part of the nursing profession (Briggs, 1972; Jay, 1979). The Briggs Report (Briggs, 1972) recommended that a new profession needed to evolve and replace mental handicap nursing. In the following decade, a long debate about the future of mental handicap nursing did not result in a new profession, as recommended in the Briggs Report. Barbara Castle in her capacity as Secretary of State for Health in 1975 set up The Jay Committee (Jay, 1979) to review mental handicap nursing and the care mental handicap nurses provided. The Jay Report (Jay, 1979) was published just before the 1979 general election that brought Margaret Thatcher's conservative government to power. The key recommendation of the Jay Report (Jay 1979) was that a social care profession should replace mental handicap nursing. This recommendation was rejected by the government, which proposed joint training by the GNC and the Central Council for the Education and Training of Social Work (CCETSW) for staff working in mental handicap services (DOHSS, 1980). While mental handicap nurses' roles involved working with people who were not generally physically and mentally ill, such nurses' pre-registration training was based on a medical model of sickness and learning disability.

Appearing in the press in 1967 were allegations made by a nursing assistant of abuse and cruelty at the Ely Hospital in Cardiff in a unit for people with learning disabilities. The Howe (1969) report confirmed longstanding abusive treatment of people with learning disabilities. The revelations about this scandal, and others reported in the 1960s and 1970s, presented a publicity problem for the whole nursing profession, but particularly so for learning disability nursing. These scandals and discredited institutions raised further questions about the appropriateness of learning disability nursing being part of the nursing profession.

FROM MENTAL HANDICAP NURSING TO LEARNING DISABILITY NURSING

In 1991 Stephen Dorrell, then Health Minister, announced in the House of Commons that the term *'mentally handicapped'* would be changed to *'people with a learning disability'*. However, the United Kingdom Central Council for Nursing, Midwifery and Health Visiting (UKCC) (predecessor to the NMC) was reluctant to change the nursing qualification title to *'registered nurse for people with a learning disability'* from *'registered nurse for the mentally handicapped'* (UKCC, 1997).

Research articles published in the mid to late 1990s on empowerment (Sines, 1995), advocacy (Holmes, 1995), human rights issues (Carr, 1995), access to health care and discriminatory processes, which served to exclude individuals from receiving services on the basis of their learning disability (Bollard, 1999), and stigmatization of people with learning disabilities in general hospitals (Shanley and Guest, 1995; Slevin, 1995) raised fundamental questions about the philosophical basis and values of the care of people with learning disabilities. A study by Clifton et al. (1992) could not identify a single nursing skill that was specific to learning disability nursing. However, their conclusion was that the combination of the specific and unique knowledge of the needs of people with learning disabilities and their nursing skills was unique to the profession. This conclusion was consistent with the observation made by Raynes et al. (1994), who noted a *'quality effect'* of learning disability nurses. However, Moulster and Turnbull (2004) challenged this focus on the uniqueness of the knowledge of learning disability nurses, arguing that the focus on knowledge was more positivist and ignored the intuitiveness of learning disability nursing. A study by Turnbull (2005) noted that the uniqueness of learning disability nurses was inherent in their relationships with people with learning disabilities, which resulted in a demand for learning disability nurses in a wide range of services.

While the academic discourse focused on the place of people with learning disabilities in mainstream society, and the uniqueness of the knowledge of learning disability nurses, the government was undecided and questioned the future role of learning disability nurses in the nursing profession. The publication of *Signposts for Success* (DH, 1995a), which detailed the extent and complexity of the health and health care needs of people with a learning disability, led to a change in the government's position. The publication of *Continuing the Commitment* (DH, 1995b) emphasised a strong future role for learning disability nursing.

> ### Learning Activity 2.2: Origins of learning disability nursing
>
> Consider the origins of learning disability nursing and reflect on one positive lasting effect on the provision of nursing care to people with learning disabilities.
> Consider the origins of learning disability nursing and reflect on one negative lasting effect on the provision of nursing care to people with learning disabilities.

STRENGTHENING THE COMMITMENT

Strengthening the Commitment: The Report of the UK Modernising Learning Disability Nursing Review (DH, DHSSPS, Welsh Government and The Scottish Government, 2012) has highlighted the four countries of the United Kingdom's commitment to ensuring that people with learning disabilities will have access to the expert learning disability nursing they need throughout their lifespan for the foreseeable future. This commitment focuses on strengthening the capacity and capability of learning disability nurses. In addition, there is recognition of the need for clear leadership to clearly articulate roles of learning disability nurses in complex, multi-professional, and inter-organisational environments in which learning disability nurses will practice in the future (Abbott, 2007). Strong leadership will be crucial to ensuring that the recommendations made in *Strengthening the Commitment* move forward and that learning disability nurses across the United Kingdom continue to provide a powerful platform from which to celebrate, promote, and develop their unique health and health care contribution to the lives of people with learning disabilities in a wide range of care settings. It is clear across the four countries of the United Kingdom that learning disability nursing will focus on ensuring equitable access to health care for people with learning disabilities, promoting community-based services, developing a service ideology based on the social model of learning disabilities, promoting independence, promoting social inclusion and citizenship, and developing services that are person-centred.

Through the Nursing and Midwifery Council, the United Kingdom has retained specific training toward registration of Registered Nurse (Learning Disabilities) (NMC, 2010). There has been recent recognition that learning disability nurses continue to play an important role in transforming the models of care of people with learning disability from institutional models of care to community-based models. As a result, learning disability nurses of today and the future require a wide range of *"traditional"* nursing skills and *"non-traditional"* nursing skills alongside learning-disability-specific clinical, behavioural, and psychological intervention skills. These skills are important for learning disability nurses to facilitate health improvement through tackling the health inequalities that people with learning disabilities experience. To achieve this, learning disability nurses need to take responsibility for defining and shaping the future of their roles (Stewart and Todd, 2001). The shift toward preventive health will likely lead to major new roles for learning disability nurses. The challenge for learning disability nurses in both clinical practice and nurse education is to be proactive in developing evidence-based practice that is relevant to meeting the needs of people with learning disabilities.

HISTORY OF INTELLECTUAL DISABILITY NURSING IN IRELAND

According to Robbins (2000), service provision for people with intellectual disabilities in the Irish Republic evolved differently than in the United Kingdom. At the time of the Mental Deficiency Act 1913, the present-day Irish Republic was part of the United Kingdom. However, the Mental Deficiency Act 1913 was implemented only in England, Scotland, and Wales. Following the war of independence, and the subsequent civil war (1920–1923), economic difficulties forced the new Irish government to rely on religious orders, county homes, and mental asylums for the provision of care for people deemed to be mentally deficient, among many other poor groups of people.

Consequently, until the 1950s, the nature of mental handicap overshadowed the development of a specialist workforce, because of differing medical and religious views. During the 1940s, Catholic religious orders developed and managed specialist residential homes and schools for people with intellectual disabilities (as learning disabilities are known in the Republic of Ireland). At the time, the Irish General Nursing Council was against the involvement of medicine in nurse education. As a result, the Royal Medico-Psychological Association provided government-funded mental deficiency nurse training. The support of the government for mental deficiency nurse training signaled a significant shift toward people with intellectual disabilities, which resulted in distinct and separate provision for people with intellectual disabilities from generalist health care and mainstream psychiatric care in the late 1940s. In the 1950s, despite initial resistance from An Bord Altranais (successor to the General Nursing Council of Ireland), mental deficiency nurse training and registration was transferred from the Royal Medico-Psychological Association to An Bord Altranais. Divergent conceptions of training versus treatment led to tensions in syllabus development during the 1960s, with an enduring impact on a workforce situated at the margins of the discipline of nursing.

MODERN-DAY DRIVERS FOR LEARNING DISABILITY NURSING PRACTICE IN THE UNITED KINGDOM

Health needs

In the United Kingdom and internationally, the population of people with learning disabilities is increasing. According to Emerson and Hatton (2009) the population of people is projected to grow by 14% between 2001 and 2021. This increase in the population is expected across the lifespan (RCN, 2011). Just as important to note as the increasing population of people with learning disabilities is the increased proportion of individuals with severe, profound, multiple, and complex health and health care needs (Parrott et al., 2008; Emerson and Baines, 2010). Like the rest of the population, people with learning disabilities are living longer. However, for people with learning disabilities, there are higher incidence rates of age-related conditions such as dementia (Torr and Davis, 2007). Mencap (2007, 2012; Mansell and Wilson, 2010) have demonstrated the vulnerability of people with learning disabilities when they are accessing generic health services in the United Kingdom. Because of this vulnerability, people with learning disabilities are increasingly at higher risk of poor physical and mental health and early mortality.

This demographic shift requires learning disability nurses to develop skills essential for delivering health and health care to people with learning disabilities from birth to end of life. Increasingly, learning disability nurses work with people with learning disabilities with a wide range of complex social and health care needs in a wide range of services providing generalist and highly specialised nursing care. As a result, learning disability nurses require a wide range of basic and specialist nursing, behavioural, and psychological intervention skills.

Policy

In the United Kingdom, health and social care services continue to undergo significant strategic, structural, and economic changes. Recently, there has been an increased focus on localisation and integration of services. Furthermore, and particularly in England, there have been significant changes to how learning disability services are commissioned and delivered. In the NHS there has been a significant emphasis on outcomes. Learning disability nurses and other health care professionals who work with people with learning disabilities need to adapt to these changes to meet the increasing complexity of the health and health care needs of people with learning disabilities (Table 2.1).

Service modernisation policies across the four countries of the United Kingdom are broadly similar and aim at the following

a. Promoting choice, independence, social inclusion and citizenship
b. Developing services influenced by the social model of disabilities that are values-based, rights-based, and person-centred
c. Progressing integration of health and social care services
d. Promoting community-based primary care services
e. Ensuring access to health and health care services

Table 2.1 Modern-day policy drivers of learning disability nursing practice in the United Kingdom

Author	Year	England	Northern Ireland	Scotland	Wales
Scottish Executive	2000			The Same as You? A review of services for people with learning disabilities	
Department of Health	2001	Valuing People: A new strategy for learning disability for the 21st century - A White Paper			
Department of Health	2002	Action for Health, Health Action Plans and Health Facilitation: Detailed good practice guidance on implementation for learning disability partnership boards			
Scottish Executive	2002			Promoting Health, Supporting Inclusion: The national review of the contribution of nurses and midwives to the care and support of people with learning disabilities	
National Assembly for Wales	2002				Inclusion, Partnership and Innovation

(continued)

Author	Year	England	Northern Ireland	Scotland	Wales
Department of Health/ Department for Children, Schools and Families	2003	Together from the Start: Practical guidance for professionals working with disabled children (birth to third birthday) and their families			
NHS Health Scotland	2004			Health Needs Assessment Report: People with learning disabilities in Scotland	
Welsh Assembly Government	2004				Learning Disability Strategy. Section 7: Guidance on service principles and service responses
Department of Health, Social Services and Public Safety	2005		Equal Lives: Review of policy and services for people with a learning disability in Northern Ireland: The N. I. Bamford Review		
Department of Health, Social Services and Public Safety	2005		A Healthier Future: A twenty-year vision for health and well-being in Northern Ireland 2005–2025		
Department of Health, Social Services and Public Safety	2006		The Bamford Review of Mental Health and Learning Disability (NI): Forensic services		
NHS Quality Improvement Scotland	2006			Best Practice Statement: Promoting access to healthcare for people with learning disabilities	
Department of Health	2007	Good Practice in Learning Disability Nursing			
Department of Health, Social Services and Public Safety	2007		Complex Needs: The nursing response to children and young people with complex physical healthcare needs		

Author	Year	England	Northern Ireland	Scotland	Wales
Scottish Government	2007			Equally Well: The report of the Ministerial Task Force on Health Inequalities	
Welsh Assembly Government	2007				Statement on Policy and Practice for Adults with Learning Disabilities
Department of Health	2008	Healthcare for All: Report of the independent inquiry into access to healthcare for people with learning disabilities			
Scottish Government	2008			Better Health, Better Care: Action plan. What it means for you	
Scottish Government	2008			Achieving our Potential: A framework to tackle poverty and income inequality in Scotland	
Department of Health	2009	Valuing People Now: A new three-year strategy for people with learning disabilities			
Department of Health	2009	World Class Commissioning for the Health and Wellbeing of People with Learning Disabilities			
Department of Health	2009	The Bradley Report: Lord Bradley's review of people with mental health problems or learning disabilities in the criminal justice system			
Department of Health/ Department for Children, Schools and Families	2009	Healthy Lives, Brighter Futures. The strategy for children and young people's health			

(continued)

Author	Year	England	Northern Ireland	Scotland	Wales
Department of Health, Social Services and Public Safety	2009		Delivering the Bamford Vision. The response of the Northern Ireland Executive to the Bamford Review of Mental Health and Learning Disability action plan (2009–2011)		
Department of Health, Social Services and Public Safety	2009		Integrated Care Pathway for Children and Young People with Complex Physical Healthcare Needs		
Department of Health, Social Services and Public Safety	2009		Autism Spectrum Disorder (ASD) Strategic Action Plan 2008/09–2010/11		
NHS Quality Improvement Scotland	2009			Tackling Indifference: Healthcare services for people with learning disabilities national overview	
Welsh Assembly Government	2009				A Community Nursing Strategy for Wales
Welsh Assembly Government	2009				Post Registration Career Framework for Nurses in Wales
Welsh Assembly Government	2009				We Are on the Way. A policy agenda to transform the lives of disabled children and young people
Department of Health	2010	Raising Our Sights: Services for adults with profound intellectual and multiple disabilities. A report by Professor Jim Mansell			
Nursing and Midwifery Council	2010	Standards for pre-registration nursing 2010	Standards for pre-registration nursing 2010	Standards for pre-registration nursing 2010	Standards for pre-registration nursing 2010

Author	Year	England	Northern Ireland	Scotland	Wales
Department of Health, Social Services and Public Safety	2010		Living Matters, Dying Matters: A strategy for palliative and end of life care for adults in Northern Ireland		
Department of Health, Social Services and Public Safety	2010		A Partnership for Care: Northern Ireland strategy for nursing and midwifery 2010–2015		
Guidelines and Audit Implementation Network	2010		Guidelines: Caring for people with a learning disability in general hospital settings		
Scottish Government	2010			Getting it Right for Every Child	
Scottish Government	2010			The Healthcare Quality Strategy for NHS Scotland	
Scottish Government	2010			Towards an Autism Strategy for Scotland	
Welsh Assembly Government	2010				Setting the Direction: Primary and community services strategic delivery programme
Gates, B.	2011	Learning Disability Nursing. Task and finish group: Report for the Professional and Advisory Board for Nursing and Midwifery			
Emerson, E., Baines, S., Allerton, L., and Welch, V.	2011	Health Inequalities & People with Learning Disabilities in the UK: 2011			
Department of Health, Social Services and Public Safety	2011		Improving Dementia Services in Northern Ireland: A regional strategy		

(continued)

Author	Year	England	Northern Ireland	Scotland	Wales
Department of Health, Social Services and Public Safety	2011		Learning Disability Service Framework. Consultation document		
Learning Disability Implementation Advisory Group and Welsh Assembly Government	2011				Practice Guidance on Developing a Commissioning Strategy for People with Learning Disabilities
Public Health Wales and Welsh Government	2011				Good Practice Framework for People with Learning Disabilities Requiring Planned Secondary Care
Welsh Government	2011				Together for Health. A five-year vision for the NHS in Wales
DH, DHSSPS, Welsh Government and the Scottish Government	2012	Strengthening the commitment: The report of the UK Modernising Learning Disability Nursing Review	Strengthening the commitment: The report of the UK Modernising Learning Disability Nursing Review	Strengthening the commitment: The report of the UK Modernising Learning Disability Nursing Review	Strengthening the commitment: The report of the UK Modernising Learning Disability Nursing Review

MODERN-DAY PROFESSIONAL REQUIREMENTS OF LEARNING DISABILITY NURSES

The debate about the contribution of learning disability nurses to the health and health care of people with learning disabilities is as old as the profession itself. In the recent past, this debate intensified somewhat with the shift to a social model of service provision for people with learning disabilities. However, in the United Kingdom, the contributions of learning disability nurses remain an important and integral part of the health care workforce. The four countries of the United Kingdom (DH, DHSSPS, Welsh Government and the Scottish Government, 2012), and the Nursing and Midwifery Council (NMC, 2010) have demonstrated that learning disability nurses will continue to be an integral part of the nursing profession for the foreseeable future. Well-prepared learning disability nurses are essential to the delivery of high-quality health and health care for people with learning disabilities. However, to achieve better outcomes for people with learning disabilities, learning disability nurses need to have the knowledge and skills to work in partnership with other nurses and a wide range of other health and social care professionals.

The NMC (2010) standards require nursing graduates to be able to deliver essential support to those in their care, including people with learning disabilities. This emphasis places an onus on nurse training institutions to ensure that the care of people with learning disabilities is a key component of nurse education in the United Kingdom. People with learning disabilities receive health and health care from a wide range of professionals and agencies. This requires inter-professional and inter-agency collaboration. An important requirement of the new pre-registration nursing education is that all nursing graduates are competent in meeting the needs of vulnerable groups, including people with learning disabilities, irrespective of the field of nursing practice. All registered nurses should deliver safe, effective, and compassionate immediate care for people with learning disabilities, where necessary, before referring them to specialist services (NMC 2010). The NMC (2010) standards identify four sets of generic and field-specific competencies.

CURRENT SERVICES IN THE UNITED KINGDOM

The closure of long-stay NHS hospitals and large residential campuses has led to the relocation of people with learning disabilities into the community. Consequently, primary health care services are now the main health and health care provider for people with learning disabilities. This requires that those with learning disabilities acknowledge and are willing to receive treatment for health concerns. However, Treat Me Right (Mencap, 2004), Death by Indifference (Mencap, 2007), the Michael Report (2008), Six Lives (Parliamentary and Health Service Ombudsman, 2009), and Death by Indifference: 74 and Counting (2012), have revealed that primary and generic tertiary health care providers need to improve significantly on the care and treatment of people with health issues and learning disabilities. Learning disability nurses will need to play a significant role by developing and delivering appropriate education and training of other nurses and health care professionals. The development and maintenance of acute-liaison roles and strategic health facilitators who are capable of providing leadership in designing and implementing health action plans, and providing educational and training opportunities for generic staff health care professionals in primary and tertiary settings, is therefore important (Michael, 2008).

WIDER LEARNING DISABILITY NURSING ROLES

Currently in the United Kingdom, learning disability nurses work in a wide range of services, including acute assessment and treatment services for people with learning disabilities and mental illnesses, primary and community services, continuing care services, the education sector, community mental health or acute services, and, more recently, the criminal justice system, meeting the generalist and specialist health and health care needs of people with learning disabilities. Changing patterns of service provision across the United Kingdom means that most learning disability nurses no longer work in long-stay institutions. Learning disability nursing roles are now widely geographically dispersed. These roles are increasingly focused on interdisciplinary and inter-agency activities in the wider community. Given the morbidity rates in the population of people with learning disabilities, the demographic changes to this population, and the re-orientation of United Kingdom health and health care policy toward prevention, working learning disability nurses will increasingly assimilate new roles, such as health facilitator and health liaison roles.

> ## Learning Activity 2.3: The role of the learning disability nurse in assessing the needs of people with profound and multiple disabilities
>
> Mandy has profound learning and multiple disabilities. In addition, she has epilepsy, type-2 diabetes and dysphagia. Mandy's support workers are concerned that she might be losing weight. They have noticed that in the past few months her clothes have become too big for her. Because of her physical disability, the staff has not been able to measure her weight. Her seizures appear to be increasing in frequency and duration, and she has had several episodes of hypoglycemia in the fast few weeks. Staff has also noticed that Mandy has not had a bowel motion for one week.
>
> Identify and explore the role of the community learning disability nurse in this situation. What assessments can a learning disability nurse undertake?

These roles will need to focus on effectively identifying and meeting the health needs of people with learning disabilities, reducing health inequalities and improving access through the promotion and implementation of reasonable adjustments in primary and tertiary settings, and promoting improved health outcomes. In fulfilling their roles in the current demographic and policy contexts, learning disability nurses need to be aware of the broader nursing roles (see Figure 2.2).

SPECIALIST LEARNING DISABILITY NURSING ROLES

Learning disability nurses working in appropriate specialist services can provide critical early intervention and crisis resolution that can reduce unnecessary admissions to acute hospitals by providing expert assessment, care planning, implementation of planned interventions, and evaluations of care.

Specialist assessment and treatment roles

The specialist role of learning disability nurses may involve working with people with learning disabilities who have complex mental health and behavioural needs in inpatient assessment and treatment services, or in the community. In low-secure inpatient assessment and treatment units, learning disability nurses may provide assessment and treatment for people with learning disabilities who may have forensic histories. The skills required to undertake effective roles in these settings include cognitive behavioural therapy, positive behaviour support, functional assessments, staff training, developing proactive and reactive behavioural strategies, and development of skills that would minimise the risk of reoffending by people with learning disabilities. A significant proportion of people with learning disabilities (7%, compared with 2.5% in the mainstream population) are involved with the criminal justice system (DH, 2010). Consequently learning disability nurses are increasingly working in these services, using their specialist assessment, planning, and liaison skills to meet the health, health care, and social care needs of people with learning disabilities.

In the community, learning disability nurses can deliver behavioural family therapy. In addition, such nurses are increasingly involved in crisis intervention services through cognitive behavioural therapy, positive behaviour support, functional assessments, staff training, development of proactive and reactive behavioural strategies, and development of skills to support people with learning

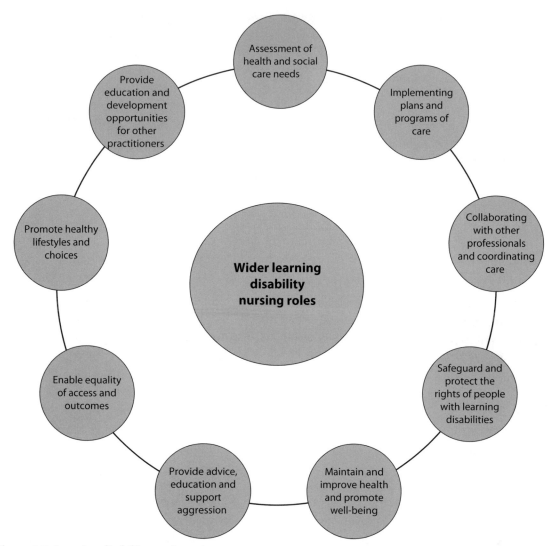

Figure 2.2 Learning disability nursing roles.

disabilities, to prevent admission to generic mental health in-patient services or specialist assessment and treatment services. There is a growing evidence base around psychological therapies and their benefits for people with learning disabilities (Brown and Marshall, 2006; Coiffait and Marshall, 2011). Consequently, learning disability nurses will require specialist skills to ensure that the assessment and treatment, and delivery of care to people with learning disabilities is timely in order to reduce hospital admissions.

Public health roles

Mafuba and Gates (2013) have recently identified health education, health prevention, health protection, facilitating access to preventative health, health promotion, and health surveillance as important specialist public health roles of learning disability nurses. They also noted in their study a significant increase in community learning disability nurses' involvement in health promotion and health screening roles. Barr (2006) has also previously noted the increasing involvement

> **Learning Activity 2.4: The specialist roles of the learning disability nurse in meeting the health and health care needs of people with profound and multiple disabilities**
>
> Refer to Mandy in Learning Activity 2.3 above.
>
> Having read the previous section on specialist learning disability nursing roles, identify those specialist roles that might be relevant in addressing Mandy's health needs.
>
> Explore how learning disability nurses could develop their knowledge and skills to undertake these roles.
>
> How would Mandy, her family, and her carers benefit from receiving support from a specialist learning disability nurse undertaking the roles identified?

of community learning disability nurses with health promotion and health screening. Mafuba and Gates (2013) observed that 94% of community learning disability nurses were involved with facilitating access to health and health care services. The roles of learning disability nurses are becoming more facilitatory, and they are increasingly expected to be involved in implementing public health initiatives for people with learning disabilities through health liaison and facilitation roles. It is important to note that the context in which learning disability nurses' public health roles evolve is undergoing fundamental change, particularly in England, with the transfer of the "public health" function of the NHS to local authorities. At the same time, the re-organisation of the NHS in England is resulting in some learning disability nursing roles being transferred to acute NHS trusts, specialist mental health and learning disability NHS organisations, local authorities, and social enterprises. These changes will affect learning disability nursing roles.

Non-medical prescribing

Epilepsy nurse specialists can undertake a non-medical prescribing course, which can enhance how learning disability nurses deliver nursing care to people with learning disabilities. The role of the epilepsy specialist nurse is varied in that it involves clinical management of cases, education and training of other professionals, and practice development to enhance the care of people with learning disabilities who live with epilepsy. This role provides opportunities to give advice and change medication rather than patients having to wait for an appointment with a medical doctor in a specialist epilepsy clinic. This allows the provision of timely and effective treatment of epilepsy, which reduces health risks by preventing seizures or adverse effects of medication.

FUTURE LEARNING DISABILITY NURSING ROLES

Learning disability nurses' roles are highly valued by people with learning disabilities, their families, and their carers. Learning disability nursing is based on the provision of safe and compassionate care, underpinned by human rights. These values and attitudes underlie the core skills learning disability nurses and all health professionals require to deliver safe and compassionate care in the future. Current practice changes and policy developments provide opportunities for learning disability nurses to undertake new, advanced, and extended roles in line with advances and role extensions in other fields of nursing practice. Evidence from *Strengthening the*

Commitment (DH et al., 2012) suggests that learning disability nurses need to focus particularly on developing competences in acute health liaison nursing, non-medical prescribing, psychological therapies such as cognitive behaviour therapy, telehealth, new roles supporting children and families through school nursing/health visiting/child, and adolescent mental health services, and forensic nursing of people with learning disabilities within the criminal justice system and specialist assessment and treatment services. The Health Equalities Framework (Atkinson et al., 2013) has detailed the determinants of health inequalities that people with learning disabilities experience. This provides opportunities for learning disability nurses to develop new roles focused on reducing premature death in the population of people with learning disabilities. The Confidential Inquiry into Premature Deaths of People with Learning Disabilities (CIPOLD) (Heslop et al., 2013) has made important recommendations for reducing such premature deaths. These include, but are not limited to, the following

  i. Clear identification of people with learning disabilities on the NHS record systems
  ii. A named health care coordinator to be allocated to people with complex or multiple health needs, or two or more long-term conditions
  iii. Standardisation of Annual Health Checks and a clear pathway between Annual Health Checks and Health Action Plans
  iv. Prioritisation of advanced health and care planning

These recommendations have clear implications for the present and future wider and specialist roles of learning disability nurses. These roles will become increasingly more complex and focused on health needs (see Figure 2.3).

CONCLUSION

There are a number of lessons that learning disability nurses of today can learn from the history of the profession to enhance their professional standing, in order to improve the health and health care outcomes of people with learning disabilities. The increasing complexity of health care needs of people with learning disabilities will require learning disability nurses to possess higher levels of both skills and knowledge to meet the needs of people with learning disabilities. Although the medical model of learning disability nursing was insufficient for meeting the holistic needs of people with learning disabilities, present and future roles of learning disability nurses will require a new repertoire of generic nursing skills and competences.

It is important for learning disability nurses to understand contemporary learning disability nursing in the light of the history of nurse education. In the United Kingdom and Ireland, the past development of learning disability nursing and its association with mental health nursing has had a significant impact on the registration of nursing since the beginning of the twentieth century. Learning disability nursing remains a separate and valued pre-registration course. Historical and contemporary debates about learning disability nurse education have concentrated somewhat on survival of the profession. There is a need for learning disability nurses, and rightly so, to focus the debates on the profession's contribution to the health and health care outcomes of people with learning disabilities.

Learning disability nursing has survived constant re-examination and change since its inception as a specialty within nursing. The continued survival of learning disability nursing will no doubt

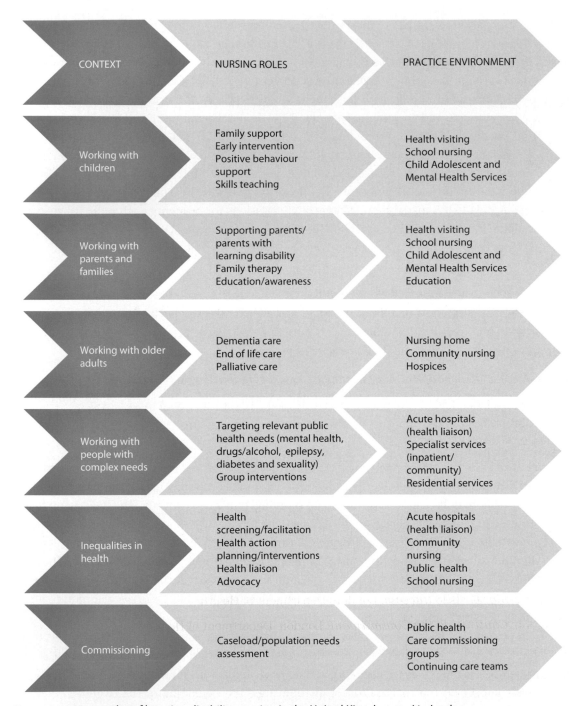

Figure 2.3 Future roles of learning disability nursing in the United Kingdom and Ireland.

depend on learning disability nurses' ability to improve existing roles and to assimilate new roles in line with the needs of people with learning disabilities, government policy, and the evidence concerning the needs of people with learning disabilities. Learning disability nursing role changes are essential to ensure that such nurses are able to provide immediate and long-term care to people with learning disabilities.

REFERENCES

Abbott, S. 2007. Leadership across boundaries: A qualitative study of the nurse consultant role in English primary care. *Journal of Nursing Management*, 15(7):703–710.

An Bord Altranais. 2005. *Requirements and Standards for Nurse Registration Education Programmes* (3rd ed.). Dublin: An Bord Altranais.

An Bord Altranais. 2013. A day in the life: Intellectual disability nurse. Dublin: An Bord Altranais. (Online). Available at http://www.nursingboard.ie/en/day_life-intel_disability_nurse.aspx (accessed September 13, 2013).

Atkinson, D., Boulter, P., Hebron, C., Moulster, G., Giraud-Saunders, A., and Turner, S. 2013. The Health Equalities Framework (HEF) - An outcomes framework based on the determinants of health inequalities. http://www.ndti.org.uk/uploads/files/The_Health_Equality_Framework.pdf (accessed August 19, 2014).

Barr, O. 2006. The evolving role of community nurses for people with learning disabilities: Changes over an 11-year period. *Journal of Clinical Nursing*, 15:72–82.

Bollard, M. 1999. Improving primary health care for people with learning disabilities. *British Journal of Nursing*, 8(18):1216–1221.

Briggs, A. 1972. *Report of the Committee on Nursing. Cmnd 5115*. London: HMSO.

Brown, M., and Marshall, K. 2006. Cognitive behaviour therapy and people with learning disabilities: Implications for developing nursing practice. *Journal of Psychiatric and Mental Health Nursing*, 13:234–241.

Carr, L.T. 1995. Sexuality and people with learning disabilities. *British Journal of Nursing*, 4(19):1135–1140.

Clifton, M., Shaw, M., and Brown, J. 1992. *Transferability of Mental Handicap Nursing Skills from Hospital to Community*. York: University of York Department of Social Policy and Social Work.

Coiffait, F.M., and Marshall, K. 2011. How to recognise and respond to mental health needs. *Learning Disability Practice*, 14(3):23–28.

DH. 1995a. *Signposts to Success*. London: Department of Health.

DH. 1995b. *Continuing the Commitment*. London: Department of Health.

DH. 2007. *Good Practice in Learning Disability Nursing*. London: Department of Health.

DH. 2010. *Positive Practice Positive Outcomes: A Handbook for Professionals Working with Offenders with a Learning Disability*. London: Department of Health.

DH, DHSSPS, Welsh Government and The Scottish Government. 2012. *Strengthening the Commitment: The Report of the UK Modernising Learning Disability Nursing Review*. Edinburgh: The Scottish Government.

DoHSS. 1980. Government's response to Jay Report. Press Release 80/189.

Dingwall, R., Rafferty, A.M., and Webster, C. 1988. *An Introduction to the Social History of Nursing*. London: Routledge.

Emerson, E., Baines, S., Allerton, L. and Welch, V. 2011. *Health Inequalities & People with Learning Disabilities in the UK: 2011*. http://www.improvinghealthandlives.org.uk/securefiles/140211_1103//IHaL%202011-09%20HealthInequality2011.pdf (accessed August 19, 2014).

Emerson, E., and Baines, S. 2010. *The Estimated Prevalence of Autism among Adults with Learning Disabilities in England*. London: DH.

Emerson, E., and Hatton, C. 2009. *Estimating Future Numbers of Adults with Profound Multiple Learning Disabilities in England*. Lancaster: Centre for Disability Research, Lancaster University.

General Nursing Council. 1926. *Shorthand Notes of the Mental Nursing Committee*. 1925–1926, Public Records Office, DT6/98.

Herringham, W. 1926. *Letter to Ministry of Health 2.2. 1926*. Public Records Office. DT48/158.

Heslop, P., Blair, P., Fleming, P., Hoghton, M., Marriott, A., and Russ, L. 2013. *The Confidential Inquiry into Premature Deaths of People with Learning Disabilities (CIPOLD)*. Bristol: Norah Fry Research Centre.

Holmes, A. 1995. Self-advocacy in learning disabilities. *British Journal of Nursing*, 4(8):448–450.

Howe Report. 1969. *Report of the Committee of Inquiry into Allegations of Ill Treatment of Patients and Other Irregularities at the Ely Hospital, Cardiff. Cm 3975*. London: HMSO.

Jay, P. 1979. *Report on the Committee of Enquiry into Mental Handicap Nursing and Care*, Cmnd 7468.

Mansell, I., and Wilson, C. 2010. 'It terrifies me the thought of the future': Listening to current concern of informal carers of people with a learning disability. *Journal of Intellectual Disability*, 14(1):21–31.

Mafuba, K., and Gates, B. 2013. An investigation into the public health roles of community learning disability nurses. *British Journal of Learning Disability*. DOI: 10.1111–bld.12071

Mencap. 2004. *Treat Me Right! Better Health for People with Learning Disabilities*. London: Mencap.

Mencap. 2007. *Death by Indifference*. London: Mencap.

Mencap. 2012. *Death by Indifference: 74 deaths and counting*. London: Mencap.

Michael, J. 2008. *Healthcare for All: Report of the Independent Inquiry into Access to Healthcare for People with Learning Disabilities*. London: Department of Health.

Mitchell, D. 1998. Learning disability nursing: Reflections on history. *Journal of Learning Disabilities for Nursing, Health Social Care*, 2:45–49.

Mitchell, D. 2004. Parallel stigma? Nurses and people with learning disabilities. *British Journal of Learning Disabilities*, 28:78–81.

Moulster, G., and Turnbull, J. 2004. The purpose and practice of learning disability nursing. In: Turnbull, J. (ed.), *Learning Disability Nursing*. Oxford: Blackwall Science.

NMC. 2010. *Standards for Pre-Registration Nurse Education*. London: Nursing and Midwifery Council.

Parliamentary and Health Service Ombudsman and Social Services Ombudsman. 2009. *Six Lives: The Provision of Public Services to People with Learning Disabilities*. London: TSO.

Parrott, R., Tilley, N., and Wolstenholme, J. 2008. Changes in demography and demand for services from people with complex needs and profound and multiple learning disabilities. *Tizard Learning Disability Review*, 13(3):26–34.

Raynes, N. V., Wright, K., Shiell, A., and Pettipher, C. 1994. *The Cost and Quality of Community Residential Care*. London: Fulton.

Robbins, J. 2000. *Nursing and Midwifery in Ireland in the Twentieth Century*. Dublin: An Bord Altranais.

RCN. 2011. *Meeting the Health Needs of People with Learning Disabilities*. London: Royal College of Nursing.

Shanley, E., and Guest, C. 1995. Stigmatization of people with learning disabilities in general hospitals. *British Journal of Nursing*, 4(13):759–760.

Slevin, E. 1995. Student nurses' attitudes towards people with learning disabilities. *British Journal of Nursing*, 4(13):761–768.

Sines, D.T. 1990. 'Valuing the Carers: An Investigation of Support Systems Required by Mental Handicap Nurses Working in Residential Services in the Community'. Unpublished PhD thesis. Southampton: University of Southampton.

Sines, D. 1995. Empowering consumers: The caring challenge. *British Journal of Nursing*, 4(8):445–448.

Stewart, D., and Todd, M. 2001. Role and contribution of nurses for learning disabilities: A local study in a county of Oxford-Anglia region. *British Journal of Learning Disabilities*, 29(4):145–150.

Torr, J., and Davis, R. 2007. Ageing and mental health problems in people with intellectual disability. *Current Opinion in Psychiatry*, 29(5):467–471.

Turnbull, J. 2005. 'In Search of the Accomplished Practitioner'. Unpublished PhD thesis. Reading: University of Reading.

UKCC. 1997. *Registrar's Letter 20/1997*. London: United Kingdom Central Council for Nursing, Midwifery and Health Visiting.

Wolfensberger, W. 1972. *The Principle of Normalization in Human Services*. Toronto: National Institute on Mental Retardation.

FURTHER READING

An Bord Altranais. 2005. Requirements and Standards for Nurse Registration Education Programmes (3rd ed). Dublin: An Bord Altranais.

Atkinson D., Boulter, P., Hebron, C., Moulster, G., Giraud-Saunders, A., and Turner, S. 2013. The Health Equalities Framework (HEF) - An outcomes framework based on the determinants of health inequalities. http://www.ndti.org.uk/uploads/files/The_Health_Equality_Framework.pdf.

DH. 2007. *Good Practice in Learning Disability Nursing*. London: Department of Health.

DH, DHSSPS, Welsh Government and the Scottish Government. 2012. *Strengthening the Commitment: The Rreport of the UK Modernising Learning Disability Nursing Review*. Edinburgh: The Scottish Government.

Gates, B. 2011. *Learning Disability Nursing: Task and Finish Group: Report for the Professional and Advisory Board for Nursing and Midwifery*. London: Department of Health.

Heslop, P., Blair, P., Fleming, P., Hoghton, M., Marriott, A., and Russ, L. 2013. *The Confidential Inquiry into Premature Deaths of People with Learning Disabilities (CIPOLD)*. Bristol: Norah Fry Research Centre.

NMC. 2010. *Standards for Pre-Registration Nurse Education*. London: Nursing and Midwifery Council.

RCN. 2012. *Going Upstream: Nursing's Contribution to Public Health: Prevent Promote and Protect*. London: Royal College of Nursing.

USEFUL RESOURCES

An Bord Altranais: http://www.nursingboard.ie/en/reqs_stds_reg.aspx

BILD: http://www.bild.org.uk/

Contact a Family: http://www.cafamily.org.uk/medical-information/conditions/

Enable Scotland: http://www.enable.org.uk/Pages/Enable_Home.aspx

Foundation for People with Learning Disabilities: http://www.learningdisabilities.org.uk/

Inclusion Ireland: http://www.inclusionireland.ie/

Intellectual Disability Info Web Pages: http://www.intellectualdisability.info/

Mencap: http://www.mencap.org.uk/

Mencap Northern Ireland: http://www.mencap.org.uk/northern-ireland

Mencap Wales: http://www.mencap.org.uk/wales

Nursing and Midwifery Council: http://standards.nmc-uk.org/Pages/Welcome.aspx

3 Learning disability nursing throughout the lifespan

Kay Mafuba and Bob Gates

INTRODUCTION

In this chapter, students of nursing will explore the nature of learning disabilities throughout the lifespan and its relationship to learning disability nursing. This will be contextualised within the Nursing and Midwifery Council for the United Kingdom (2010) and An Bord Altranais (2005) standards for competence.

A learning disability is a lifelong condition, and it is therefore not unusual for learning disability nurses to work with, or offer support to, people with learning disabilities throughout their lifespans, quite literally from the cradle to the grave. Holistic approaches in learning disability nursing seek to promote interventions that adopt a whole-person-centred approach. This means providing nursing that responds to the various dimensions of being, and these typically include attention to the physical, emotional, social, economic, and spiritual needs of people.

Therefore, this chapter will focus on the knowledge and kinds of practical skills that learning disability nurses will need when working with people with learning disabilities across their lifespans. The role of the learning disability nurse during the childhood and adolescence of people with learning disabilities is explored in the context of diagnosing learning disability, parenting children with learning disabilities, transition, psychological and physical changes during adolescence, and transition into adulthood. The lifestyle and health needs of adults and older adults with learning disabilities, employment and retirement, personal relationships, and parenting needs of adults with learning disabilities will be explored. The chapter concludes by exploring end-of-life care needs, and palliative care for people with learning disabilities.

This chapter will focus on the following issues:

- Childhood
  - Diagnosis of a learning disability
  - Parenting
  - Starting school
- Adolescence
  - Transition issues
  - Psychological and physical changes
  - The role of the learning disability nurse

- Adulthood
  - Maintaining healthy lifestyles and health
  - Employment
  - Personal relationships
  - Parents with learning disabilities
- Older adults with learning disabilities
  - Retirement
  - Health needs of older adults with learning disabilities
  - Loss
- End-of-life care
  - Breaking news
  - End-of-life decisions
  - Palliative care and people with learning disabilities

Competences

NMC Competences and Competencies

Domain 1: Professional values - Field standard for competence and competencies –
1.1; 2.1; 3.1; 4.1.
Domain 2: Communication and interpersonal skills - Field standard for competence
and competencies – 1.1; 2.1; 3.1.
Domain 3: Nursing practice and decision-making - Field standard for competence and
competencies – 1.1; 3.1; 5.1; 8.1.
Domain 4: Leadership, management and team working – Field standard for competence and competences – 1.1; 1.2; 6.1.

An Bord Altranais Competences and Indicators

Domain 1: Professional/ethical practice – 1.1.1; 1.1.2; 1.1.8.
Domain 2: Holistic approaches to care and the integration of knowledge – 2.2.1; 2.3.2;
2.3.3; 2.3.4.
Domain 3: Interpersonal relationships – 3.1.2; 3.1.3; 3.2.1; 3.2.2.
Domain 4: Organisation and management of care – 4.1.2; 4.1.3; 4.3.1.

CHILDHOOD

Diagnosis of a learning disability

Pregnancy and the subsequent birth of any child leads to new circumstances that require parents and other family members to make significant changes to their lifestyles. This process of change and adaptation becomes more significant and complex if the unborn or new baby is diagnosed with, or suspected of having a learning disability (Barr and Millar, 2003). Prospective parents, and parents of a child with, or suspected of having learning disabilities will seek answers. This requires effective liaison, and multiagency cooperation between specialist services, primary care services, learning disabilities specialist services, and the family. During this stressful time, parents and families of children with learning disabilities will require coordinated and integrated support that will facilitate access to all the essential services. Figure 3.1 outlines key elements of an integrated care pathway that may be used to support families during this process of diagnosis.

The National Service Framework for Children, Young People and Maternity Services (DH/DfES, 2004) has highlighted the importance of multiagency care pathways for children with long-term conditions, such as those with learning disabilities, in order to improve their health and health care outcomes. Providing an effective care pathway for children and young people with learning disabilities and complex needs is difficult. However, defined care pathways are important in defining and identifying services that families of children with learning disabilities can identify and access easily. Defined care pathways for children with learning disabilities and complex needs provide opportunities for joining processes and agencies together.

It is important to note that

> **At the point of diagnosis of a child's disability, a parent's first question is hardly likely to be about the local early childhood intervention services. These families are frightened, disturbed, upset, grieving and constantly vulnerable. The role of the professionals involved with them is to catch them when they fall, listen to their sorrow, dry their tears of pain and anguish, and, when the time is right, plan the pathway forward.**

(Carpenter, 2005, p. 181)

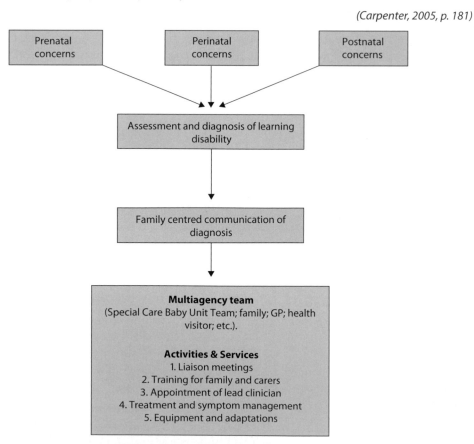

Figure 3.1 Pathways for assessment and diagnosis of a learning disability.

> ## Box 3.1 *Communicating diagnosis of a learning disability*
>
> Provide unlimited time for face-to-face discussion of diagnosis and prognosis.
>
> Breaking the news must be undertaken in a location and place that ensures complete privacy.
>
> Parents should receive the news together from a lead clinician, and preferably in the presence of a relative or friend who would be able to provide support.
>
> Written materials explaining the diagnosis and prognosis should be provided.
>
> Where English is not the first language of both or one of the parents, professional interpretation services should be made available.
>
> Information about how best to support the child must be provided.
>
> Parents must be provided with a key liaison professional with the Special Care Baby Unit.

The National Service Framework for Children, Young People and Maternity Services (DH/DfES 2004) has set out four key standards for the provision of integrated care pathways for children with complex needs. Guidance is provided about how to communicate the diagnosis of a learning disability to the parents and the family (see Box 3.1).

After breaking the news to the family regarding the diagnosis of a learning disability, and prognosis planning for discharge from hospital, transfer of care to primary care services needs to be commenced. A lead professional (normally a clinician) must be identified and allocated to coordinate the process in partnership with the parents and carers. The lead professional will need to inform all relevant community health and social care services. The lead professional should also begin coordinating a discharge plan, which takes into account the needs of the family. During the discharge planning, the child's general practitioner will need to be invited to the discharge planning meeting, and clear plans should be put in place for shared social and medical care before discharge from hospital. A detailed needs assessment should be undertaken, which will include identification of essential adaptations, equipment, and any supplies, and should be in place before discharge. Necessary training for the parents and other carers should be arranged, and provided prior to discharge. There should be clear channels of communication in the absence of the lead clinician, and the family may need to be provided with an emergency contact number that should ideally be available 24 hours a day. Following discharge from hospital, a home visit by the lead clinician, and other relevant professionals should be arranged within three days of transfer (DH/DfES, 2004). A multiagency team, which includes all appropriate health and social care professionals, will need to be set up. The team is responsible for carrying out a detailed assessment, which focuses on identifying long-term medical, health care, developmental, and social care needs of the child. In addition, the needs of the family, and any environmental adaptations need to be identified (see Figure 3.2).

Parenting

In general, parenting is a challenging task, and it may be all the more difficult if a child has a learning disability. Parents and families of children with learning disabilities are likely to face and experience parenting challenges that extend beyond idealised or mainstream expectations (Gray, 2002). Rogers (2011) has argued that prospective parents experience pressures from internalised norms and societal expectations to produce 'perfect' children. When a child with a learning disability is

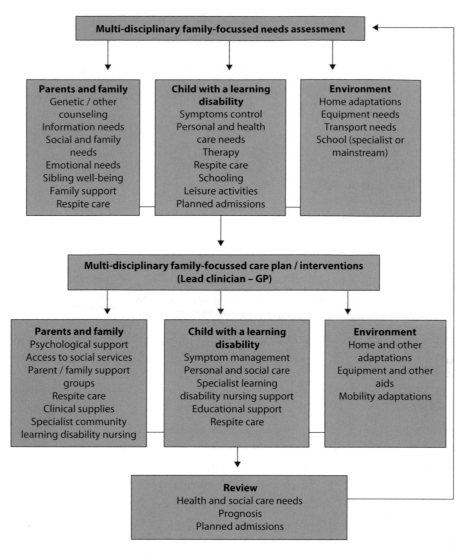

Figure 3.2 Pathways for managing children with learning disabilities in the community.

expected or born, parents are likely to experience shock, loss, disappointment, and bereavement. In most cases, if no adequate support is provided, these initial reactions are likely to result in denial, anxiety, parental and family conflicts, conflicts between professionals, and conflicts between the family, professionals, and agencies. Subsequently, the right levels of support, both formal and informal, are important for families of children with learning disabilities.

McConkey et al. (2008), in a study that investigated the impact of bringing up a child with a learning disability observed that mothers of children with learning disabilities experienced high levels of stress, poor health, and poor family relationships. The study concluded that care pathways for children with learning disabilities need to be family focused. Figure 3.2 illustrates a care pathway for managing children with learning disabilities in the community.

Adequately caring for children with learning disabilities is often challenging and stressful, and can significantly impact on the family relationships for all family members across the lifespan of the person with learning disabilities. In a study investigating the psychological problems of and marital adjustments needed by families caring for children with learning disabilities, Kilic et al. (2013) concluded that the continued provision of education and support for families is of vital importance. The presence of a learning disability in a child is likely to result in other parental needs that are dependent on the degree of the child's learning disability and cultural background, as well as the social and economic circumstances of the family.

Health care agencies and health care professionals need to adopt family-centered approaches and care pathways to adequately meet the health and social care needs of children with learning disabilities and complex needs. Family-focused interventions and care pathways are important because parents' and families' positive attitudes and psychological well-being are important in the intellectual, psychological, and social development of children with learning disabilities (Shobana and Saravanan, 2014).

Health care professionals, such as community learning disability nurses, need not only take account of the health and social care needs of the families of children with learning disabilities, but their cultural needs in order to design appropriate and multidisciplinary interventions. There is also a need to recognise the variation between the needs of fathers, mothers, siblings, and wider family that may result from having a child with a learning disability (Verma and Kishore, 2009). It is also important to note that the needs of a family of a child with a learning disability will not remain static across the lifespan but will vary with the gender, age, and level of impairment of the child with a learning disability.

Starting school

In 2011 in England, 89% of children with moderate learning disabilities, 24% of children with severe learning difficulties, and 18% of children with profound and multiple learning disabilities were being educated in mainstream schools (Emerson et al., 2011). For parents and carers of children with learning disabilities, deciding on an appropriate school may be difficult and could require professional support. In addition to the developmental limitations due to learning disabilities, other related conditions are likely to play a significant role in the schooling of a child with a learning disability. For example, Emerson et al. (2010), in a study of the mental health of young children with learning disabilities, observed that they experienced significantly higher rates of mental health problems when compared to children without learning disabilities. In addition, children with learning disabilities are prone to increased risk of attention deficit hyperactivity disorder

---

Learning Activity 3.1

Consider the needs assessment and care planning required for managing children with learning disabilities and complex needs (refer to Figure 3.2).

What is the role of the learning disability nurse who may be involved in the assessment process?

What could the positive outcomes of the involvement of learning disability nurses be in assessment, planning, and delivery of care for children with learning disabilities and complex needs?

(ADHD) (Hastings et al., 2005). Furthermore, children with autism and learning disabilities are at increased risk of developing challenging behaviour (Griffith et al., 2010). Worse still, epilepsy is the most common neurological disorder in children with learning disabilities and can have a significant impact on a child's schooling (Reilly and Ballantine, 2011).

Interventions to support children with learning disabilities in schools should focus on the management of additional health needs. The conditions highlighted previously may have minimal effect on some children's schooling, but these conditions may require significant support from a wide range of professionals. Individualised approaches within school environments and close collaboration among schools, parents, and health care professionals are in place to meet a child's needs. Learning disability nurses working in school nursing teams, child and adolescent mental health services, and community learning disability teams can provide useful interventions that could contribute to meeting the schooling needs of children with learning disabilities.

ADOLESCENCE

In England, 23,776 children in 2012 were identified as having a learning disability, representing 0.21% of the total child population (Emerson, 2013). Children with learning disabilities are likely to have poorer health and health outcomes than children without learning disabilities. There is a body of evidence which shows that people with learning disabilities have much greater health needs than those of comparable age groups who do not have learning disabilities (NHS Executive, 1998; Backer et al., 2009). For example, according to Linna et al. (1999) people with learning disabilities experience higher rates of mental health disorders as compared to the general population. In addition Dekker et al. (2002) reported that approximately 40% of children and adolescents with learning disabilities are likely to have a diagnosable mental health problem. These high rates of mental health problems among adolescents with learning disabilities are important for a number of reasons during this transition into adulthood. Adolescence is a time of intense emotional and social change, and mental health problems can have significant negative impact on the life opportunities, social inclusion, and well-being of children with learning disabilities (Quilgars et al., 2005). In addition, Hatton and Emerson (2003) and Baker et al. (2005) have reported that mental health problems in adolescents with learning disabilities negatively impact the general well being of their families and carers. Furthermore, Emerson and Hatton (2007) have reported that the mental health problems of adolescents with learning disabilities are likely to lead to group residential home placements.

Transition issues

Emerson et al. (2013) have reported that at the end of Key Stage 2, children with learning disabilities, perhaps not unexpectedly, achieve significantly lower than children who do not have learning disabilities. For example, in 2011, only 15% of children with moderate learning disabilities, 3% of children with severe learning disabilities, and 2% of children with profound and multiple learning disabilities attained the expected levels in English and Mathematics versus 74% of the children who did not have learning disabilities. These low levels of attainment mean that adolescents with learning disabilities will require purposeful and planned transfer from education and other child services to adult social and health care services.

Bloomquist et al. (1998) have reported that 90% of children with disabilities now survive into adulthood. This means there is now a growing need for specialised transition services to ensure that there is seamless transfer and transition from children's to adult health care and social care services. Currently in the United Kingdom, there is no specific national provision for transition for adolescents with learning disabilities. Currently, children with learning disabilities stay in children's services perhaps longer than is required or appropriate. Current transfers are abrupt and inappropriate, with some children becoming invisible by default, or voluntarily.

Multidisciplinary working is essential for adolescents with learning disabilities going through transition from children's to adult services. The *National Service Framework for Children and Young People's Continuing Care* (DH, 2010) recognised that transition for children with continuing health and social care needs need to be guided, educational, and therapeutic instead of administrative. For transition services for adolescents with learning disabilities to be effective, professionals and health and social care services need to be aware that these adolescents will be undergoing broader changes beyond their clinical needs. These adolescents, regardless of their learning disabilities, will desire and strive for autonomy and involvement in decision making about their lives. It is therefore important to involve families and carers in the transition process. Effective transition services require leadership, collaboration, cross-boundary working, resources, a skilled and knowledgeable workforce, effective administration support, and clearly defined pathways. The Royal College of Nursing (RCN, 2004) has suggested a transition pathway for adolescents with learning disabilities (see Figure 3.3).

Psychological and physical changes

As discussed earlier in this chapter, adolescents with learning disabilities have high rates of mental health problems (see Chapter 5) and behavioural difficulties (see Chapter 9). Adolescence is a time of emotional change, and for those with learning disabilities intellectual impairment reduces their capacity to adapt creatively to life's challenges. According to Hatton and Emerson (2004), adolescents with learning disabilities are more likely to experience poverty and social disadvantage, which, in turn, is likely to contribute to complexity in their lives. Ammerman et al. (1994) have reported that adolescents with learning disabilities experience higher rates of stressful life events, including physical and sexual abuse, as compared with those without learning disabilities. The presence of mental illness and experience of stressful life events result in increased levels of behaviours likely to challenge services.

In addition, adolescents experience comorbid disorders, such as epilepsy, autism, and ADHD (Allington-Smith, 2006), which impact on their experiences during this period of their lives. Furthermore, long-term physical conditions such as epilepsy, diabetes, and obesity are common in adolescents with learning disabilities. It is also important to recognise that some genetic conditions, such as Prader–Willi, Down, and Asperger syndromes, are associated with adolescents with learning disabilities. The treatment and management of health and social conditions resulting from these syndromes require careful planning.

Communication difficulties, and additional sensory disabilities such as hearing impairments, reduce adolescents' ability to interact with others or contribute meaningfully to their transition from children's to adult services. For some adolescents with learning disabilities, a lack of coping strategies is likely to result in a reliance on aberrant behaviours such as shouting, screaming, or aggression. Adolescents with learning disabilities may also have low self-esteem and may experience

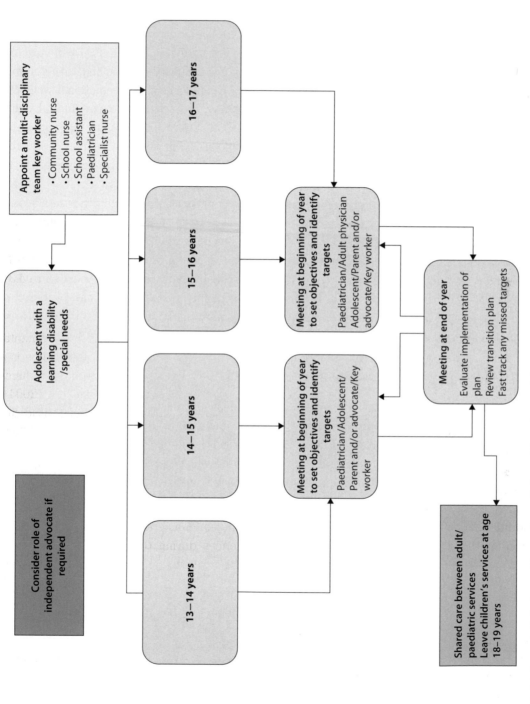

Figure 3.3 Adolescent clinical transition pathway (Adapted from RCN, *Adolescent Transition Care: Guidance for Nursing Staff*, London: Royal College of Nursing, 2004.)

stigmatization by others. This can result in depression and anxiety, particularly in older children with learning disabilities as the ability gap between them and their non-disabled peers widens.

The role of the learning disability nurse

As more people with learning disabilities grow into adulthood, learning disability nurses need to develop skills to recognise and manage disorders in adolescents with learning disabilities. This requires them to work in a wide range of multidisciplinary health teams. The ultimate outcome for the involvement of learning disability nurses with adolescents with learning disabilities should be supporting in order to achieve their full potential in terms of ability, physical, psychological, and emotional well-being. Learning disability nurses need to be aware that this will always require them to work in multiagency settings such as education, health, and social services. The RCN (2004) has suggested that meeting the needs of adolescents with learning disabilities during transition to adult services could be facilitated by using a competency-based framework covering self-advocacy, health care behaviours, sexual health, psychosocial support, educational and vocational planning, and health and lifestyles.

Pre-registration and post-registration nurses working in primary, acute, and other settings, and across a wide range of agencies require training to be able to care for and support adolescents with learning disabilities during transition to adulthood. Involving practitioners from all agencies in interprofessional learning is essential to facilitate the establishment of effective transition policies and processes that incorporate all aspects of the wider health and social care needs of adolescents with learning disabilities. Such interprofessional needs include transitional care, adolescents' perspectives, mental health and behavioural problems, communication, leadership, and interprofessional and interagency working.

ADULTHOOD

Donelly (2008) has reported that only 1% of people with learning disabilities live in owner-occupied accommodation as compared with 79% of the general population of the United Kingdom. Ericson et al. (2013) have reported that, as of 2012, across the adult age groups of adults with learning disabilities in England, 79.4% of residential accommodation was provided by the independent sector (the most common form of residential support was the independent sector), with the rest living in adult placements or local authority-staffed residential care homes. However, research has shown that adults with learning disabilities have a negative view of shared housing and would prefer support to live autonomously (Gorfin and McGlaughlin, 2003). A study by Kirkpatrick (2011) has demonstrated that the relocation of people with complex support needs has led to better quality of life and improved outcomes in appropriate community accommodation. Whatever the model of community residential accommodation adults with learning disabilities opt for, it is important to remember that their health and social support needs will need to be taken into account.

Maintaining healthy lifestyles and health

Unhealthy lifestyles, poor dietary habits, and physical inactivity among adults with learning disabilities have been widely reported (Robertson et al., 2000; Emerson, 2005; McGuire et al., 2007). The lives of adults with learning disabilities are characterised by poor diet and physical inactivity. Such sedentary lifestyles contribute to an increased prevalence of obesity in adults with learning disabilities (van Schrojenstein Lantman-de Valk et al., 2000). A study by Messent et al.

Box 3.2   Risks of sedentary lifestyles

- Reduced cardiovascular fitness
- Hypertension
- Obesity
- Chronic health conditions
- Cardiovascular disease
- Hypercholesterolemia
- Type-2 diabetes
- Osteoarthritis

(1998) suggested that people with learning disabilities have alternatives to living sedentary lives. A study by Robertson et al. (2000) reported that 84% of men and 88% of women with learning disabilities living in residential settings led sedentary lifestyles. Physical inactivity is a risk factor for hypertension, obesity, chronic health conditions, cardiovascular disease, hypercholesterolemia, type-2 diabetes, and osteoarthritis (DH, 2007; Rimmer and Yamaki, 2006; Fontaine et al., 2003), and these are significantly more prevalent in adults with learning disabilities. Poor cardiovascular fitness levels contribute to higher morbidity and mortality rates in adults with learning disabilities.

The benefits of active lifestyles have been well documented: Improved cardiovascular fitness and reduced levels of obesity (Kyle et al., 2004; Melzer et al., 2004), reduced risk of depression and anxiety, and improved mood and self-esteem (DH, 2005). Adults with learning disabilities will require personal support to reduce levels of inactivity. Learning disability nurses can contribute to the improvement of health outcomes for adults with learning disabilities by engaging in health promotion activities that focus on their dietary habits and physical activity. In addition, learning disability nurses need to work flexibly in advocating that reasonable adjustments be made for adults with learning disabilities for the widely acknowledged barriers to improved lifestyles (Messent et al., 1999) to be addressed.

In addition to the impact of sedentary lifestyles, adults with learning disabilities are known to experience poorer health than those of comparable age groups who do not have learning disabilities (Backer et al., 2009). Mental health disorders (Linna et al., 1999), visual impairments (Barr et al., 1999), epilepsy (Ryan and Sunada, 1997), hypothyroidism (Barr et al., 1999), health inequalities

---

Learning Activity 3.2

Consider the risks presented by the sedentary lifestyles of adults with learning disabilities (refer to Box 3.1 and the *Health Equalities Framework* [Atkinson et al., 2013]).

- What roles could learning disability nurses undertake to address these risks?
- What could the positive outcomes of the involvement of learning disability nurses be in addressing these risks?

(Melville et al., 2006; Atkinson et al., 2013), poor access to health care (Brown et al., 2010), unequal access to health services (Kerr, 2004), poor uptake of public health initiatives (Wood and Douglas, 2007), and reduced access to health screening and health promotion services (Kerr et al., 1996) are common in adults with learning disabilities and contribute to their poorer health and life experiences.

Employment

Emerson et al. (2013) reported that 7.1% of adults with learning disabilities in England were in some form of paid employment, with the majority working in part-time roles. Employment is an indicator of health, and health inequity for people with learning disabilities (Atkinson et al., 2013 - HEF). Adults with learning disabilities experience significant barriers to employment. In the United Kingdom, these barriers have social and psychological origins. Rose et al. (2010) have concluded that the system of benefits paid to adults with learning disabilities in the United Kingdom is a considerable disincentive for them to get work. The level of learning disability, difficulties in concentrating, limited communication skills, inability to learn new skills, and long-term health problems negatively impact the employability of adults with learning disabilities (McConkey and Mezza, 2001). Furthermore, adults with learning disabilities are likely to suffer discrimination when seeking employment (Huffman and Cohen, 2004). Studies both in the United Kingdom and United States have indicated that people with learning disabilities predominantly work in sheltered employment settings, despite employment policies that encourage employment of people with learning disabilities in mainstream settings (Kaehne and Beyer, 2013; Migliore et al., 2007, 2008). Peer support, safety concerns, transportation, long-term work commitments, inflexible working hours, social environment, and work skills issues have been shown to influence the ability of people with learning disabilities to be employed outside of sheltered settings (Kaehne and Beyer, 2013; Migliore et al., 2007, 2008).

A study by Barreira et al. (2011) observed a positive correlation between mainstream employment, peer contact, and satisfaction with social life. Ross and Mirowsky (1995) have reported that employment has a significant effect on the mental and physical health of adults. On the other hand, unemployment has been shown to have adverse psychological and health effects (Wilson and Walker, 1993). Currently in the United Kingdom, learning disability nurses have no direct involvement in the employment of people with learning disabilities. However, learning disability nurses can play an important role in directing people with learning disabilities to appropriate agencies.

Personal relationships

Adults with learning disabilities continue to experience social and cultural barriers to personal and sexual expression, despite relatively recent ideological shifts in attitudes towards the normalisation of their lives (Karellou, 2003). This is also despite studies which show that adults with learning disabilities can have an understanding of their relationship and sexual rights, and the social and environmental barriers that impact these rights (Healy et al., 2009; Evans et al., 2009). The personal and sexual relationships of people with learning disabilities can be dominated by their families and their carers. This is more significant where people with learning disabilities have limited ability to demonstrate independence of choice, self-determination, and social competence. In addition, the cultural background and norms of adults with learning disabilities are important in determining their level of personal and sexual engagement with others. Some adults with learning disabilities might lack the capacity to give informed sexual consent or distinguish between abusive and non-abusive relationships. This leaves them vulnerable to opportunistic or intentional sexual abuse (Murphy, 2003).

Despite the societal ideological changes about the sexuality of people with learning disabilities, relatives, carers, and service providers of people with learning disabilities are known to limit the sexual expression of adults with learning disabilities. (Abbott and Howarth, 2007). This means that the relationship and sexual needs of people with learning disabilities are routinely ignored. Studies have shown wide variations in attitudes toward the sexual needs of adults with learning disabilities (Karellou, 2003; Bazzo et al., 2007). In addition, the legal requirements and ethical considerations on carers and service providers to safeguard vulnerable adults with learning disabilities may conflict with an individual's right to personal and sexual relationships. Such ethical and legal dilemmas are likely to limit the discussion of the sexual needs of adults with learning disabilities. These attitudes and the lack of clarity of legal and ethical considerations may result in limited sex education of adults with learning disabilities, resulting in sexual vulnerability and sexual disinhibitions of some people with learning disabilities.

A study by Murphy (2003) has suggested that a very limited number of adults with learning disabilities received sex education. This is despite evidence to show that they can benefit from such education (Dukes and McGuire, 2009). Learning disability nurses have an important role in providing health education about sexual health, safe(r) sexual practices, consent, pregnancy, abuse, and choices of sexual orientation to adults with learning disabilities, their families, and their carers. In addition, safeguarding issues are incredibly important here, given the increased vulnerability of adults with learning disabilities, and this also represents an important role of learning disability nurses (Jenkins and Davies, 2011).

Parents with learning disabilities

Existing studies suggest that families of people with learning disabilities experience high levels of stress (Emerson, 2003; Blacher et al., 2005; Gerstein et al., 2009). A study by Gerstein et al. (2009) highlighted significant differences between the mothers' and fathers' levels of stress, with mothers experiencing higher levels of stress. Baker et al. (2003) have suggested that the presence of comorbid behaviour problems in a child with a learning disability contributes to parental stress. In addition, Neece et al. (2008) concluded that a child with learning disability's degree of learning disability, behaviour problems, and lack of social skills were correlated to levels of parental stress. On the other hand, parental loci of control, parenting satisfaction, and family support have all been shown to moderate parental stress induced by a child's behavioural difficulties.

People with learning disabilities can have relationships and can get married, and have children (Llewellyn, 2013). However, in many countries, questions and concerns still remain about the rights to parenthood and parenting skills of adults with learning disabilities. This is particularly so when there are health issues such as mental illness or epilepsy. Concerns can also arise if the children have health issues and need significant levels of support to access services. Emerson and Brigham (2013) have observed that parents with learning disabilities are likely to experience mental illness, substance abuse, and smoking. Studies by Azar et al. (2012) and Mayes and Llewellyn (2012) have shown that children born to parents with learning disabilities are much more likely to end up in child protection services.

A study by Aunos et al. (2003) has shown that the presence of a learning disability by itself is not a reliable indicator of poor parenting and that it is possible for some parents with learning disabilities to have adequate parenting skills. Training, modeling, visual manuals, and audio guidance have all been shown to enhance the parenting skills of adults with learning disabilities (Feldman et al., 1986; Feldman and Case, 1999).

Parents with learning disabilities do benefit from professional help with their parenting (Wade et al., 2008; Glazemakers and Deboutte, 2013). The learning disability nurse's role here can include the provision of professional guidance and support, teaching parenting skills and strategies, and teaching child behaviour management skills.

OLDER ADULTS WITH LEARNING DISABILITIES

Globally, increasing numbers of people with learning disabilities are now living into older age (Fisher and Kettl, 2005; Walker and Ward, 2013; Hole et al., 2013; Doody et al., 2013a), and increasing numbers are outliving their parents or family carers (Bibby, 2013). Currently, the life expectancy of people with learning disabilities is 70 years (Emerson and Hatton, 2008), and the majority of those aged 60 or older are not known to health or social care services (Emerson et al., 2012). This is primarily because, for example, in England, more than two-thirds of this population lives with aging family carers (Emerson and Hatton, 2008). Emerson et al. (2012) estimated that in 2011 there were 204,985 people with learning disabilities in England age 60 or older, representing 23% of the total English population of people with learning disabilities. The increasing numbers of adults with learning disabilities transitioning into older adults is significant to health and social care roles of learning disability nurses in the context of radical shifts in policy and practice in the United Kingdom. As with the general population, as people increase in age, issues regarding work, retirement, loss and bereavement, and reduced health and social care support may occur (Glaesser and Perkins, 2013). This presents challenges and difficulties for older people with learning disabilities who may require continuing lifelong support with routine activities of daily living.

Ageing is a significant life transition. However, it is viewed negatively. For older people with learning disabilities, because of their negative and limited life experiences and opportunities, this transition may progress without even being noticed or recognised (Jenkins, 2010). It is important that health and social care services proactively develop and respond to the changing profile and needs of older people with learning disabilities through developing collaborative working practices across agencies and professions (Doody et al., 2013a). In addition, this will require effective planning and delivery of services for older adults with learning disabilities (Doody et al., 2013b). For learning disability nurses to contribute effectively to meeting the health and social care needs of older adults with learning disabilities, such nurses' roles need to focus on addressing causes of health inequalities, such as housing, and facilitating and delivering inclusive service-user focused care and support. In addition to appropriate housing, older adults with learning disabilities will need to be able to access a wide range of community care and support services, including personal assistance necessary to prevent social isolation (Shaw et al., 2011).

Retirement

In the United Kingdom, the promotion of rights, choice, inclusion, and independence have been essential values of health and social care service provision for people with learning disabilities for a considerable time. As previously outlined, people with learning disabilities tend to work in supported employment schemes (Parmenter, 1999; Macali, 2009; Mcdermott and Edwards, 2012). There is very limited support for older people with learning disabilities working in these supported employment schemes to make intentional and informed decisions about their retirement. It is important that transition planning from sheltered or other forms of supported employment that takes account of the health and social care needs of older adults with learning disabilities is implemented. Policy makers need to make provisions for flexible programmes of retirement for older adults with learning disabilities (Bigby, 2008), and take into account the varying needs of older adults with learning disabilities. Systems to enable successful transition to retirement for older adults with learning disabilities will need to focus on person-centred planning that supports people in making informed choices about their retirement. Learning disability nurses working with older adults with learning disabilities have a significant role in promoting and facilitating active ageing for older adults with learning disabilities. In addition, nurses at all levels of health and social care can play a useful role in informing policies and strategies that need to be implemented to ensure that appropriate services are delivered to older adults with learning disabilities.

Health needs of older adults with learning disabilities

Older adults with learning disabilities experience chronic and long-term health problems that are similar to older adults without learning disabilities. However, there is a significant body of evidence to show that older adults with learning disabilities have a predisposition to increased prevalence rates of age-related, pre-existing, and complex health conditions (Haverman et al., 2010; Glaesser and Perkins, 2013).

Older adults with learning disabilities experience significantly high levels of physical frailty from age 50 years (Evenhuis et al., 2012). This is predominantly associated with age, genetic conditions like Down syndrome, early onset dementia, motor disability, and severe and profound learning disabilities. This means that older adults with learning disabilities may lose skills for independent living, social skills, and decision making, and consequently lose their autonomy much earlier than older adults who do not have a learning disability (Lehmann et al., 2013).

Although older adults learning disabilities experience chronic and long-term conditions similar to older adults without learning disabilities, a study in Ireland by McCarron et al. (2013) reported multi-morbidity rates as high as 63% in the study sample. Increased levels of anxiety and depressive disorders associated with long-term conditions such as heart failure, stroke, chronic obstructive pulmonary disease, coronary artery disease, diabetes, and cancer have been reported (Hermans and Evenhuis, 2013). In addition, sedentary lifestyles, cataracts, hearing impairments, type-2 diabetes, hypertension, osteoarthritis, osteoporosis, allergies, and epilepsy are all prevalent in older adults with learning disabilities (Haverman et al., 2011).

Inequalities in health and health disparities experienced by adults with learning disabilities continue into old age. This is particularly common with underdiagnosed or inadequately managed preventable health conditions (Haverman et al., 2011), which in many cases lead to premature deaths. As the population of older adults with learning disabilities increases, learning disability nurses need to play a significant role in early diagnosis of preventable conditions, symptomatic treatment of manageable long-term conditions, facilitating access to services, and promoting the health and well-being of older adults with learning disabilities (Dixon-Ibarra et al., 2013; Krinsky-McHale and Silverman, 2013).

Loss

As discussed previously, people with learning disabilities are living longer and in some cases outliving their parents and or carers. There is now a likelihood that older adults with learning disabilities will experience significant loss due to the death of their parents or carers (Blackman, 2002). End-of-life issues such as the impact of old age, terminal illness, death, grief, mourning, and bereavement are becoming increasingly important in the lives of older adults with learning disabilities, along with their families, housemates, and carers (Botsford, 2000).

Historically, people with learning disabilities have been excluded from end-of-life services. It is, however, important to recognise that people with learning disabilities will go through the grieving process like any other person who has suffered the loss of a close relation. It could be argued that perhaps because of cognitive limitations, older adults' ability to cope with loss would require more support. Like any other older adult, older adults with learning disabilities have a fundamental human right to be supported to know about death and dying (Wiese et al., 2013). Older adults with learning disabilities will need to be prepared physically, emotionally, and psychologically to adjust to the age-related losses and stressors that may result in alterations to their thinking, experiences, and actions (Kessel et al., 2002).

Coping with and minimising the impact of aging and loss that may lead to emotional and psychological problems for older adults with learning disabilities will require

- End-of-life education from appropriately trained professionals
- Grief counseling
- Bereavement services
- Responsive end-of-life care services

Case Study 3.1

John Jacobs is a 53-year-old man with a mild learning disability, epilepsy, and type-2 diabetes. His parents, who have been his sole carers for most of his life, are both now well into their 80s and require health and social care support. Since he was 25 years old and until recently, John was working in a local sheltered employment scheme. John was making a small contribution into his pension.

John was discharged from the local hospital following a period of hospitalisation after having a mild stroke. The stroke left him paralyzed on his left side and incontinent of urine. He was discharged into a group residential home with three other males who are older than him. The majority of his carers have been employed for a number of years and are experienced in supporting people with learning disabilities with similar health and social care needs.

John is still receiving physiotherapy, but he is finding the loss of personal and social skills difficult to cope with and staff are concerned that he is getting depressed. They are also concerned that the level of his health needs requires him to be in a nursing home rather than a residential home. Staff has recently contacted the local community team for people with learning disabilities for support and help, and a learning disability nurse has been identified as the key worker.

Learning disability nurses have important roles in providing training and support for care staff working directly with older adults with learning disabilities. Learning disability nurses will need to develop adequate coordination skills to ensure that older adults with learning disabilities experiencing the various effects of ageing are appropriately supported.

Student Activity 3.3

a. Given John's age, consider the challenges the key worker will have to address if John is assessed as needing to be cared for in a nursing home rather than a residential home.
b. Given what you have learned so far in this chapter, explore the role a learning disability nurse will play in meeting John's health and social care needs. You need to consider this in the wider context of the complex health and health care needs of older adults with learning disabilities (see Figure 3.4).
c. Identify and describe the roles of the health and social care professionals who may need to be involved in this case.

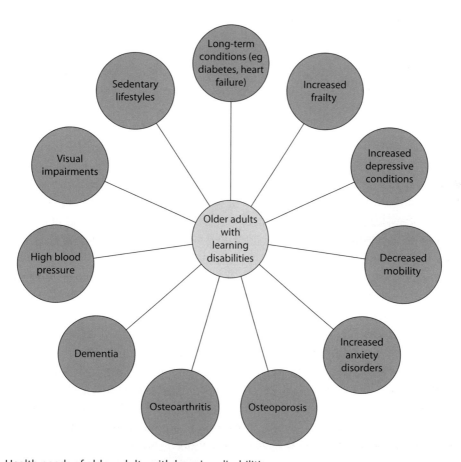

Figure 3.4 Health needs of older adults with learning disabilities.

END-OF-LIFE CARE

The majority of the 500,000 deaths that occur in England each year are associated with chronic illness (Department of Health, 2008). Although most people with long-term conditions identify their home as their preferred place of death, only a minority of those with such long-term conditions do die at home, due to the institutionalisation of the process of dying (Brumley et al., 2003). How and where people die affects the quality of experiences and satisfaction with the process of dying. For people with life-limiting illnesses, including people with learning disabilities, good end-of-life care and palliative care are essential elements of high-quality care that is delivered with compassion. It is important that any approach to palliative and end-of-life care focuses on offering people who are living with long-term illnesses who are terminally ill informed choices about the place and type of end-of-life care. People with learning disabilities who want to die at home need to be supported, and admissions to acute settings should be minimised wherever possible.

End-of-life care is becoming an important aspect of caring for and supporting those who are terminally ill. Death is an inevitable part of life, and this is no different for people with learning disabilities. It is important for carers to understand the spiritual, physical, and psychological aspects surrounding care planning for people with learning disabilities at the ends of their lives.

End-of-life care and people with learning disabilities

Globally, the philosophy of the palliative care movement has been focused on improving the quality of life of people who are terminally ill and their families, through the prevention and relief of suffering by ensuring that pain is assessed and treated, as well as ensuring psychological and spiritual well-being (WHO, 2002). Accurate assessment of terminal illness, good communication, appropriate symptom management and control, and psychological and spiritual support need to form the basis of end-of-life care for people with learning disabilities.

There is a growing body of knowledge about end-of-life care for people with learning disabilities. However, the current NHS framework for palliative care does not have specific guidance on meeting the end-of-life needs of people with learning disabilities. People with learning disabilities with life-limiting illnesses are as entitled to receive good end-of-life care in places of their choice as any other terminally ill individual (Reddall, 2010). However, it is important to acknowledge that providing end-of-life care for people with learning disabilities can be complex and challenging for both the professionals and relatives involved (Read, 1998). Limited verbal communication skills on the part of people with learning disabilities and lack of competence in using alternative or augmentative communication methods by professionals has been sighted as a significant negative factor in how end-of-life care is provided to people with learning disabilities (Jones et al., 2007). In addition, it has been observed that health care professionals caring for terminally ill people with learning disabilities are generally unaware of the meaning of end-of-life care in practice or how they can support people with learning disabilities to access palliative care support (Reddall, 2010). Learning disability nurses and other health care professionals caring for terminally ill or potentially terminally ill people with learning disabilities will find 'the dying trajectory' useful (Brown et al., 2005) (see Figure 3.5).

'The dying trajectory' is important in that it provides a framework for assessing the possibility of terminal illness where there is significant alteration of a person with a learning disability's health status. In light of evidence from a study by Ng and Li (2003) showing that 50% of the professionals who had cared for terminally ill people with profound learning disabilities were unable to identify

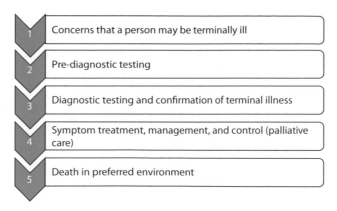

1. Concerns that a person may be terminally ill

2. Pre-diagnostic testing

3. Diagnostic testing and confirmation of terminal illness

4. Symptom treatment, management, and control (palliative care)

5. Death in preferred environment

Figure 3.5 **The dying trajectory.** (Adapted from Brown, M. et al., *Journal Research in Nursing*, 15(4)–361, 2010.)

signs and symptoms of end of life, this framework is an indispensable tool for professionals, such as learning disability nurses, working in a variety of settings. The use of this framework is likely to prevent the delay in the diagnosis of terminal illness that may impact the provision of appropriate palliative care in the right environment. Health care professionals who work with people with learning disabilities who require end-of-life care have advocated the availability of appropriate frameworks and guidelines (Morton-Nance and Schafer, 2012). Successful provision of end-of-life and palliative care for people with learning disabilities will require person-centred modifications of current approaches. The Confidential Inquiry into Premature Deaths of People with Learning Disabilities (Heslop et al., 2013) highlighted the need to address inequalities experienced by people with learning disabilities with life-limiting conditions through improved joint working and coordination, reasonable adjustments, advance planning, shared decision making, and proactive assessments (Marriott et al., 2013).

Breaking the news

Hearing that an illness is terminal can be a frightening experience for anyone, including those with learning disabilities (McEnhill, 2013). Like anyone else, people with learning disabilities are likely to experience a range of emotions, such as shock, fear, anger, resentment, denial, helplessness, sadness, frustration, relief, and acceptance. However, it is important to be aware of cognition and communication issues that may be associated with some individuals with learning disabilities. Communicating with people with learning disabilities that they have a terminal illness is likely to be complex and challenging for health and social care professionals. However, professionals, such as learning disability nurses, are expected to communicate directly with people with learning disabilities with life-limiting conditions who require end-of-life and palliative care.

For some people with a learning disability, and particularly those with significant communication difficulties, and those who have been in long-term institutions, communicating effectively the concepts of terminal illness, palliative care, and death may not be possible (McEnhill, 2008). To ensure that people with learning disabilities with communication difficulties receive adequate support, sign language, augmentative communication, and communication professionals such as speech and language therapists need to be involved to enhance communication. Translation services for those whose first language is not English need to be used. Although the involvement of carers can be useful in facilitating communication, it is important to be aware that this can be useful in the short term because of the negative emotions the carers may be experiencing.

Despite the challenges previously noted, professionals need not make assumptions about people with learning disabilities' understanding of terminal illness and death. Before discussing a diagnosed terminal illness with a person with a learning disability, it is important to be familiar with a person's previous experiences of terminal illness, which led to death of a person with whom he or she was familiar. Any approach for breaking the news about terminal illness needs to take into account the cognitive impairments of the individual with a learning disability (Tuffrey-Wijne and McEnhill, 2008).

End-of-life decisions

Following the diagnostic testing and confirmation of a terminal illness, decisions need to be made about the preferences, priorities, and place of death for the person with a learning disability. Involving people with learning disabilities in such an important but difficult decision can be complex and challenging. Wagemans et al. (2013) have identified the factors that professionals, such as learning disability nurses, need to consider when supporting people with learning disabilities and their carers to make informed end-of-life decisions (see Figure 3.6).

First, where there is an absence of mental capacity, health care professionals need to ensure that relatives or informal or formal carers are involved in decision making. It is important that the express wishes of the relatives or informal or formal carers are respected where there is an absence of mental capacity and informed consent cannot be obtained. In addition, health care professionals will need to ensure that assessment of quality-of-care decisions is delegated to the relatives or informal or formal carers. Furthermore, professionals need to ensure that they build consensus

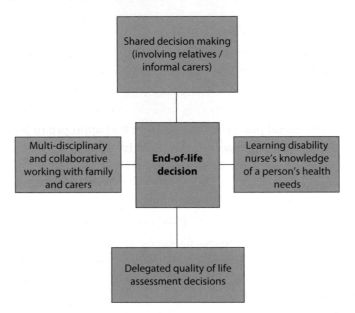

Figure 3.6 Factors affecting end-of-life decisions for people with learning disabilities. (Adapted from Wagemans, A. et al., *Journal of Intellectual Disability Research*, 57(4):380–389, 2013.)

with relatives or informal or formal carers, and delegate best-interest decisions. Finally, professionals involved in end-of-life decisions need to have knowledge and experience of the health care needs and preferences of the person with learning disabilities.

This process of shared decision making is important because it provides an inclusive framework, which ensures that the person with a learning disability, his or her family, and his or her carers are central to the end-of-life and palliative care interventions. It is important that learning disability nurses and other health care professionals involved are knowledgeable about the preferences of people with learning disabilities, their families, and their carers. Prioritising and honouring the preferences and priorities of people with learning disabilities who are dying requires knowledge and understanding of those preferences (Davies and Higginson, 2004).

Palliative care and people with learning disabilities

Inadequacies of the current approaches to end-of-life and palliative care for people with learning disabilities have been recently noted (Ryan et al., 2010). The Confidential Inquiry into Premature Deaths of People with Learning Disabilities (Heslop et al., 2013) has recommended good practice in the end-of-life care of people with learning disabilities (Marriot et al., 2013). At the centre of effective palliative care for people with learning disabilities needs to be collaborative working between health care professionals, a person with a learning disability, and his or her family and carers.

Palliative care involves the management and control of symptoms such as pain. Although not all people who are terminally ill will experience pain, it is a common feature in end-of-life care. For people with learning disabilities and particularly those with communication problems, it may be complex and challenging to assess pain. Relatives and carers may be able to assist with pain assessment. Where pain is assessed or suspected, learning disability nurses caring for people with learning disabilities receiving end-of-life care need to collaborate with general practitioners and other palliative care specialists to ensure that appropriate pain relief is provided. Learning disability nurses need to be aware of alternative approaches to pain relief, such as physiotherapy, massage, reflexology, or other complementary therapies that can facilitate relaxation.

Other complications associated with end of life include constipation and loss of appetite. Learning disability nurses providing end-of-life care to people with learning disabilities need to ensure that the diets of such individuals are high in fiber. Where constipation is an issue, learning disability nurses need to liaise with general practitioners to ensure that appropriate laxatives are prescribed and administered. As end of life approaches, the digestive system may slow down and this may result in reduced or loss of appetite. Medication can also contribute to loss of appetite. Dysphagia can also be a feature of end of life.

The use of opioid analgesics will result in chemical imbalance of the brain and this can cause confusion or hallucinations. This may result in restlessness, verbal aggression, or physical aggression. This can be particularly difficult to assess where such behaviours already existed prior to terminal illness. As end of life approaches, it is likely that a person will become tired and drowsy and will spend more time sleeping. Breathing is likely to become irregular and noisy because of increased mucus in the lungs. Blood circulation will reduce, resulting in cyanosis. Learning disability nurses who provide end-of-life care will require wide ranging knowledge, and physical nursing skills to facilitate appropriate end-of-life and palliative care.

CONCLUSION

There are a number of lessons that learning disability nurses of today and tomorrow can learn from a cradle-to-the-grave approach to nursing those with learning disabilities, in order to improve the health and health care outcomes for people with learning disabilities. The increasing complexity of the health and health care needs of people with learning disability and the increasing complexity of health and social care provision will require learning disability nurses to possess higher levels of knowledge about the changing, complex needs of people with learning disabilities. In meeting the holistic needs of people with learning disabilities across the lifespan, present and future roles of learning disability nurses will require a wide range of nursing skills and competences across the lifespan of people with learning disabilities.

It is important for learning disability nurses to understand contemporary learning disability nursing in the context of the normal lifespan of people with learning disabilities. Learning disability nurses need to be aware that the diagnosis of a learning disability in a child has a significant and often long-term impact on the family and wider society. Learning disability nurses will require the knowledge, skills, competence, and sensitivity to support parents as they respond to and face significant challenges. Effectively supporting adolescents with learning disabilities is complex and challenging. Learning disability nurses will need to work in partnership and collaborate with other agencies and professionals to improve access to appropriate services, to improve the health and health care outcomes of this vulnerable group. The lifestyles, health, and health care needs of people with learning disabilities are often complex and challenging. This is more so today than ever before because of an increased life expectancy for people with learning disabilities. To meet the changing needs of this population, learning disability nurses will need to develop and continue to develop new ways of working with people with learning disabilities, their families and their carers, and other professionals across a wide range of agencies and organisations. People with learning disabilities are now living longer with complex and often long-term conditions in a wide range of community-based residential facilities. Learning disability nurses working in these settings and other NHS community-based services will need to develop their knowledge and skills to enhance the care experience of people with learning disabilities, especially in end-of-life care. While this may be a new and complex area for many learning disability nurses, efforts can be focused on building relationships with people with learning disabilities, their families and carers, and other professionals and palliative care organisations to enhance end-of-life care experiences for people with learning disabilities.

REFERENCES

Abbott, D., and Howarth, J. 2007. Still off-limits? Staff view on supporting gay, lesbian and bisexual people with intellectual disabilities to develop sexual and intimate relationships. *Journal of Applied Research in Intellectual Disabilities*, 20(2):116–126.

Allington-Smith, P. 2006. Mental health of children with learning disabilities. *Advances in Psychiatric Treatment,* 12:130–140.

Ammerman, R.T., Hersen, M., van Hasselt, V.B., Lubetsky, M.J., and Sieck, W.R. 1994. Maltreatment in psychiatrically hospitalized children and adolescents with developmental disabilities: Prevalence and correlates. *Journal of the American Academy of Child & Adolescent Psychiatry*, 33(4) 567–576.

Association for Children's Palliative Care. 2007. *Integrated Multi-Agency Care Pathways for Children with Life-Threatening and Life Limiting Conditions.* Bristol: Association for Children's Palliative Care.

Aunos, M., Feldman, M., and Goupil, G. 2008. Mothering with intellectual disabilities: Relationship between social support, health and well-being, parenting and child behaviour outcomes. *Journal of Applied Research in Intellectual Disabilities*, 21(4):320–330.

Azar, S.T., Stevenson, M.T., and Johnson, D.R. 2012. Intellectual disabilities and neglectful parenting: Preliminary findings on the role of cognition in parenting risk. *Journal of Mental Health Research in Intellectual Disabilities*, 5(2):94–129.

Backer, C., Chapman, M., and Mitchell, D. 2009. Access to secondary healthcare for people with learning disabilities: A review of the literature. *Journal of Applied Research in Intellectual Disabilities*, 22(6):514–525.

Baker, B.L., Blacher, J., and Olsson, M.B. 2005. Preschool children with and without developmental delay: Behavioural problems, parents' optimism and well being. *Journal of Intellectual Disability Research*, 49:575–590.

Barr, O. and Millar, R. 2003. Parents of children with intellectual disabilities: Their expectations and experience of genetic counseling. *Journal of Applied Research in Intellectual Disabilities,* 16(3):189.

Barr, O., Gilgunn, J., Kane, T. and Moore, G. 1999. Health screening for people with learning disabilities by a community learning disabilities nursing service in Northern Ireland. *Journal of Advanced Nursing,* 29(6):1482–1491.

Barreira, P.J., Tepper, M.C., Gold, P.B., Holley, D., and Macias, C. 2011. Social value of supported employment for psychosocial program participants. *Psychiatric Quarterly*, 82(1):69–84.

Bibby, R. 2013. 'I hope he goes first': Exploring determinants of engagement in future planning for adults with a learning disability living with ageing parents. What are the issues? *British Journal of Learning Disabilities*, 41(2):94–105.

Bigby, C. 2008. Beset by obstacles: A review of Australian policy development to support ageing in place for people with intellectual disability. *Journal of Intellectual and Developmental Disability*, 33(1):76–86.

Blacher, J., Neece, C. L., and Paczkowski, E. 2005. Families and intellectual disability. *Current Opinion in Psychiatry,* 18:507–513.

Blackman, N.J. 2002. Grief and intellectual disability: A systemic approach. *Journal of Gerontological Social Work*, 38(1/2):253–263.

Bloomquist, K.B., Brown, G., Peerson, A., and Presler, E.P. 1998. Transitioning to independence: Challenges for young people with disabilities and their caregivers. *Orthopaedic Nursing*, May/June, pp. 27–35.

Botsford, A.L. 2000. Integrating end of life care into services for people with an intellectual disability. *Social Work in Health Care*, 31(1):35–48.

Brown., M., MacArthur., J., McKechanie., A., Hayes., M., and Fletcher, J. 2010. Equality and access to general healthcare for people with learning disabilities: Reality or rhetoric? *Journal of Research in Nursing,* 15(4):351–361.

Brumley, R.D., Enguidanos, S., and Cherin, D.A. 2003a. Effectiveness of a home-based palliative care program for end-of-life. *Journal of Palliative Medicine*, 6(5):715–724.

Carpenter, B. 2005. Early childhood intervention: Possibilities and prospects for professionals, families and children. *British Journal of Special Education*, 32(4):176–183.

Chadwick, D.D., Jolliffe, J., and Goldbart, J. 2002. Carer knowledge of dysphagia management strategies. *International Journal of Language and Communication Disorders*, 27(3):135–144.

Davies, E. and Higginson, I.J. (Eds.) 2004. *The Solid Facts: Palliative Care*. Copenhagen: World Health Organization.

Dekker, M.C., Koot, H.M., van-der-Ende, J., and Verhulst, F.C. 2002. Emotional and behavioral problems in children and adolescents with and without intellectual disability. *Journal of Child Psychology and Psychiatry and Allied Disciplines*, 43:1087–1098.

DH. 2004. *National Service Framework for Children, Young People and Maternity Services*. London: Department of Health.

DH. 2005. *Choosing Activity: A Physical Activity Action Plan.* London: Department of Health.

DH. 2007. *Obesity General Information.* London: Department of Health.

DH. 2010. *National Framework for Children and Young People's Continuing Care*. London: Department of Health.

Dixon-Ibarra, A., Lee, M., and Dugala, A. 2013. Physical activity and sedentary behavior in older adults with intellectual disabilities: A comparative study. *Adapted Physical Activity Quarterly*, 30(1):1–19.

Donelly, V. 2008. Housing options for people with learning disabilities. *Learning Disability Practice*, 11(10):26–26.

Doody, C.M., Markey, K., and Doody, O. 2013a. Future need of ageing people with an intellectual disability in the Republic of Ireland: Lessons learned from the literature. *British Journal of Learning Disabilities,* 41(1):13–21.

Doody, C., Markey, K., and Doody, O. 2013b. The experiences of registered intellectual disability nurses caring for the older person with intellectual disability. *Journal of Clinical Nursing,* 22(7/8):1112–1123.

Dukes, E. and McGuire, B.E. 2009. Enhancing capacity to make sexuality-related decisions in people with an intellectual disability. *Journal of Intellectual Disability Research*, 53(8):727–734.

Emerson, E. 2003. Mothers of children and adolescents with intellectual disability: Social and economic situation, mental health status, and the self-assessed social and psychological impact of the child's difficulties. *Journal of Intellectual Disability Research. Special Issue on Family Research*, 47(4-5):385–399.

Emerson, E. 2005. Underweight, obesity and exercise among adults with intellectual disabilities in supported accommodation in Northern England. *Journal of Intellectual Disability Research*, 49(2):134–143.

Emerson, E. and Brigham, P. 2013. Health behaviours and mental health status of parents with intellectual disabilities: Cross sectional study. *Public Health (Elsevier)*, 127(12):1111–1116.

Emerson, E. and Hatton, C. 2007. *The Mental Health of Children and Adolescents with Learning Disabilities in Britain.* Lancaster: Institute for Health Research, Lancaster University.

Emerson, E. and Hatton, C. 2008. *People With Learning Disabilities in England, CeDR Research Report.* Lancaster: University of Lancaster.

Emerson, E., Einfeld, S., and Stancliffe, R. 2010. The mental health of young children with intellectual disabilities or borderline intellectual functioning. *Social Psychiatry & Psychiatric Epidemiology*, 45(5):579–587.

Emerson, E., Hatton, C., Robertson, J., Baines, S., Christie, A. and Glover, G. 2013. People with learning disabilities in England 2012. Learning Disabilities Observatory, University of Lancaster. Available at http://www.improvinghealthandlives.org.uk/securefiles/140217_0333// IHAL2013-10%20People%20with%20Learning%20Disabilities%20in%20England%202012v3.p (accessed August 19, 20014).

Emerson, E., Hatton, C., Robertson, J., Roberts, H., Baines, S., Evison, F. and Glover, G. (2012) *People with Learning Disabilities in England 2011.* Lancaster: Learning Disabilities Observatory, University of Lancaster.

Evans, D.S., McGuire, B.E., Healy, E., and Carley, S.N. 2009. Sexuality and personal relationships for people with an intellectual disability. Part II: Staff and family carer perspectives. *Journal of Intellectual Disability Research*, 53(11):913–921.

Evenhuis, H.M., Hermans, H., Hilgenkamp, T.I.M., Bastiaanse, L.P., and Echteld, M.A. 2012. Frailty and disability in older adults with intellectual disabilities: Results from the healthy ageing and intellectual disability study. *Journal of the American Geriatrics Society*, 60(5):934–938.

Fisher, K. and Kettl, P. 2005. Aging with mental retardation: Increasing population of older adults with MR require health interventions and prevention strategies. *Geriatrics*, 60:26–29.

Fontaine, K.R., Redden, D.T., Wang, C., Westfall, A.O., and Allison, D.B. 2003. Years of life lost due to obesity. *Journal of American Medical Association*, 289(2):187–193.

Gerstein, E.D., Crnic, K.A., Blacher, J., and Baker, B.L. 2009. Resilience and the course of daily parenting stress in families of young children with intellectual disabilities. *Journal of Intellectual Disability Research*, 53(12):981–997.

Glaesser, R.S. and Perkins, E.A. 2013. Self-injurious behavior in older adults with intellectual disabilities. *Social Work*, 58(3):213–221.

Glazemakers, I. and Deboutte, D. 2013. Modifying the 'Positive Parenting Program' for parents with intellectual disabilities. *Journal of Intellectual Disability Research*, 57(7):616–626.

Gray, D.E. 2002. Everybody just freezes. Everybody is just embarrassed: Felt and enacted stigma among parents of children with high functioning autism. *Sociology of Health and Illness*, 24(6):734–749.

Gorfin, L. and McGlaughlin, A. 2003. Housing for adults with a learning disability: 'I want to choose, but they don't listen'. *Housing, Care & Support*, 6(3):4–8.

Griffith, G.M., Hastings, R.P., Nash, S., and Hill, C. 2010. Using matched groups to explore child behavior problems and maternal well-being in children with Down syndrome and autism. *Journal of Autism & Developmental Disorders*, 40(5):610–619.

Hallawell, B., Stephens, J., and Charnock, D. 2012. Physical activity and learning disability. *British Journal of Nursing*, 21(1):609–612.

Hassall, R., Rose, J., and McDonald, J. 2005. Parenting stress in mothers of children with an intellectual disability: The effects of parental cognitions in relation to child characteristics and family support. *Journal of Intellectual Disability Research*, 49(6):405–418.

Hastings, R.P., Beck, A., Daley, D., and Hill, C. 2005. Symptoms of ADHD and their correlates in children with intellectual disabilities. *Research in Developmental Disabilities*, 26(5):456–468.

Hatton, C. and Emerson, E. 2003. Families with a person with intellectual disabilities: Stress and impact. *Current Opinion in Psychiatry*, 16:497–501.

Hatton, C. and Emerson, E. 2004. The relationship between life events and psychopathology amongst children with intellectual disabilities. *Journal of Applied Research in Intellectual Disabilities*, 17(2):109–117.

Haverman, M., Heller, T., Lee, L., Maaskant, M., Shooshtari, S., and Strydom, A. 2010. Major health risks in aging persons with intellectual disabilities: An overview of recent studies. *Journal of Policy and Practice in Intellectual Disabilities*, 7(1):55–69.

Haverman, M., Perry, J., Salvador-Carulla, L., Walsh, P.N., Kerr, M. Van Schrojenstein Lantman-de Valk, H., Van Hove, G., Berger, Dasa, M., Azema, B., Buono, S., Cara, A.C., Germanavicius, A., Linehan, C., Määttä, T., Tossebro, J., and Weber, G. 2011. Ageing and health status in adults with intellectual disabilities: Results of the European POMONA II study. *Journal of Intellectual and Developmental Disability*, 36(1):49–60.

Healy, E., McGuire, B.E., Evans, D.S., and Carley, S.N. 2009. Sexuality and personal relationships for people with an intellectual disability. Part I: Service-user perspectives. *Journal of Intellectual Disability Research*, 53(11):905–912.

Hermans, H. and Evenhuis, H.M. 2013. Factors associated with depression and anxiety in older adults with intellectual disabilities: Results of the healthy ageing and intellectual disabilities study. *International Journal of Geriatric Psychiatry*, 28 (7):691–699.

Heslop, P., Blair, P., Fleming, P., Hoghton, M., Marriott, A., and Russ, L. 2013. *Confidential Inquiry into premature deaths of people with learning disabilities (CIPOLD)*. Bristol: University of Bristol.

Hole, R.D., Stainton, T., and Wilson, L. 2013. Ageing adults with intellectual disabilities: Self-advocates' and family members' perspectives about the future. *Australian Social Work*, 66(4):571–589.

Huffman, M. L. and Cohen, P. N. 2004. Wage inequality: Job segregation and devaluation across U.S. labor markets. *The American Journal of Sociology,* 109(4), 902–937.

Jenkins, R. 2010. How older people with learning disabilities perceive ageing. *Nursing Older People,* 22(6):33–37.

Jenkins, R. and Davies, R. 2011. Safeguarding people with learning disabilities. *Learning Disability Practice*, 14(1):32–39.

Jones, A., Tuffrey-Wijne, I., Bernal, J., Butler, G., and Hollins, S. 2007. Meeting the cancer information needs of people with learning disabilities: Experiences of paid carers. *British Journal of Learning Disabilities,* 35:12–18.

Kaehne, A. and Beyer, S. 2013. Supported employment for young people with intellectual disabilities facilitated through peer support: A pilot study. *Journal of Intellectual Disabilities*, 17(3):236–251.

Karellou, J. 2003. Laypeople's attitudes towards the sexuality of people with learning disabilities in Greece. *Sexuality and Disability*, 21(1):65–84.

Kerr, M. 2004. Improving the general health of people with learning disabilities. *Advances in Psychiatric Treatment*, 10:200–206.

Kerr, M., Richards, D., and Glover, G. 1996. Primary care for people with a learning disability—a group practice survey. *Journal of Applied Research in Intellectual Disability*, 9(4):347–352.

Kessel, S., Merrick, J., Kedem, A., Borovsky, L., and Carmeli, E. 2002. Use of group counseling to support aging-related losses in older adults with intellectual disabilities. *Journal of Gerontological Social Work,* 38(1/2):241–251.

Kilic, D., Gencdogan, B., Bag, B., and Arican, D. 2013. Psychosocial problems and marital adjustments of families caring for a child with intellectual disability. *Sexuality & Disability*, 31(3):287–296.

Kirkpatrick, K. 2011. A home of my own—progress on enabling people with learning disabilities to have choice and control over where and with whom they live. *Health*, 107:153–162.

Krinsky-McHale, S.J. and Silverman, W. 2013. Dementia and mild cognitive impairment in adults with intellectual disability: Issues of diagnosis. *Developmental Disabilities Research Review*, 18(1):31–42.

Kyle, U.G., Morabia, A., Schutz, Y., and Pichard, C. 2004. Sedentarism affects body fat mass index and fat-free mass index in adults aged 18 to 98 years. *Nutrition*, 20(3):255–260.

Lacy, P and Ouvry, C. (Eds) 1998. *People with Profound and Multiple Learning Disabilities: A Collaborative Approach to Meeting Complex Needs.* London: David Fulton.

Lehmann, B.A., Bos, A.E.R., Rijken, M., Cardol, M., Peters, G.J.Y., Kok, G., and Curfs, L.M.G. 2013. Ageing with an intellectual disability: The impact of personal resources on well-being. *Journal of Intellectual Disability Research*, 57(11):1068–1078.

Li, S. and Ng, J. 2008. End-of-life care: Nurses' experiences in caring for dying patients with profound learning disabilities—a descriptive case study. *Palliative Medicine*, 22:949–955.

Linna, S.L., Moilanen, I., Ebeling, H., Piha, J., Kumpulainen, K., Tamminen, T., and Almqvist, F. 1999. Psychiatric symptoms in children with intellectual disability. *European Child and Adolescent Psychiatry*, 8(suppl. 4):77–82.

Llewellyn, G. 2013. Parents with intellectual disability and their children: Advances in policy and practice. *Journal of Policy & Practice in Intellectual Disabilities*, 10(2):82–85.

Macali, L. 2009. Contemporary disability employment policy in Australia: How can it best support transitions from welfare to work? *Australian Bulletin of Labour*, 32(3):227–239.

Mafuba, K. and Gates, B. 2013. An investigation into the public health roles of community learning disability nurses. *British Journal Learning Disability*, DOI: 10.1111-bld.12071.

Marriott, A., Marriott, J., and Heslop, P. 2013. Good practice in helping people cope with terminal illnesses. *Learning Disability Practice,* 16(6):22–25.

Mayes, R. and Llewellyn, G. 2012. Mothering differently: Narratives of mothers with intellectual disability whose children have been compulsorily removed. *Journal of Intellectual & Developmental Disability*, 37(2):121–130.

McCarron, M., Swinburne, J., Burke, E., McGlinchey, E., Carroll, R., and McCallion, P. 2013. Patterns of multimorbidity in an older population of persons with an intellectual disability: Results from the intellectual disability supplement to the Irish longitudinal study on aging (IDS-TILDA). *Research in Developmental Disabilities*, 34(1):521–527.

McConkey, R. and Mezza, F. 2001. Employment aspirations of people with learning disabilities attending day centres. *Journal of Learning Disabilities*, 5(4):309–318.

McConkey, R., Truesdale-Kennedy, M., Chang, M., Jarrah, S., and Shukri, R. 2008. The impact on mothers of bringing up a child with intellectual disabilities: A cross-cultural study. *International Journal of Nursing Studies*, 45(1):65–74.

Mcdermott, S. and Edwards, R. 2012. Enabling self-determination for older workers with intellectual disabilities in supported employment in Australia. *Journal of Applied Research in Intellectual Disabilities*, 25(5):423–432.

McEnhill, L. 2008. Breaking bad news of cancer to people with learning disabilities. *British Journal of Learning Disabilities*, 36(3):157–164.

McEnhill, L. 2013. *Widening access to palliative care for people with learning disabilities.* London: Health the Hospices.

McGuire, B.E., Daly, P., and Smyth, F. 2007. Lifestyle and health behaviours of adults with an intellectual disability. *Journal of Intellectual Disability Research*, 51(7):497–510.

Melville, C.A., Cooper, S.A., Morrison, I.J., Finlayson, J., Allan, L., Robinson, N., Burns, E., and Martin, G. 2006. The outcomes of an intervention study to reduce the barriers experienced by people with intellectual disabilities accessing primary healthcare services. *Journal of Intellectual Disability Research*, 50(1):11–17.

Melzer, K., Kayser, B., and Pichard, C. 2004. Physical activity: The health benefits outweigh the risks. *Current Opinion in Clinical Nutrition and Metabolic Care*, 7(6):641–647.

Messent, P.R., Cooke, C.B., Long, J. 1999. Primary and secondary barriers to physically active healthy lifestyles for adults with learning disabilities. *Disability & Rehabilitation,* 21(9):409-419.

Messent, P.R., Cooke, C.B. and Long, J. 1998. Daily physical activity in adults with mild and moderate learning disabilities: Is there enough? *Disability & Rehabilitation,* 20(11):424–427.

Migliore, A., Mank, D., Grossi, T., and Rogan, P. 2007. Integrated employment or sheltered workshops: Preferences of adults with intellectual disabilities, their families, and staff. *Journal of Vocational Rehabilitation,* 26(1):5–19.

Migliore, A., Mank, D., Grossi, T., and Rogan, P. 2008. Why do adults with intellectual disabilities work in sheltered workshops? *Journal of Vocational Rehabilitation,* 28(1):29–40.

Murphy, G.H. 2003. Capacity to consent to sexual relationships in adults with learning disabilities. *Journal of Family Planning and Reproductive Health Care,* 29(3):148–149.

Neece, C. and Baker, B. 2008. Predicting maternal parenting stress in middle childhood: The roles of child intellectual status, behaviour problems and social skills. *Journal of Intellectual Disability Research,* 52(12):1114–1128.

Ng, J. and Li, S. 2003. A survey exploring the educational needs of care practitioners in learning disability (LD) settings in relation to death, dying and people with learning disabilities. *European Journal of Cancer Care,* 12:12–19.

Parmenter, T.R. 1999. Implications of social policy for service delivery: The promise and the reality. *Journal of Intellectual and Developmental Disability,* 24(4):321–331.

Quilgars, D., Searle, B., and Keung, A. 2005. Mental health and well-being. In: Bradshaw, J., and Mayhew, E., (Eds.). *The Well-Being of Children in the UK.* London: Save the Children, pp.134–160.

RCN 2004. *Adolescent Transition Care: Guidance for Nursing Staff.* London: Royal College of Nursing.

Read, S. 1998. Learning disabilities. The palliative care needs of people with learning disabilities. *International Journal of Palliative Nursing,* 4(5):246–251.

Read, S. 2005. Learning disabilities and palliative care: Recognizing pitfalls and exploring potential. *International Journal of Palliative Nursing,* 11:15–20.

Reddall, C. 2010. A palliative care resource for professional carers of people with learning disabilities. *Journal of Cancer Care,* 19(4):469–475.

Reilly, C. and Ballantine, R. 2011. Epilepsy in school-aged children: More than just seizures? *Support for Learning,* 26(4):144–151.

Rimmer, J.H. and Yamaki, K. 2006. Obesity and intellectual disability. *Mental Retardation and Developmental Disability Research Review,* 12(1):22–27.

Robertson, J., Emerson, E. and Gregory, N., Hatton, C., Turner, S., Kessissoglou, S. and Hallam, A. 2000. Lifestyle related risk factors for poor health in residential settings for people with intellectual disabilities. *Research in Developmental Disability,* 21(6):469–486.

Rogers, C. 2011. Disabling a family? Emotional dilemmas experienced in becoming a parent of a child with learning disabilities. *British Journal of Special Education,* 34(3):136–143.

Rose, J., Perks, J., Fidan, M., and Hurst, M. 2010. Assessing motivation for work in people with developmental disabilities. *Journal of Intellectual Disabilities,* 14(2):147–155.

Ross, C. and Mirowsky, J. 1995. Does employment affect health? *Journal of Health and Social Behaviour,* 36(3):230–243.

Ryan, K., McEvoy, J. Guerin, S., and Dodd, P. 2010. An exploration of the experience, confidence and attitudes of staff to the provision of palliative care to people with intellectual disabilities. *Palliative Medicine,* 24(6):566–572.

Ryan, R. and Sunada, K. 1997. Medical evaluations of persons with mental retardation referred for psychiatric assessment. *General Hospital Psychiatry,* 19(4):274–280.

Seymour, S. and C. Ingleton 2008. Transitions into the terminal phase: Overview. In, Payne, S., Seymour, J. and Ingleton, C. *Palliative Care Nursing: Principles and evidence for practice.* Glasgow: Bell and Bain, pp. 181–211.

Shaw, K., Cartwright, C., and Craig, J. 2011. The housing and support needs of people with an intellectual disability into older age. *Journal of Intellectual Disability Research,* 55(9):895–903.

Shobana, M. and Saravanan, C. 2014. Comparative study on attitudes and psychological problems of mothers towards their children with developmental disability. *East Asian Archives of Psychiatry,* 24(1):16–22.

Tuffrey-Wijne, I. and McEnhill, L. 2008. Communication difficulties and intellectual disability in end of life care. *International Journal of Palliative Nursing,* 14(4):189–194.

Turner, M. 2008. *Preferred Place of Care Project 2005–2007 Final Report: 1-8. Updated 2011.* (Online). Available at http://tinyurl.com/cokyt4s (accessed April 28, 2014).

Van Schrojenstein Lantman-de Valk H.M.J., Metsemakers, J.F.M., Haveman, M.J., and Crebolder, H.F.J.M. 2000. Health problems in people with intellectual disability in general practice: A comparative study. *Family Practice,* 17(5):405–407.

Verma, R.K. and Kishore, M.T. 2009. Needs of Indian parents having children with intellectual disability. *International Journal of Rehabilitation Research,* 32(1):71–76.

Wade, C., Llewellyn, G., and Matthews, J. 2008. Review of Parent Training Interventions for Parents with Intellectual Disability. *Journal of Applied Research in Intellectual Disabilities,* 21(4):351–366.

Wagemans, A., Van Schrojenstein Lantman-De Valk, H., Proot, I., Metsemakers, J., Tuffrey-Wijne, I., and Curfs, L. 2013. The factors affecting end-of-life decision-making by physicians of patients with intellectual disabilities in the Netherlands: A qualitative study. *Journal of Intellectual Disability Research,* 57(4):380–389.

Walker, C. and Ward, C. 2013. Growing older together: Ageing and people with learning disabilities and their family carers. *Tizard Learning Disability Review,* 18(3):112–119.

Wiese, M., Dew, A., Stancliffe, R.J., Howarth, G., and Balandin, S. 2013. 'If and when?'—the beliefs and experiences of community living staff in supporting older people with intellectual disability to know about dying. *Journal of Intellectual Disability Research*, 57(10):980–992.

Wilson, L. & Walker, G. 1993. Unemployment and health: A review. *Public Health*, 107(3):153–162.

Wood, R. and Douglas, M. 2007. Cervical screening for women with learning disability: Current practice and attitudes within primary care in Edinburgh. *British Journal of Learning Disabilities*, 35(2):84–92.

World Health Organisation. 2002. *WHO definition of palliative care.* http://www.who.org.

FURTHER READING

Brown, H., Burns, S., and Flynn, M. 2005. *Dying matters. A workbook on caring for people with learning disabilities who are terminally ill*. London: The Mental Health Foundation.

Emerson, E., Hatton, C., Robertson, J., Baines, S., Christie, A. and Glover, G. 2013. *People with learning disabilities in England 2012*. Learning Disabilities Observatory, University of Lancaster. Available at http://www.improvinghealthandlives.org.uk/securefiles/140217_0333//IHAL2013-10%20People%20with%20Learning%20Disabilities%20in%20England%202012v3.p

Heslop, P., Blair, P., Fleming, P., Hoghton, M., Marriott, A., and Russ, L. 2013. *Confidential Inquiry into premature deaths of people with learning disabilities (CIPOLD)*. Bristol: University of Bristol.

RCN (2004) *Adolescent transition care: Guidance for nursing staff*. London: Royal College of Nursing.

USEFUL RESOURCES

BILD (British Institute of Learning Disabilities): http://www.bild.org.uk

Foundation for People with Learning Disabilities: http://www.learningdisabilities.org.uk/publications/mh-children-adolescents/

Improving Health and Lives – Learning Disability Observatory: http://www.improving-healthandlives.org.uk

General information: www.learningdisabilties.org.uk

NHS Choices – End of life care: http://www.nhs.uk/planners/end-of-life-care/pages/end-of-life-care.aspx

NHS Choices – Learning disability: http://www.nhs.uk/Livewell/Childrenwithalearningdisability/Pages/Childrenwithalearningdisabilityhome.aspx

Palliative Care of People with Learning Disabilities Network: http://www.pcpld.org

4 Role of the learning disability nurse in promoting health and well-being

Kay Mafuba

INTRODUCTION

In this chapter, students of nursing will explore the role of the learning disability nurse in promoting the health and well-being of people with learning disabilities. This will be contextualised within the Nursing and Midwifery Council for the United Kingdom (2010) and An Bord Altranais (2005) standards for competence.

This chapter incorporates key concepts and policies in public health, and includes the key policy drivers that are refocusing nursing interventions to be centrally concerned with prevention. The role of learning disability nurses in helping people with learning disabilities plan for good health and well-being will be explored. We will also explore learning disability nurses' public health roles, and, in particular, the importance of health promotion in care planning, health facilitation, and health action planning will be addressed, as well as newer roles such as health liaison nursing in primary care and acute settings. These roles are explored in the context of well-known health issues, such as cardiovascular fitness, obesity, epilepsy, mental ill health, sexuality, diet, and smoking. Many of these conditions will require learning disability nurses to develop careful and imaginative ways of constructing nursing interventions to improve or maintain the health status of people with learning disabilities.

This chapter will focus on the following issues:

- Key concepts and policies
  - What is public health?
- Health promotion
  - Why health promotion?
  - Characteristics of successful health promotion
- Health facilitation
  - Why health facilitation?
  - Essential skills for health facilitation

- Health action planning
  - Why health action planning?
- Health liaison
  - Why health liaison?
- Public health policies
  - England
  - Scotland
  - Northern Ireland
  - Wales
  - U.K. frameworks
- Learning disability public health nursing practice
- Current public health roles of learning disability nurses
  - Facilitating access to health care
  - Health screening and health surveillance
  - Health promotion and health education
  - Health protection and health prevention
- Factors that influence learning disability nurses' public health practice
  - Public health role clarity
  - Demographic intelligence
  - Interprofessional and interagency collaboration
  - Leadership
  - Resources
  - Politics

Competences

NMC Competences and Competencies

Domain 1: Professional values - Field standard for competence and competencies – 1.1; 2.1; 3.1; 4.1.

Domain 2: Communication and interpersonal skills - Field standard for competence and competencies – 1.1; 2.1; 4.1.

Domain 3: Nursing practice and decision-making - Field standard for competence and competencies – 1.1; 3.1; 5.1; 8.1.

Domain 4: Leadership, management and team working - Field standard for competence and competencies – 1.1; 1.2; 2.1; 6.1; 6.2.

(continued)

KEY CONCEPTS AND POLICIES

What is public health?

The concept of public health is contentious (Dawson and Verweij, 2007). There is no agreed definition of what 'public health' means (Baggott, 2011; Kaiser and Mackenbach, 2008). The lack of an agreed dialogical definition is not surprising, given that the meaning of 'health' itself is a subject of endless debate (Blaxter, 2004). An all-encompassing definition of public health (Baggott, 2011) is problematic, and a source of significant confusion (Griffiths and Hunter, 1999). Recent efforts have been made to develop conceptual models of public health in an effort to clarify the concept. The most notable model was developed by Griffiths et al. (2005). The framework has three inter-related domains of *'health prevention'*, *'health, improvement'*, and *'health service delivery and quality'*. What is not disputed in the literature is that public health refers to the health of identified populations (WHO, 1986). The contention about defining public health was partly explained by Rosen's observations that health is interconnected with social life (Rosen, 1993).

According to Winslow

> **Public health is the science and the art of preventing disease, prolonging life and promoting physical health and efficiency through organised community efforts for the sanitation of the environment, the control of community infections, the education of the individual in principles of personal hygiene, the organisation of medical and nursing service for the early diagnosis and preventative treatment of disease, and the development of social machinery which will ensure to every individual in the community a standard of living adequate for the maintenance of health.**

(Winslow, 1920, p. 23)

This approach to public health highlights the importance of public health roles, including those of learning disability nurses in meeting the public health needs of people with learning disabilities.

The Acheson Report has described public health as

> **...the science and art of preventing disease, prolonging life and promoting health through organised efforts of society.**

(Acheson, 1988, p. 27)

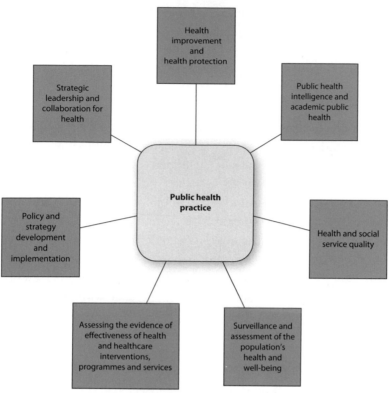

Figure 4.1 Key areas of public health practice. (Adapted from Faculty of Public Health, *What is public health?* [Online], 2013. Available at http://www.fph.org.uk/what_is_public_health [accessed July 17, 2013].)

The U.K. public health policy adopts the Acheson (1988) definition (Chief Medical Officer, 2007). Another notable influence on our understanding of the meaning of U.K. public health is the Faculty of Public Health (FPH). The equivalent organisation in the Republic of Ireland is the Institute of Public Health (IPH). The FPH is the standard setting body for professionals and specialists in public health in the United Kingdom. The FPH organises public health practice into three domains (health improvement, health protection, and improving services) (Faculty of Public Health, 2012). These domains are similar to Griffiths et al.'s model (Griffiths et al., 2005). In addition to the three domains, the FPH identifies nine key areas of public health practice, and these are given in Figure 4.1.

HEALTH PROMOTION

Health promotion is a process of enabling people to have control over the determinants of their health in order to improve their health and well-being (WHO, 1986). As a concept and set of practical strategies, it remains an essential guide in addressing the major health challenges that people with learning disabilities face, including communicable and non-communicable diseases, and issues related to their human development and health. Health promotion is a process directed toward enabling people with learning disabilities to take action. Health promotion is therefore not something that is done on or to people with learning disabilities; it is done by, with, and for people with learning disabilities either as individuals or as groups. The purpose of health promotion is to strengthen the skills and capabilities of individuals with learning disabilities to take action and the capacity of groups or communities to act collectively to exert control over the determinants of their health and achieve positive change. The health promotion role of learning disability nurses is concerned with making healthier choices easier choices for people with learning disabilities. Health promotion involves the overlapping activities of health education, health protection and prevention.

Why health promotion?

Broadly, health promotion focuses on prolonging healthy life, reducing inequalities in health, and reducing pressure on health services. People with learning disabilities have increased comorbidity, communication difficulties, a high prevalence of serious conditions such as epilepsy, and specific patterns of health needs associated with the aetiology of their disability. Unfortunately, this combination of need is mirrored by a consistent picture of poor health promotion uptake, inadequate care for serious morbidity, unrecognised health needs, and poor access to health care.

There is a great disparity between the health of people with learning disabilities and that of the general population (Howells, 1986; Beange and Bauman, 1990; Wilson and Haire, 1990; Michael, 2008; Ombudsman, 2009). These studies or reviews (from Wales, Australia, and England) suggest that examination of any community-based population of people with learning disabilities consistently uncover serious health problems such as

- Untreated, yet treatable, medical conditions
- Untreated specific health issues related to the individual's disability
- A lack of uptake of generic health promotion such as blood-pressure screening

For people with learning disabilities, health promotion is important because there is a disparity between the health and health care needs of this group of people compared to that of the general population (Kerr, 2004; DH, 2001). It is important to recognise that these disparities in health and health outcomes are avoidable (Straetmans et al., 2007). These disparities could be improved through appropriate interventions (Oullette-Kuntz, 2005). For people with learning disabilities, these disparities result from poor access to health services, limited options in lifestyle, and poor living standards (Whitehead, 1992).

Health promotion is important for people with learning disabilities because international studies have shown poor uptake of public health initiatives by people with learning disabilities (Beange et al., 1995; Beange and Bauman, 1990; Jacobson et al., 1989; Kerr et al., 1996; Stein and Allen, 1999; Jones and Kerr, 1997; Sullivan et al., 2003; Wood and Douglas, 2007). Other studies have shown that people with learning disabilities have reduced access to health screening and health promotion services (Kerr et al., 1996; Whitfield et al., 1996). Lennox et al. (2000) have noted the need for effective health advocacy for people with learning disabilities from relevant health professionals. Kerr et al. (2003) have observed that health care outcomes are dependent on individuals' ability to seek appropriate care. The role of learning disability nurses in promoting the health of people with learning disabilities is therefore important.

A significant proportion of people with learning disabilities and their carers will need professional support to be able to access public health and other health care services. Codling and Macdonald (2011) have pointed to a lack of evidence that shows the involvement of people with learning disabilities in addressing their health care needs. This suggests that people with learning disabilities can be passive participants in their health and health care, and that they may be dependent on others for their health and health care outcomes (Robertson et al., 2001; Campbell and Martin, 2009; Keywood et al., 1999). In the past few decades, efforts to depathologise learning disabilities have gathered pace, resulting in people with learning disabilities having to access generic health services.

Delivering effective public health and health promotion services for people with learning disabilities is challenging (Thomas and Kerr, 2011). Research suggests that the provision of public health services for people with learning disabilities, in most cases, is opportunistic (McIlfatrick et al., 2011). This is despite evidence that points to a need for targeted activities that focus on promoting the health and health care needs of people with learning disabilities (Chauhan et al., 2010). Opportunistic approaches to preventive health for people with learning disabilities are not adequate in meeting the health care needs of this population (Lennox et al., 2000). Felce et al. (2008) have suggested that in the absence of people with learning disabilities' ability to self-refer for health care, it is logical that provision of health services for this population be proactive rather than reactive. Learning disability nurses have an important role in developing and implementing health promotion strategies that meet the health needs of people with learning disabilities (Table 4.1). Recent international studies have demonstrated that preventive interventions such as health screenings are effective in identifying the health needs of people with learning disabilities in the United Kingdom (Baxter et al., 2006; Cooper et al., 2006; Emerson and Glover, 2010; Emerson et al., 2011); in Australia (Beange et al., 1995); and in New Zealand (Webb and Rogers, 1999).

In the United Kingdom the introduction of the Quality Outcomes Framework (QOF) in 2004, and the later introduction of Directed Enhanced Services (DES) in England (*Scottish Enhanced Services Programme* [SESP] in Scotland), placed the responsibility of preventive health service provision for people with learning disability on general practitioners. There has been a longstanding debate as to whether this role belongs to primary care or to learning disability nurses working community teams for people with learning disabilities (Matthews and Hegarty, 1997; Curtice and Long, 2002).

Table 4.1 Approaches to health promotion

Approach	Objective	Activity	Examples
Education	To provide information and create well-informed people. To empower choice and foster personal growth through provision of knowledge. To prevent disease by persuading people to adopt lifestyles that promote freedom from disease. To raise awareness of the need for health policy, to stimulate people to tackle the social, environmental, and political influences on health.	Information giving regarding cause of illnesses and effect of lifestyles. Develop knowledge and skills for people to be able to make healthier choices. Educate people to change attitudes and behaviour and adopt healthier lifestyles.	Persuasive education. Provision of education (one to one, groups, peers, media, etc.).
Protection	To influence individuals' choices. To modify individuals' risks. To modify the environment.	Political and social action.	Public health policy development. Changes to the environment.
Prevention	*Primary prevention* - Seeks to prevent onset of disease. *Secondary prevention* - Aims to halt the progression of disease. *Tertiary prevention* - Rehabilitation to minimise risk.	Diagnosis and treatment.	Screening. Diagnostic tests. Medical or surgical intervention.

Characteristics of successful health promotion

Effectively promoting the health and well-being of people with learning disabilities requires

- Knowledge and competence of the health promotion workforce that includes learning disability nurses and others
- Knowledge-based public health and health promotion practice
- Evidence-based public health and health promotion practice
- Integrated and seamless local and national health promotion policies
- Intergrated health-promoting services
- Active participation by people with learning disabilities
- Healthy local and national public policy
- Structures and systems that are effective in putting healthy public policy into practice
- Strengthening and empowering local community actions and strategies
- Reorientation of health services from treatment to prevention
- Strengthening structures and processes in all sectors, to create supportive environments that promote the health and well-being of people with learning disabilities
- Funding and availability of resources specifically targeted at meeting the public health needs and promoting the health and well-being of people with learning disabilities

HEALTH FACILITATION

Health facilitation involves both case work to help people access mainstream services and also development work within mainstream services to help parts of the NHS to develop the necessary skills for other health care professionals. The impetus for both is to help ensure that good health care is delivered in primary and secondary care, as needs to as by specialist learning disability services (DH, 2002). Health facilitation needs to occur on a number of levels, e.g., individual, operational, and strategic. Ultimately, health facilitation is about ensuring healthier lives and better health for people with learning disabilities (DH, 2002). Health facilitation is important because good health care needs to be delivered by ordinary services, as well as specialist learning disability services. Health facilitation includes working directly with people with learning disabilities and their carers to

- Undertake holistic health needs assessments
- Trace individual problems to their source and seek their resolution
- Develop the ability of people with learning disabilities to recognise and address their own health needs

Health facilitation also includes working with a wide range of health services services to help them plan better to meet people with learning disabilities' health needs (DH, 2002). The purpose of health facilitation is to facilitate and advocate better acess to resources for people with learning disabilities to gain full access to the health care they need in both primary and secondary NHS services (Jukes 2002).

Why health facilitation?

People with learning disabilities experience unequal access to health services (Kerr, 2004; DRC, 2006; Iacono and Davis, 2003; Janicki et al., 2002; Scheepers et al., 2005; Mencap, 2004). People with learning disabilities experience inadequate diagnosis of treatable conditions (Hollins et al., 1998; Mencap, 2007; DH, 2007a; DH, 2007b; Durvasula et al., 2002). In the United Kingdom, access to public health is primarily through the primary health care system. Current literature shows that a significant proportion of health inequalities in people with learning disabilities are linked to poor quality health care provision (Michael, 2008; Mencap, 2012; Parliamentary Health Ombudsman and Social Services Ombudsman, 2009). This rather suggests that these inequalities are preventable. U.K. government policy has focused on improving people with learning disabilities' access to generic and preventive health services for some considerable time (DH, 1992; DH, 1995; NHS Executive, 1998; DH, 2001; DH, 2009; Ruddick, 2005). However, the continuing disparities in health in people with learning disabilities suggest that policies alone are not enough.

Barriers to accessing services contribute to health inequalities for people with learning disabilities. A significant number of barriers that contribute to failure in meeting the health care needs of people with learning disabilities have been identified (Melville et al., 2006; Barr et al., 1999; Bollard, 1999; NHS Health Scotland, 2004). Lack of role clarity of the professionals working with people with learning disabilities has been consistently identified as one of the most common barriers (Thornton, 1996; Powrie, 2003; NHS Health Scotland, 2004; Phillips et al. 2004). The importance of primary health care services in meeting the health needs of people with learning disabilities has been highlighted (Lennox and Kerr, 1997; Phillips et al. 2004). Effective health facilitation is therefore important in ensuring that people with learning disabilities can access appropriate health care.

Essential skills for health facilitation

Appropriate subject knowledge: Successful health facilitation requires relevant background knowledge regarding the health and social care needs of people with learning disabilities.

Clinical skills: To function effectively as a health facilitator, learning disability nurses will have to be competent in complex and comprehensive health needs assessments and risk assessments to be able to assist with screening or assessment and clinical procedures, in a wide range of clinical settings in which they practice.

Health and social care needs: Knowledge of health and social care needs of people with learning disabilities is indispensable for learning disability nurses to be able to provide advice and share their knowledge and expertise with other health and social care professionals.

Determinants of health: The impact of the wider determinants of health and their impact on people with learning disabilities was discussed earlier. Knowledge of wider determinants of health and barriers to services experienced by people with learning disabilities is important for learning disability nurses to be able to develop systems and protocols that are essential to meeting the health and social care needs of people with learning disabilities.

Communication and multidisciplinary team (MDT) working: Health facilitation involves a wide range of stakeholders. Learning disability nurses will require effective communication and negotiation skills in dealing with other professionals, agencies, carers, and people with learning disabilities. These skills are also vital in developing partnership working arrangements with other agencis and professionals. In addition, to fulfill their roles as health facilitators, learning disability nurses need to be familiar with health services in the areas in which they practice, in order to facilitate access to appropriate services. Appropriate experience of how health services opperate is also important for learning disability nurses to fulfill this role.

HEALTH ACTION PLANNING

Health action plans provide details of the actions essential to maintaining and improving the health of people with learning disabilities and the support required for the implementation of the plans, where required. Health action planning links people with learning disabilities to a wide range of health services and support mechanisms necessary for attaining better health. For health action plans to work, reasonable adjustments may need to be made. Health action plans are produced in partnership with people with learning disabilities. Health action plans are important for educating people with learning disabilities, and their carers, about their health and how they can maintain and improve it. In addition, health action plans are important for influencing health care services to inform changes that are important in developing systems and structures that positively impact the health and health care of people with learning disabilities.

Points to note

- Health action plans are simply plans about what people can do to be fit and healthy.
- Health action plans list any help and support that might be needed to achieve and maintain good health.
- Health action plans are not, but can be, dependent on other forms of care planning such as person-centred planning or a Care Programme Approach.
- Health action plans may be reactive or proactive, or both reactive and proactive. They aim to
  - Ensure that individual medical needs, including those relating to specific syndromes with health consequences, are properly addressed for people with learning disabilities.
  - Address the wider determinants of health.
  - Remove the barriers to good health for people with learning disabilities.
  - Support the mainstream health agenda and the drive to reduce health inequalities.

Why health action planning?

People with learning disabilities are known to have much greater health needs than those of comparable age groups who do not have learning disabilities (NHS Executive, 1998; DH, 1999; Cancer Research UK, 2008; Backer et al., 2009). In addition, people with learning disabilities experience higher rates of mental health problems as compared to the general population (Wilson and Hare, 1990; Linna et al., 1999). Furthermore, people with learning disabilities experience higher rates of visual impairments (Beange et al., 1995; Barr et al., 1999); epilepsy (Ryan and Sunada, 1997; McDermott et al., 1997; Whitfield et al., 1996); hypertension and hypothyroidism (Barr et al., 1999); and obesity (van Schrojenstein Lantman-de Valk et al., 2000). People with learning disabilities are more likely to die from preventable causes (Hollins and Sinason, 1998; Mencap, 2007; DH, 2007a; DH, 2007b; Durvasula et al., 2002; Nissen and Havemann, 1997; Pawar and Akuffo, 2008; van Schrojenstein Lantman-de Valk et al., 2000). Studies have shown that the health problems that people with learning disabilities experience are commonly and widely undiagnosed, misdiagnosed, and untreated (Wilson and Hare, 1990; Bailey and Cooper, 1997). Although the life expectancy of people with learning disabilities has increased with that of the general population (McLoughlin, 1988), overall life expectancy still remains lower, and mortality rates remain significantly higher than those of the general population (Durvasula et al., 2002;

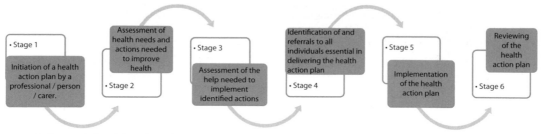

Figure 4.2 Stages in health action planning.

Hollins and Sinason, 1998). It is therefore important in the context of public health that learning disability nurses have an understanding of the risk factors associated with learning disabilities in order to prevent premature deaths (Durvasula et al., 2002). If used appropriately, health action planning could improve the health and health care outcomes for people with learning disabilities (see Figure 4.2).

HEALTH LIAISON

The focus of health liaison is to provide a service to people with learning disabilities when they are admitted in a general or mainstream hospital in accident and emergency departments, inpatient wards, or outpatient departments. The key focus of health liaison is to

- Support and assist other professionals with mental capacity assessment of people with learning disabilities in order for them to consent to treatment
- Assist with diagnosis and treatment
- Support the management of patients with learning disabilities who are receiving assessments or treatment for physical health conditions
- Provide advice on discharge planning or the need for continuing care
- Support health and health care agencies to make reasonable environmental and system adjustments.

In their role as health liaison nurses, learning disability nurses liaise with other services and professionals such as the medical team who will be treating the person with a learning disability, care managers, and primary care services. To effectively undertake the health liaison role, liaison nurses need to have a visible and accessible hospital base (Brown et al., 2011). In addition, there is a need for collaboration between learning disability specialist services, primary care, and acute services.

Why health liaison?

Health liaison is important for learning disability nursing because people with learning disabilities experience health inequalities (Scheepers et al., 2005; Melville et al., 2006), and poor access to health care (DH, 1999; DH, 2001; NPSA, 2004; Mencap, 2004; DRC, 2006; Whitehead, 1992; Nocon et al., 2008; Brown et al., 2011). Studies have shown that people with learning disabilities are considered a low priority by health care professionals (Aspray et al., 1999). In addition, international studies have highlighted widespread concerns about the inequalities in health for people with learning disabilities (Janicki, 2001; Scheepers et al., 2005; WHO, 2003). Existing evidence

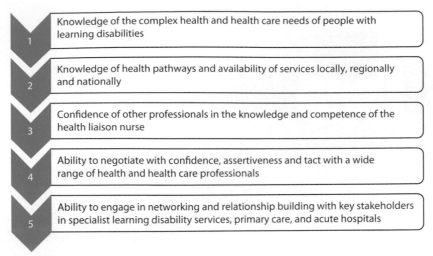

1	Knowledge of the complex health and health care needs of people with learning disabilities
2	Knowledge of health pathways and availability of services locally, regionally and nationally
3	Confidence of other professionals in the knowledge and competence of the health liaison nurse
4	Ability to negotiate with confidence, assertiveness and tact with a wide range of health and health care professionals
5	Ability to engage in networking and relationship building with key stakeholders in specialist learning disability services, primary care, and acute hospitals

Figure 4.3 Skills for health liaison.

suggests that the disparities in health and health outcomes for people with learning disabilities are attributable to people with learning disabilities themselves, health organisations, and health service systems. Straetmans et al. (2007) identified communication difficulties and limited understanding of the diagnostic and treatment issues for people with learning disabilities. In addition, Lennox and Diggins (1999) have noted that health care professionals have limited augmentative communication skills, which further limits their ability to diagnose and treat people with learning disabilities appropriately. For people with learning disabilities themselves, communication and practical difficulties of navigating in hospitals and other health care facilities can limit their ability to access services. People with learning disabilities have complex health needs, and comorbidity is common. Messent et al. (1999) identified lifestyle-related comorbidity as a significant contributory factor to disparities in health for people with learning disabilities. Cognitive impairments limit people with learning disabilities' ability to access public health and other preventive health initiatives (Jones and Kerr, 1997). Learning disability nurses have important roles in facilitating communication between people with learning disabilities and health services.

To effecively liaise with other professionals and agencies, learning disability nurses require specialist health liaison skills (see Figure 4.3). Brown et al. (2011) have suggested a conceptual model of learning disability liaison nursing (see Figure 4.4).

PUBLIC HEALTH POLICIES

Each of the four countries of the United Kingdom has different public health policies, and this divergence has been increasing recently (Greer, 2009).

England

In England, *Choosing Health* (DH, 2004) identified six key priority areas for public health: reducing the number of people who smoke, reducing obesity and improving diet and nutrition, increasing exercise, encouraging and supporting sensible drinking, improving sexual health, and improving mental health. Since then, a series of other public health policy initiatives has been adopted, including *Delivering Choosing Health* (DH, 2005); *Our Health, Our Care, Our Say* (DH, 2006a);

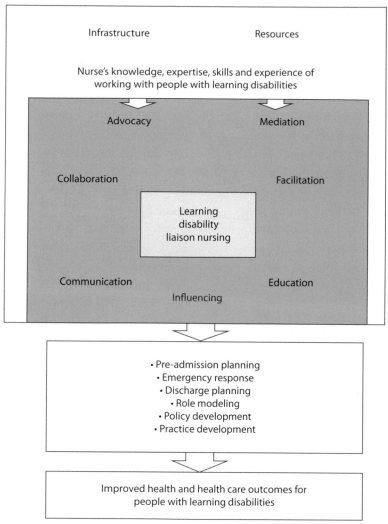

Figure 4.4 Conceptual model of learning disability liaison nursing service. (Adapted from Brown, M., et al. *Journal of Intellectual Disability Research*, doi: 10.1111/j.1365-2788.2011.01511.x, 2011.)

Health Challenge England (DH, 2006b); *Tackling Health Inequalities* (DH, 2007a), and, more recently, *Healthy Lives, Healthy People* (DH, 2010).

Scotland

There has been a distinct public health approach in Scotland for a considerable time (Greer, 2009; Donnelly, 2007). *Scotland's Health: A Challenge to Us All* (Scottish Office, 1992) identified coronary heart disease and cancer as key public health targets. Since then, a series of other policies have emerged, including *Our National Health: A Plan for Action, a Plan for Change* (Scottish Executive, 2000a), *Improving Health in Scotland* (Scottish Executive, 2003), *Better Health, Better Care: Action Plan* (Scottish Government, 2007), and *Equally Well* (Scottish Government, 2008). Like in England, none of these policies specifically addressed the public health needs of people with learning disabilities, but they applied to the whole population.

Case study 4.1

Tim is a 30-year-old man with moderate learning disabilities and Prader–Willi syndrome. He lives at home with his parents and attends a supported employment project for four days each week. He has limited social contacts and therefore relies on his immediate family for social support. He is severely overweight and diabetic, and has epilepsy, which is managed by medication. He has not been receiving any support from the local community team for people with learning disabilities.

It is clear that Tim has a long history of weight-management problems associated with his Prader–Willi syndrome. Prader–Willi syndrome is a genetic condition where there is an associated fixation with food, which can become an obsession. The syndrome is complex, and there are a range of characteristics present that include episodes of mental illness and challenging behaviours (see Chapter 1).

Tim was returning home from supported employment with his support worker on the bus. Tim managed to get off the bus without his support worker realising it, and then made his way to a supermarket, and began to randomly open packets of biscuits and cakes and eat them. He was approached by staff and challenged. Tim 'lashed' out at them, which resulted in the police being called. While waiting for the police to arrive Tim became increasingly anxious and restless and began to masturbate. His speech became increasingly incoherent and when the police arrived, he could not give an account of himself and was unable to give the name of a family contact. The police recognised that Tim might have some form of mental disorder and escorted him to a local assessment and treatment unit for people with learning disabilities for assessment. You are a student nurse on the unit and your mentor has asked you to carry out an assessment on Tim.

On the day of this assessment Tim is visibly agitated and restless and threatening to harm those around him. He is unable to give the name of an immediate contact; he cannot state where he lives or with whom. When pressed for this information he begins to masturbate, talk to himself, and rock back and forth.

Student Activity 4.1

Describe how you would use health promotion to support Tim in managing his weight-management problems.

Using a recognised model, construct a health action plan for managing Tim's diabetes.

Explore how you would use health facilitation to meet Tim's health and social care needs.

Discuss the role(s) of other professionals in the assessment process.

Explore the role of health liaison nursing while Tim is in an acute assessment and treatment unit.

Identify relevant NMC/An Bord Altranais competencies that are applicable in this scenario.

Northern Ireland

Northern Ireland has adopted a much more focused and sustained public health policy approach (Wilde, 2007; NI Executive, 2008). Since the 1990s, key policy documents have emerged, including *Health and Wellbeing: Towards the New Millennium* (DHSSNI, 1996), *Well in 2000* (DHSSNI, 1997), *Investing for Health* (DHSSPSNI, 2002), and *A Healthier Future* (DHSSPS, 2004). Recent work led by the Public Health Agency has strengthened this position for people with learning disabilities (Public Health Agency, 2011; Slevin et al., 2011).

Wales

Wales was the first U.K. country to develop a comprehensive and inclusive public health strategy (Welsh Office NHS Directorate, 1989; 1992) that was quite distinct (Greer, 2009; Coyle, 2007). The identified priority areas were cancer, maternal and child health, emotional health, respiratory illness, cardiovascular diseases, learning disabilities, mental distress and illness, injuries, healthy environments, and physical disabilities. Since then, a series of other public health policy initiatives emerged and include *Better Health, Better Wales* (Welsh Office, 1998), *Improving Health in Wales* (NAfW, 2001), *Wellbeing in Wales* (Welsh Assembly Government, 2002), *Wales—A Better Country* (Welsh Assembly Government, 2003), and *Designed for Life* (Welsh Assembly Government, 2005).

Other developments

The U.K.-wide general practitioner contract specifies three distinct groups of services: essential services (compulsory – consultations), additional services (optional – immunisation and screening), and enhanced services (optional – specialised services). There were originally 10 indicators on the *Quality Outcomes Framework* (QOF), and this has been repeatedly revised, and has included learning disabilities since 2006. In 2008, additional payment for the provision of *Clinical Directed Enhanced Services* (NHS Employers, 2014) for people with learning disabilities was introduced. This was intended to improve access to generic public health services by people with learning disabilities at the primary health care level.

Valuing People: A New Strategy for Learning Disability for the 21st Century (DH, 2001) highlighted the need to improve the health of people with learning disabilities in England and Wales (*The Same as You* in Scotland) (Scottish Executive, 2000b). The complexity of the health care needs of people with learning disabilities is acknowledged, and the inadequacies of existing models of health care provision for people with learning disabilities in generic health care settings highlighted. In Scotland, the *Health Needs Assessment Report: People with Learning Disabilities in Scotland* (NHS Health Scotland, 2004) highlighted the needs of people with learning disabilities and provided guidance to health care professionals about how these could be met.

Since *Valuing People* was published in 2001 (DH, 2001), there have been other notable developments which have affected the implementation of public health policy for people with learning disabilities. Although these are not discussed at this point in any detail, they are worth noting in order for students and practitioners to widen their understanding of the practice environment. These notable developments include the *Treat Me Right* report (Mencap, 2004), which highlighted the health needs of people with learning disabilities and suggested how access to services could be improved. *Equal Treatment: Closing the Gap* (DRC, 2006) revealed an inadequate response from the NHS and the English and Welsh governments to the major physical health inequalities experienced by people with mental health needs and people with learning disabilities. *Death by Indifference* (Mencap, 2007) alleged institutional discrimination within the NHS, which resulted in people with learning disabilities receiving ineffective health care. The report presented the stories of six people who the authors believe died unnecessarily as a result of health care professionals' lack of understanding of the complexity of the health care needs of people with learning disabilities. *Healthcare for All* (Michael, 2008) highlighted the high levels of unmet health needs of people with learning disabilities, poor access to services, and ineffectiveness of the treatment they received. *Valuing People Now* (DH, 2009) outlined the English government's response to the *Healthcare for All* report (Michael, 2008). *Six Lives* (Parliamentary and Health Service Ombudsman and Social Services Ombudsman, 2009) was the government's response to *Death by Indifference* (Mencap, 2007). *Death by* Indifference: 74 *Deaths and Counting* (Mencap, 2012) has reported further avoidable deaths of people with learning disabilities. *Confidential Inquiry into Premature Deaths of People with Learning Disabilities (CIPOLD)* concluded that the effectiveness and quality of health care provided to people with learning disabilities was inadequate and recommended proactive interventions to address these deficiencies (Helsop et al., 2013).

LEARNING DISABILITY PUBLIC HEALTH NURSING PRACTICE

Brief history of public health roles of learning disability nurses

Jukes (1994) has traced to the 1960s the origins of the learning disability nurse's involvement with public health for people with learning disabilities. Several attempts have been made to identify and clarify the contribution of learning disability nurses to health promotion (Elliot-Cannon, 1981). The Griffiths Report (Griffiths, 1988), and the NHS and Community Care Act (DH, 1990) emphasised the *'health'* contribution of learning disability nursing. More recently, the Department of Health has clearly emphasised the public health role of the learning disability nurse in England (DH, 2001; DH, 2007c). However, defining the public health role of learning disability nurses has been difficult (Mobbs et al., 2002). As a result, the public health role of learning disability nurses has evolved differently across the United Kingdom (Mobbs et al., 2002). Primary care and social care services have a conflicting understanding of the role and contribution of learning disability nurses to the delivery of public health services to people with learning disabilities (McGarry and Arthur, 2001). There is very little research into the learning disability nurse's role, practice, and contribution to public health services for people with learning disabilities (Boarder, 2002). Recent research on the role of learning disability nurses has concentrated on their broader professional roles such as advocacy (Gates, 1994; Jukes, 1994; Mobbs et al., 2002; Llewellyn and Northway, 2007), and generic community nursing roles (Holloway, 2004; Melville et al., 2005; Boarder, 2002; Powell et al., 2004).

Learning disability nurses have a key public health role in a number of key areas, including contributing to public health policy development, planning public health policy implementation, and taking a lead role in the implementation and delivery of public health policy for people with learning disabilities (Mafuba and Gates, 2013).

CURRENT PUBLIC HEALTH ROLES OF LEARNING DISABILITY NURSES

Recent studies have noted increasing involvement of learning disability nurses with public health in England (Boarder, 2002; Mobbs et al., 2002; Barr, 2006; Barr et al., 1999). McConkey et al. (2002) have reported the increasing involvement of community learning disability nurses with health promotion and health screening of people with learning disabilities in Northern Ireland. The public health roles of learning disability nurses are changing as a result of recent policy initiatives such as health facilitation and health action planning (Scottish Executive, 2000b; DH, 2001; DHSSPS, 2004). Learning disability nursing students and practitioners need to be aware that the influences on how they undertake their public health roles are likely to be complex and may not necessarily be consistent with the descriptions provided here.

A recent study by Mafuba and Gates (2013) has demonstrated that learning disability nurses are involved with health care delivery, health education, health prevention and protection, facilitating access to health, health promotion, and health surveillance in meeting the public health needs of people with learning disabilities.

Facilitating access to health care

Facilitating access to health care is the most common public health role of learning disability nurses (Bollard, 2002; Marshall and Moore, 2003; Barr et al., 1999; Abbott, 2007; Mafuba and Gates, 2013). It is clear that the public health roles of learning disability nurses are becoming more facilitatory as a result of recent policy initiatives (Scottish Executive, 2000b; DH, 2001; DHSSPS, 2004). For detailed discussion on the facilitatory roles of learning disability nurses, refer to the section on health liaison.

Health screening and health surveillance

Health screening is an important role for learning disability nurses in improving the health and health care of people with learning disabilities. First, the number of health problems among people with learning disabilities has been estimated to be 2.5 times greater than among people without a learning disability, and mortality rates are higher than those of the general population. People with learning disabilities are disproportionately affected by respiratory disease, epilepsy, dysphagia, constipation, mental health problems, communication difficulties, visual impairments, dental problems, coronary heart disease, diabetes, and obesity. Mortality from these conditions is preventable, and learning disability nurses play an important role in assessing these needs. Causes for higher mortality rates are diverse and complex but include co-morbid conditions, reduced access and barriers to services, and poor diagnosis and poor treatment by health professionals. People with learning disabilities experience poor access to mainstream public health and health promotion services, such as health screening and health protection services and immunisation programmes. The involvement of learning disability nurses with health screening and health surveillance across the United Kingdom and Northern Ireland is varied. One explanation could be that health screening is part of the general practitioner contract, and learning disability nurses' involvement in this area is only through collaboration with general practitioners who might not see these activities as a priority. Another explanation could be that U.K. health has been target-driven in the recent past (Bevan, 2006), resulting in people with learning disabilities being part of the national statistics. The recent incorporation of the Improving Health and Lives Learning Disabilities Observatory into Public Health England has highlighted the importance of detailed health screening and health surveillance for people with learning disabilities. Similarly in Northern Ireland, public health services for people with learning disabilities have been the remit of the Public Health Agency since 2009.

Health promotion and health education

Health promotion involves enabling people with learning disabilities to increase control over their health to improve their experience of health and health care. In undertaking health promotion, learning disability nurses work with people with learning disabilities and their carers to deal with

- Factors that influence health, such as lifestyle and health care-seeking behaviours
- Broader determinants of health, which are outside the control of people with learning disabilities, such as their living environment, employment, and the provision and availability of and accessibility of health services

In this role learning disability nurses work with individuals with learning disabilities and their families to provide knowledge, values, and skills that are essential for them to take positive and preventive health actions.

In undertaking health education learning disability nurses focus on influencing the attitudes to determinants of health, health, and health care of individuals with learning disabilities and their carers. The focus of health education is to use the health experiences of people with learning disabilities and their communities to increase health literacy necessary for health improvement.

Health protection and health prevention

Health protection involves important activities of public health practice that affect whole populations, such as food, hygiene, water, environmental health, medicines control, and a wide range of other activities. The aim of these activities is to minimise the risk of adverse impact to health of environmental determinants of health.

Health prevention involves immunisation, health screening, and other public health activities that focus on the prevention and early detection of learning disability, disease, and illness. Health prevention programmes are implemented in communities and primary and acute health care care settings. For people with learning disabilities, health prevention may include annual health checks and screening tests. According to Gordon (1987) health prevention activities occur at three levels

- *Universal health prevention:* Focuses on providing information, knowledge, and skills to a whole population to prevent lifestyles or promote lifestyles that affect health and health outcomes.

- *Selective health prevention:* In learning disability public health nursing practice, selective health prevention activities may involve working with individuals and groups at risk of developing specific health problems, for example, providing screening services for early onset of dementia for people with Down syndrome.

- *Indicated health prevention:* This activity involves screening programmes targeting specific individuals who exhibit early signs of specific illnesses or diseases.

FACTORS THAT INFLUENCE LEARNING DISABILITY NURSES' PUBLIC HEALTH PRACTICE

Public health role clarity

As discussed earlier, public health practice is multiprofessional and multiagency in nature; it is therefore important that learning disability nurses are clear about their public health roles within their area of practice (Wick, 2007). Public health role clarity is an important foundation of how learning disability nurses engage with public health practice to meet the public health needs of people with learning disabilities (Mafuba, 2013).

Agreed-upon dialogical definition of public health practice

As discussed earlier, the concept of public health is contentious (Dawson and Verweij, 2007). Learning disability nursing students and learning disability nurses need to be aware of a lack of '*shared knowledge*' and '*shared categorisations*' of public health problems that people with learning disabilities experience. The impact of this is likely to be organisational variations in the public health services provided to people with learning disabilities. To prevent variations in interpretation of what '*public health*' means in practice, learning disability nurses and collaborating professionals and agencies need to agree on what public health means in their area of practice.

Demographic intelligence

In the United Kingdom there is no unified central database of the population of people with learning disabilities. Local registers exist, and as previously discussed, these are important in highlighting the extent of the known and unknown health needs of the population of people with learning disabilities (Emerson and McGrother, 2010). Current, validated, and accurate registers are vital in the implementation of public health initiatives for people with learning disabilities by learning disability nurses (Turner and Robinson, 2010). Registers provide essential statistical intelligence about the populations of people with learning disabilities, which learning disability nurses require in order to fulfil their public health practice. Understanding the distribution of the population and morbidity rates of people with learning disabilities is therefore important for learning disability nurses to deliver targeted and appropriate public health services for people with learning disabilities (Mafuba, 2013). Demographic intelligence is important in the investigation and diagnosis of the epidemiological problems that affect people with learning disabilities. In addition, demographic intelligence is useful in facilitating prioritisation of public health programmes for people with learning disabilities. Furthermore, it enables better targeting of public health initiatives. Demographic intelligence is also useful for monitoring and evaluating the impact of public health programmes and strategies in the population of people with learning disabilities. The work being undertaken by the Improving Health and Lives Learning Disabilities Observatory in England (now part of Public Health England) is making significant contributions to the demographic intelligence of the population of people with learning disabilities.

Interprofessional and interagency collaboration

Interprofessional working in the delivery of health and public health programmes has been advocated (WHO, 1999; HDA, 2003; Wildridge et al., 2004; Dion, 2004; Tope and Thomas, 2007). The argument for interprofessional working in public health is based on the fact that public health problems are too complex to be met by one profession (WHO, 1999). In addition to interprofessional working, public health practice is by nature interagency (HDA, 2003; Tope and Thomas, 2007). Learning disability nurses need to be aware that interagency partnership working could be difficult to develop (Wildridge et al. 2004). This may result in interagency and philosophical tensions for a variety of reasons, including philosophical differences. Historically in the United Kingdom learning disabilities specialist services, for example, learning disability nurses have practised under the leadership of psychiatry. Psychiatry has historically prioritised psychiatric treatments rather than prevention. It is important for learning disability nurses to be aware that philosophical tensions are inevitable in an interprofessional environment such as public health practice (Bridges et al., 2007; Robinson and Cottrell, 2005).

Leadership

In providing public health services to people with learning disabilities, learning disability nurses find themselves occupying a fine line between health and social care (Mafuba, 2009). Strategic leadership in organisations which employ learning disability nurses is essential for learning disability nurses to effectively meet the public health needs of people with learning disabilities (Mafuba, 2013). The multiprofessional, and interorganisational public health environments in which learning disability nurses practice is complex, and requires clearly defined public health leadership to meet the public health needs of people with learning disabilities.

Resources

The increasing divergence between public health needs and limited financial resources has led to implicit rationing of health services, including public health services in the United Kingdom (Hunter, 1995; Ham and Coulter, 2001; Eichler et al., 2004; Greer, 2004). Ham and Coulter (2001) have noted that the impact of implicit and explicit rationing of public health services contributes to exclusion of services which are at the margins of health services, such as those for people with learning disabilities. The consequence of this is that public health organisations which employ learning disability nurses tend to focus on the bigger picture.

Politics

The nature of U.K. health service policy is that policy formulation is very much driven from the centre (Ham, 2004), with policy implementation delegated to local organisations. Political decisions by the central government constantly shift the boundaries of how learning disability nurses engage with public health practice. In addition, local public health priorities may not focus on the public health needs of people with learning disabilities (Mafuba, 2013).

Case study 4.2

Having read this chapter, read the following extract from *Healthy Lives, Healthy People: A Call to Action on Obesity in England* (DH, 2011, p. 23) and answer the questions that follow.

*As our priority is now healthy weight in adults as well as children, effective and **tailored support** for the more than 60% of adults who are already overweight or obese is essential. Successful **local strategies** will need to strike a balance between 'treatment' interventions that **help individuals to reach a healthier weight** and **sustained preventive effort** to help to make healthy weight increasingly the norm. These are not alternatives – both are vital if we are to 'shift the curve'.*

*Many local areas already commission weight management services and a range of providers are already delivering and **developing evidence-based services** aimed at different population groups. The commissioning of weight management services will remain the responsibility of local areas, but we will provide support to build local capability and support evidence-based approaches.*

Student Activity 4.2

Why is the Ottawa Charter important and what are its central themes?

What is the difference between health education and health promotion?

What role does empowerment and self-advocacy play in health promotion? Reflect on an example from your experience of working with a person with a learning disability.

Identify at least five professionals who could be involved in promoting the health and well-being of people with learning disabilities, explaining the potential roles such professionals could play.

Reflect on how what you have learned here will assist you in meeting the professional requirements for your course.

CONCLUSION

Whereas the health and life expectancy of the people in the United Kingdom has improved in recent decades, the health and life expectancy of people with learning disabilities has not improved at the same rate. People with learning disabilities still experience significant inequalities in health and health outcomes. Preventive health is pivotal in improving the health and health experience of people with learning disabilities. This means learning disability nurses will need to assimilate new public health roles and engage with public health practice in new ways to improve the health and life expectancy of people with learning disabilities.

Because of their daily contact with people with learning disabilities, it is clear that learning disability nurses will increasingly play a pivotal role in enabling people with learning disabilities to live healthy lives, reduce preventive mortality, and influence the implementation of public health policy for people with learning disabilities. The Royal College of Nursing has provided a template for the development of the public health roles of learning disability nurses in the four countries of the United Kingdom (RCN, 2012). This requires

- All nurses, regardless of their work environment, knowing and understanding the health needs of their local population
- The identification of defined populations that would enable health care teams to target individuals who would most benefit from upstream approaches
- Working in partnership with other members of health and social care organisations to influence the work on tackling the wider determinants of health
- Engaging local people and groups, including those who are not working, in upstream awareness and action
- Nurses making it their business to be informed, aware, and responsive to disease outbreaks and other threats to health nurses utilising public health evidence in everyday practice, not just evidence for treating illness
- Nurses working to a public health knowledge and skills framework based on the 'novice to expert' criteria (RCN, 2012, p.12).

REFERENCES

Abbott, S. 2007. Leadership across boundaries: A qualitative study of the nurse consultant role in English primary care. *Journal of Nursing Management*, 15(7):703–710..

Acheson, D. 1998. *Independent Inquiry into Inequalities Report*. London: TSO.

An Bord Altranais 2005. *Requirements and Standards for Nurse Registration Education Programmes* (3rd ed.) Dublin: An Bord Altranais.

Aspray, T.J., Francis, R.M., Tyrer, S.P., and Quilliam, S.J. 1999. Patients with learning disability in the community. *British Medical Journal*, 318:476–477.

Backer, C., Chapman, M., and Mitchell, D. 2009. Access to secondary healthcare for people with learning disabilities: A review of the literature. *Journal of Applied Research in Intellectual Disabilities*, 22(6):514–525.

Baggott, R. 2011. *Public Health Policy and Politics*. 2nd ed. London: Palgrave Macmillan.

Bailey, N.M. and Cooper, S.A. 1997. The current provision of specialist health services to people with learning disabilities in England and Wales. *Journal of Intellectual Disability Research*, 41(1):52–59.

Barr, O. 2006. The evolving role of community nurses for people with learning disabilities: Changes over an 11-year period. *Journal of Clinical Nursing*, 15:72–82.

Barr, O., Gilgunn, J., Kane, T., and Moore, G. 1999. Health screening for people with learning disabilities by a community learning disabilities nursing service in Northern Ireland. *Journal of Advanced Nursing*, 29(6):1482–1491.

Baxter, H., Lowe, K., Houston, H., Jones, G., Felce, D., and Kerr, M. 2006. Previously unidentified morbidity in patients with intellectual disability. *British Journal of General Practice*, 56(523):93–98.

Beange, H. and Bauman, A. 1990. Caring for the developmentally disabled in the community. *Australian Family Physician*, 19(10):1555, 1558–1563.

Beange, H., McElduff, A., and Baker, W. 1995. Medical disorders of adults with mental retardation: A population study. *American Journal of Mental Retardation*, 99(6):595–604.

Bevan, G. 2006. Setting targets for healthcare performance—lessons from a case study of the English NHS. *National Institute Economic Review*, 197(1):67–79.

Blaxter, M. 2004. *Health*. Cambridge: Polity.

Boarder, J.H. 2002. The perceptions of experienced community learning disability nurses of their roles and ways of working. *Journal of Learning Disabilities*, 6(3):281–296.

Bollard, M. 1999. Improving primary healthcare for people with learning disabilities. *British Journal of Nursing*, 8(18):1216–1221.

Bridges, J., Fitzgerald, M., and Meyer, J. 2007. New workforce roles in healthcare: Exploring the longer-term journey of organisational innovations. *Journal of Health Organisation and Management*, 21(4–5):381–392.

Brown, M., MacArthur, J., McKechanie, A., Mack, S., Hayes, M., and Fletcher, J. 2011. Learning disability liaison nursing services in south-east Scotland: A mixed-methods impact and outcome study. *Journal of Intellectual Disability Research*, doi: 10.1111/j.1365-2788.2011.01511.x.

Campbell, M. and Martin, M. 2009. Reducing health inequalities in Scotland: The involvement of people with learning disabilities as national health service reviewers. *British Journal of Learning Disabilities*, 38(1):49–58.

Cancer Research UK. 2008. *Policy Statement: Inequalities in Cancer Experienced by Those with Learning Disabilities*. London: Cancer Research UK.

Chauhan, U., Kontopantelis, E., Campbell, S., Jarrett, H., and Lester, H. 2010. Health checks in primary care for adults with intellectual disabilities: How extensive should they be? *Journal of Intellectual Disability Research*, 54(6):479–486.

Chief Medical Officer. 2007. *Public Health in England*. London: DH.

Codling, M. and Macdonald, N. 2011. Sustainability of health promotion for people with learning disabilities. *Nursing Standard*, 25(22):42–47.

Cooper, S.A., Morrison, J., Melville, C., Finlayson, J., Allan, L., Martin, G., and Robinson, N. 2006. Improving the health of people with intellectual disabilities: Outcomes of a health screening programme after 1 year. *Journal of Intellectual Disability Research*, 50(9):667–677.

Coyle, E. 2007. Public health in Wales. In: Griffiths, S. and Hunter, D. (Eds.), *New Perspectives in Public Health*. London: Routeledge, pp. 37–44.

Curtice, L. and Long, L. 2002. The health log: Developing a health monitoring tool for people with learning disabilities within a community support agency. *Journal of Learning Disabilities*, 30(2):68–72.

Dawson, A. and Verweij, M. 2007. The meaning of 'public' in 'public health'. In: Dawson, A. and Verweij, M. (Eds.), *Ethics Prevention and Public Health*. New York: Oxford University Press, pp. 13–29.

DH. 1990. *NHS and Community Care Act*. London: HMSO.

DH. 1992. *The Health of the Nation: A Strategy for Health in England*. London: HMSO.

DH. 1995. *The Health of the Nation: A Strategy for People with Learning Disabilities*. London: HMSO.

DH. 1999. *Saving Lives: Our Healthier Nation*. London: Department of Health.

DH. 2001. *Valuing People. A New Strategy for the 21st Century*. London: TSO.

DH. 2002. *Action for Health: Health Action Plans and Health Facilitation*. London: Department of Health.

DH. 2004. *Choosing Health: Making Healthy Choices Easy*. London: Department of Health.

DH. 2005. *Delivering Choosing Health*. London: Department of Health.

DH. 2006a. *Our Health Our Care Our Say: A New Direction for Community Services*. London: Department of Health.

DH. 2006b. *Health Challenge England*. London: Department of Health.

DH. 2007a. *Tackling Health Inequalities*. London: Department of Health.

DH. 2007b. *Good Practice Guide in Learning Disabilities Nursing*. London: Department of Health.

DH. 2007c. *Promoting Equality*. London: Department of Health.

DH. 2009a. *Health Action Planning and Health Facilitation for People with Learning Disabilities: Good Practice Guidance*. London: Department of Health.

DH. 2009b. *Valuing People Now: A New Three-Year Strategy for People with Learning Disabilities*. London: Department of Health.

DH. 2010. *Healthy Lives, Healthy People: Our Strategy for Public Health in England*. London: Department of Health.

DH. 2011. *Healthy Lives, Healthy People: A Call to Action on Obesity in England*. London: Department of Health.

DHSSNI. 1996. *Health and Wellbeing: Towards the New Millennium*. Belfast: DHSSNI.

DHSSNI. 1997. *Well in 2000*. Belfast: DHSSNI.

DHSSPS. 2004. *A Healthier Future*. Belfast: DHSSPSNI.

DHSSPSNI. 2002. *Investing for Health*. Belfast: DHSSPSNI.

Dion, X. 2004. A multi-disciplinary team approach to public health working. *British Journal of Community Nursing*, 9(4):149–154.

Donnelly, P. 2007. Public health in Scotland: The dividend of devolution. In: Griffiths, S. and Hunter, D. (Eds.), *New Perspectives in Public Health*. Abingdon: Radcliffe, pp. 22–29.

Disability Rights Commission (DCR) 2006. *Equal Treatment: Closing the Gap*. Stratford Upon Avon: Disability Rights Commission.

Durvasula, S., Beange, H., and Baker, W. 2002. Mortality of people with intellectual disability in northern Sydney. *Journal of Intellectual and Developmental Disability*, 27(4):255–264.

Eichler, H., Kong, S.X., Gerth, W.C., Marros, P., and Jonsson, B. 2004. Use of cost-effective analysis in healthcare resource allocation decision making: How are cost effective thresholds expected to emerge? *Value in Health*, 7(5):518–528.

Elliot-Cannon, C. 1981, Do the mentally handicapped need specialist community nursing? *Nursing Times*, 77(27):77–80.

Emerson, E. and Glover, G. 2010. Health checks for people with learning disabilities 2008/9 & 2009/10. Improving Health and Lives: Learning Disabilities. Observatory. (Online). Available at www.phine.org.uk/uploads/doc/vid_7393_health_checks.pdf (accessed March 13, 2012).

Emerson, E. and McGrother, C. 2010. The use of pooled data for learning disabilities registers: A scoping review. (Online). Available at http://www.improvinghealthandlives.org.uk/publications/951/What_Learning_Disability_Registers_can_tell_us (accessed March 11, 2012).

Emerson, E., Copeland, A., and Glover, G. 2011. The uptake of health checks for adults with learning disabilities: 2008/9 to 2010/11. (Online). Available at http://www.improvinghealthandlives.org.uk/publications/972/Health_Checks_For_People_With_Learning_Disabilities_2010-11 (accessed March 13, 2012).

Faculty of Public Health. 2012. What is public health? (Online). Available at http://www.fph.org.uk/what_is_public_health (accessed July 17, 2013).

Felce, D., Baxter, H., Lowe, K., Dunstan, F., Houston, H., Jones, G., Grey, J., Felce, J. and Kerr, M. 2008. The impact of checking the health of adults with intellectual disabilities on primary care consultation rates, health promotion and contact with specialists. *Journal of Applied Research in Intellectual Disabilities*, 21(6):597–602.

Gates, B. 1994. *Advocacy: A nurses' guide*. London: Scutari Press.

Gordon, R. 1987. An operational classification of disease prevention. In: Steinberg, J.A. and Silverman, M.M. (Eds.), *Preventing Mental Disorders*, Rockville, MD: U.S. Department of Health and Human Services.

Greer, S.L. 2009. *Territorial Politics and Health Policy*. Manchester: Manchester University Press.

Greer, S.L. 2004. *Territorial Politics and Health Policy: UK Health Policy in Comparative Perspective*. Manchester: Manchester University Press.

Griffiths, R. 1988. *Community Care: Agenda for Action. Report for the Secretary of State for Social Services*. London: HMSO.

Griffiths, S. and Hunter, D. 1999. *Perspectives in Public Health*. Oxford: Radical Medical Press.

Griffiths, S., Jewell, T., and Donelly, P. 2005. Public health in practice: The three domains of public health. *Public Health*, 119(10):907–913.

Ham, C. 2004. *Health Policy in Britain: The Politics and Organisation of the National Health Service* (5th ed.). Basingstoke: Palgrave MacMillan.

Ham, C. and Coulter, A. 2001. Explicit and implicit rationing: Taking responsibility and avoiding blame for healthcare choices. *Journal of Health Services Research and Policy*, 6(3):163–169.

HDA. 2003. *The Working Partnership*. London: Health Development Agency.

Heslop P., Blair, P., Fleming, P., Hoghton M, Marriott A., and Russ, L. 2013. *Confidential Inquiry into Premature Deaths of People with Learning Disabilities (CIPOLD)*. Bristol: Norah Fry Research Centre-University of Bristol.

Hollins, S. and Sinason, V. 1998. *I Can Get through It*. London: Gaskell.

Hollins, S., Attard, M.T., von Fraunhofer, N., McGuigan, S., and Sedgwick, P. 1998. Mortality in people with learning disability: Risks, causes, and death certification findings in London. *Developmental Medicine and Child Neurology*, 40(1):50–56.

Holloway, D. 2004. Ethical dilemmas in community learning disabilities nursing: What helps nurses resolve ethical dilemmas that result from choices made by people with learning disabilities? *Journal of Learning Disabilities*, 8(3):283–U298.

Howells, G. 1986. Are the medical needs of mentally handicapped adults being met? *Journal of the Royal College of General Practitioners*, 36(291):449–453.

HSCIC. 2014. Quality and outcomes framework. (Online) Available at http://www.hscic.gov.uk/qof (accessed August 24, 2014).

Hunter, D.J. 1995. Rationing healthcare: The political perspective. *British Medical Bulletin*, 51(4):876–884.

Iacono, T. and Davis, R. 2003. The experiences of people with developmental disability in emergency departments and hospital wards. *Research in Developmental Disabilities*, 24(4):247–264.

Jacobson, J.W., Janicki M.P., and Ackerman, L.J. 1989. Healthcare service usage by older persons with developmental disabilities living in community settings. *Adult Residential Care Journal*, 3(3):181–191.

Janicki, M.P. 2001. Toward a rationale strategy for promoting healthy ageing amongst people with intellectual disabilities. *Journal of Applied Research in Intellectual Disabilities*, 14(3):171–174.

Jones, R.G. and Kerr, M.P. 1997. A randomised control trial of an opportunistic health screening tool in primary care for people with learning disability. *Journal of Learning Disability Research*, 41(5):409–415.

Jukes, M. 2002. Health facilitation in learning disability: A new specialist role. *British Journal of Nursing*, 11(10):694–698

Kaiser., S. and Mackenbach, J.P. 2008. Public health in eight European countries: An international comparison of terminology. *Public Health*, 122(2):211–216.

Kerr, M. 2004. Improving the general health of people with learning disabilities. *Advances in Psychiatric Treatment*, 10:200–206.

Kerr, M., McCulloch, D., Oliver, K., McLean, B., Coleman, E., Law, T., Beaton, P., Wallace, S., Newell, E., Eccles, T., and Prescott, R.J. 2003. Medical needs of people with intellectual disability require regular reassessment, and the provision of client- and carer-held reports. *Journal of Intellectual Disability Research*, 47(2):134–145.

Kerr, M., Richards, D., and Glover, G. 1996. Primary care for people with a learning disability—a group practice survey. *Journal of Applied Research in Intellectual Disability*, 9(4):347–352.

Keywood, K., Fovargue, S. and Flynn, M. (1999) *Best practice? Healthcare Decision Making by, with and for Adults with Learning Disability*. Liverpool: Joseph Rowntree Foundation.

Lennox, N., Beange, H. and Edwards, N. 2000. The health needs of people with intellectual disability. *Medical Journal of Australia*, 173(6): 328–330.

Lennox, N. and Diggins, J. N. (1999) *Management Guidelines: People with Developmental and Intellectual Disabilities* Melbourne: Therapeutic Guidelines Ltd.

Lennox, N. G. and Kerr, M. P. 1997. Primary healthcare and people with an intellectual disability: The evidence base. *Journal of Intellectual Disability Research*, 41(5):365–372.

Linna, S. L., Moilanen, I., Ebeling, H., Piha, J., Kumpulainen, K., Tamminen, T., and Almqvist, F. 1999. Psychiatric symptoms in children with intellectual disability. *European Child and Adolescent Psychiatry*, 8(suppl. 4):77–82.

Llewellyn, P. and Northway, R. 2007. The views and experiences of learning disability nurses concerning their advocacy education. *Nurse Education Today*, 27(8):955–963.

Mafuba, K. 2009. The public health role of learning disability nurses: A review of the literature. *Learning Disability Practice*, 12(4):33–37.

Mafuba, K. 2013. Public health: Community learning disability nurses' perception and experience of their role. Unpublished PhD thesis, University of West London.

Mafuba, K. and Gates, B. 2013. An investigation into the public health roles of community learning disability nurses. *British Journal Learning Disability*. DOI: 10.1111-bld.12071.

Marshall, D. and Moore, G. 2003. Obesity in people with intellectual disabilities: The impact of nurse-led health screenings and health promotion activities. *Journal of Advanced Nursing*, 41(2):147–153.

Matthews, D. and Hegarty, J. 1997. The OK health check: A health assessment checklist for people with learning disabilities. *British Journal of Learning Disabilities*, 25(4):138–143.

McConkey, R., Moore, G., and Marshall, D. 2002. Changes in the attitudes of GP's to the health screening of people with learning disabilities. *Journal of Learning Disabilities*, 6(4):373–384.

McDermott, S. Platt, T., and Krishnaswami, S. 1997. Are individuals with mental retardation at risk for chronic disease? *Family Medicine*, 29(6):429–434.

McGarry, J. and Arthur, A. 2001. Informal caring in late life: A qualitative study of the experiences of older carers. *Journal of Advanced Nursing*, 33(2):182–189.

McIlfatrick, S., Taggart, L., and Truesdale-Kennedy, M. 2011. Supporting women with intellectual disabilities to access breast cancer screening: A healthcare professional perspective. *European Journal of Cancer Care*, 20(3):412–420.

McLoughlin, I.J. 1988. A study of mortality experiences in a mental handicap hospital. *British Journal of Psychiatry*, 153:645–649.

Melville, C.A., Cooper S.A., Morrison I.J., Finlayson J., Allan, L., Robinson N., Burns E., and Martin, G. 2006. The outcomes of an intervention study to reduce the barriers experienced by people with intellectual disabilities accessing primary healthcare services. *Journal of Intellectual Disability Research*, 50(1):11–17.

Mencap. 2004. *Treat Me Right! Better Health for People with Learning Disabilities*. London: Mencap.

Mencap. 2007. *Death by Indifference. Following Up the Treat Me Right Report*. London: Mencap.

Mencap. 2012. *Death by Indifference: 74 Deaths and Counting*. London: Mencap.

Messent, P.R., Cooke, C.B., and Long, J. 1999. What choice: A consideration of the level of opportunity for people with mild and moderate learning disabilities to lead a physically active healthy lifestyle. *British Journal of Learning Disabilities*, 27(2):73–77.

Michael, J. 2008. *Healthcare for All: Report of the Independent Inquiry into Access to Healthcare for People with Learning Disabilities*. London: Department of Health.

Mobbs, C., Hadley, S., Wittering, R., and Bailey, N.M. 2002. An exploration of the role of the community nurse, learning disability, in England. *British Journal of Learning Disabilities*, 30(1):13–18.

NafW. 2001. *Improving Health in Wales*. Cardiff: National Assembly for Wales.

NHS Executive. 1998. *Signposts for Success in Commissioning and Providing Health Services for People with Learning Disabilities* London: DH.

NHS Employers. 2014. Enhanced services. (Online) Available at http://www.nhsemployers. org/payandcontracts/generalmedicalservicescontract/directedenhancedservices/pages/ enhancedservices201415.aspx (accessed August 23, 2014).

NHS Health Scotland. 2004 *Health Needs Assessment Report: People with Learning Disability in Scotland.* Glasgow: NHS Health Scotland.

NI Executive. 2008. *Programme for Government.* Belfast: NIE.

Nissen, J.M. and Haveman, M.J. 1997. Mortality and avoidable death in people with severe self-injurious behaviour: Results of a Dutch study. *Journal of Intellectual Disability Research*, 41(3):252–257.

NMC. 2010. *Standards for Pre-Registration Nurse Education.* London: Nursing and Midwifery Council.

Nocon, A., Sayce, L., and Nadirshaw, Z. 2008. Health inequalities experienced by people with learning disabilities: Problems and possibilities in primary care. *Learning Disability Review*, 13(1):28–36.

NPSA. 2004. *Understanding the Patient Safety Issues for People with Learning Disabilities.* London: National Patient Safety Agency.

Ouellette-Kuntz, H. 2005. Understanding health disparities and inequities faced by individuals with intellectual disabilities. *Journal of Applied Research in Intellectual Disabilities*, 18(2):113–121.

Parliamentary and Health Service Ombudsman and Social Services Ombudsman. 2009. *Six Lives: The Provision of Public Services to People with Learning Disabilities.* London: TSO.

Pawar, D.G. and Akuffo, E.O. 2008. Comparative survey of comorbidities in people with learning disability with and without epilepsy. *The Psychiatrist*, 32:224–226.

Phillips, A., Morrison, J., and Davis, R.W. 2004. General practitioners' educational needs intellectual disability health. *Journal of Intellectual Disability Research*, 48(2):142–149.

Powell, H., Murray, G., and McKenzie, K. 2004. Staff perceptions of community learning disability nurses' role. *Nursing Times*, 100(19):40–42.

Powrie, E. 2003. Primary healthcare provision for adults with a learning disability. *Journal of Advanced Nursing*, 42(4):413–423.

Public Health Agency. 2011. Implementing Bamford: Knowledge from research. Belfast: Public Health Agency. (Online). Available at http://www.publichealth.hscni.net/sites/default/files/ Bamford_Summary_Report.pdf (accessed January 7, 2012).

RCN. 2012. *Going Upstream: Nursing's Contribution to Public Health: Prevent, Promote and protect.* London: Royal College of Nursing.

Robertson, J., Emerson., Hatton, C., Gregory, N., Kessissoglou, S., Hallam, A., and Walsh, P.N. 2001. Environmental opportunities and support for exercising self-determination in community-based residential settings. *Research in Developmental Disabilities*, 22(6):487–502.

Robinson, M. and Cottrell, D. 2005. Health professionals in multi-disciplinary and multi-agency teams: Changing professional practice. *Journal of Interprofessional Care*, 19(6):547–560.

Rosen, G. 1993. *A History of Public Health*. Expanded ed. Baltimore, MD: Johns Hopkins University Press.

Ruddick, L. 2005. Health of people with intellectual disabilities: A review of factors influencing access to healthcare. *British Journal of Health Psychology*, 10(4):559–570.

Ryan, R. and Sunada, K. 1997. Medical evaluations of persons with mental retardation referred for psychiatric assessment. *General Hospital Psychiatry*, 19(4):274–280.

Scheepers, M., Kerr, M.O., Hara, D., Bainbridge, D., Cooper, S.A., Davis, R., Fujiura, G., Heller, T., Holland, A., Krahn, G., Lennox N., Meany, J., and Wehmeyer, M. 2005. Reducing health disparity in people with intellectual disabilities: A report from Health Issues Special Interest Research Group of the International Association for the Scientific Study of Intellectual Disabilities. *Journal of Policy and Practice in Intellectual Disabilities*, 2(3–4):249–255.

Scottish Executive. 2000a. *Our National Health: A Plan for Action, A Plan for Change*. Edinburgh: Scottish Executive.

Scottish Executive. 2000b. *The Same as You*. Edinburgh: Scottish Executive.

Scottish Executive. 2003. *Improving Health in Scotland*. Edinburgh: Scottish Executive.

Scottish Government. 2007. *Better Health Better Care: Action Plan*. Edinburgh: Scottish Government.

Scottish Government. 2008. *Equally Well*. Edinburgh: Scottish Government.

Scottish Office. 1992. *Scotland's Health: A Challenge to Us All*. Edinburgh: HMSO.

Slevin, E., Taggart, L., McKonkey, R., Cousins, N., Truesdale-Kennedy, M., and Downing, S. 2011. Supporting people with intellectual disabilities who challenge or who are ageing: A rapid review of evidence Belfast: Centre for Intellectual and Developmental Disabilities—Public Health Agency and University of Ulster. (Online). Available at http://www.publichealth.hscni.net/sites/default/files/Intellectual%20Disability.pdf (accessed January 7, 2012).

Stein, K. and Allen, N. 1999. Cross sectional survey of cervical cancer screening in women with learning disabilities. *British Medical Journal*, 318(7184):641.

Straetmans, J.M.J.A.A., van Schrojenstein Lantman-de Valk, H.M.J., Schellevis, F.G., and Dinant, G.J. 2007. Health problems of people with intellectual disabilities: The impact for general practice. *British Journal of General Practice* 57(534):64–66.

Sullivan, S., Hussain, R., Slack-Smith, L.M., and Bittles, A.H. 2003. Breast cancer uptake of mammography screening services by women with intellectual disabilities. *Preventive Medicine*, 37(5):507–512.

Thomas, G. and Kerr, M.P. 2011. Longitudinal follow-up of weight change in the context of a community-based health promotion programme for adults with intellectual disability. *Journal of Applied Research in Intellectual Disabilities*, 24(4):381–387.

Thornton, C. 1996. A focus group inquiry into the perceptions of primary healthcare teams and the provision of healthcare for adults with learning disability living in the community. *Journal of Advanced Nursing*, 23(6):1168–1176.

Tope, R. and Thomas, E. 2007. *Creating an Interprofessional Workforce*. London: DH.

Turner, S. and Robinson, C. 2010. *Health Checks for People with Learning Disabilities: Implications and Actions for Commissioners*. Durham: Improving Health and Lives— Learning Disabilities Observatory.

van Schrojenstein Lantman-de Valk H.M.J., Metsemakers, J.F.M., Haveman, M.J., and Crebolder, H.F.J.M. 2000. Health problems in people with intellectual disability in general practice: A comparative study. *Family Practice*, 17(5):405–407.

Webb O.J. and Rogers L. 1999. Health screening for people with intellectual disability: The New Zealand experience. *Journal of Intellectual Disability Research*, 43(6):497–503.

Welsh Assembly Government. 2002. *Well-Being in Wales*. Cardiff: Welsh Assembly Government.

Welsh Assembly Government. 2003. *Wales: A Better Country*. Cardiff: Welsh Assembly Government.

Welsh Assembly Government. 2005. *Designed for Life: Creating World Class Health and Social Care for Wales in the 21st Century*. Cardiff: Welsh Assembly Government.

Welsh Office. 1998. *Strategic Framework: Better Health Better Wales*. Cardiff: Welsh Office.

Welsh Office NHS Directorate. 1989. *Welsh Health Planning Forum: Strategic Intent and Direction for the NHS in Wales*. Cardiff: Welsh Office.

Welsh Office NHS Directorate. 1992. *Caring for the Future*. Cardiff: Welsh Office.

Whitehead, M. 1992. The concepts and principles of equity and health. *International Journal of Health Services*, 22(3):429–445.

Whitfield M., Langan J., and Russell O. 1996. Assessing general practitioners' care of adult patients with learning disability: Case-control study. *Quality in Healthcare*, 5(1):31–35.

WHO. 1986. *First conference on health promotion: Ottawa Charter for Health Promotion November 17–21*. Ottawa: WHO/Health and Welfare Canada/Canadian Association for Public Health.

WHO. 1999. *Health 21: The Health for All Policy Framework for The WHO European Region: European Health for All—Series No 6*. Copenhagen: World Health Organisation.

WHO (2003) *The World Health Report 2003: Shaping the Future*. Geneva: WHO.

Wick, C.J. 2007 Setting the stage: Writing job descriptions that work. *Executive Housekeeping Today*, 29(7):9–11.

Wilde, J. 2007. Public health in a changing Ireland: An all-Ireland perspective. In: Griffiths, S. and Hunter, D. (Eds.), *New Perspectives in Public Health*. London: Routeledge, pp. 45–54.

Wildridge V; Childs S; Lynette Cawthra L; Madge B 2004. How to create successful partnerships: A review of the literature. *Health Information and Libraries Journal*, 21(1):3–19.

Wilson, D.N. and Haire, A. 1990. Healthcare screening for people with mental handicap living in the community. *British Medical Journal*, 301(6765):1379–1381.

Winslow, C. 1920. The untilled fields of public health. *Modern Medicine*, 2:183–191.

Wood, R. and Douglas, M. 2007. Cervical screening for women with learning disability: Current practice and attitudes within primary care in Edinburgh. *British Journal of Learning Disabilities*, 35(2):84–92.

FURTHER READING

An Bord Altranais. 2005. *Requirements and Standards for Nurse Registration Education Programmes* (3rd ed.). Dublin: An Bord Altranais.

Baggott, R. 2011. *Public Health Policy and Politics* (2nd ed.). Basingstoke: Palgrave MacMillan.

Evans, D., Coutsaftiki, D., and Fathers, C.P. 2011. *Health Promotion and Public Health for Nursing Students*. Exeter: Learning Matters Ltd.

Hubley, J. and Copeman, J. with Woodall, J. 2013. *Practical Health Promotion* (2nd ed.). Cambridge: Polity Press.

Linsley, P., Kane,R., and Owen, S. 2011. *Nursing for Public Health (Promotion, Principles, and Practice)*. Oxford: Oxford University Press.

NMC. 2010. *Standards for Pre-Registration Nurse Education*. London: Nursing and Midwifery Council.

RCN. 2012. *Going Upstream: Nursing's Contribution to Public Health: Prevent Promote and Protect*. London: Royal College of Nursing.

USEFUL RESOURCES

An Bord Altranais: http://www.nursingboard.ie/en/reqs_stds_reg.aspx

BILD: http://www.bild.org.uk/

Contact a Family: http://www.cafamily.org.uk/medical-information/conditions/

Enable Scotland: http://www.enable.org.uk/Pages/Enable_Home.aspx

Foundation for People with Learning Disabilities: http://www.learningdisabilities.org.uk/

General Medical Council: http://www.gmc-uk.org/learningdisabilities/

Inclusion Ireland: http://www.inclusionireland.ie/

Intellectual Disability Info Web Pages: http://www.intellectualdisability.info/

Learning Disabilities Observatory: https://www.improvinghealthandlives.org.uk/publications

Mencap: http://www.mencap.org.uk/

Mencap Northern Ireland: http://www.mencap.org.uk/northern-ireland

Mencap Wales: http://www.mencap.org.uk/wales

Nursing and Midwifery Council: http://standards.nmc-uk.org/Pages/Welcome.aspx

5 Learning disability nursing and mental health

Bob Gates

INTRODUCTION

It is known that people with learning disabilities are at greater risk of developing mental health problems than the general population. Because of the high prevalence of mental health problems in this population, there is a need to prepare learning disability nurses to promote good mental health and well-being, or its maintenance in those who are particularly vulnerable (Ferguson, 2009). To be explored in this chapter is the nature of, and manifestations of, good mental health, as well as manifestations of mental ill health, assessment tools used in nursing practice, and how to conduct a mental state examination. A range of approaches to treatments will be outlined, as well as the Care Programme Approach. Finally, relevant mental health legislation, and assessment of mental capacity, Independent Mental Capacity Advocates (IMCAs), Deprivation of Liberty, and safeguarding issues are outlined.

Since the introduction of the White Paper *Valuing People* (2001), many commissioners of health services are now pursuing mainstream mental health service provision for people with learning disabilities, with services being primarily driven by policies such as *No Health without Mental Health* (2011). The interface between mental health services and specialist learning disability services is fragmented, and finding good clinical protocols for care planning for people with learning disabilities with mental health problems is difficult. Therefore, this chapter will focus on the knowledge and practical skills that learning disability nurses will need to meet the mental health needs of people with learning disabilities, and this will be contextualised within the Nursing and Midwifery Council for the United Kingdom (2010) and An Bord Altranais (2005) standards for competence.

This chapter will focus on the following issues:

- Introduction
- The nature of mental health and well-being
- Manifestations of mental ill health
  - Affective disorders
  - Depression
  - Bipolar disorder
  - Anxiety
  - Suicide and deliberate self-harm (DSH)

- Schizophrenia
- Obsessive compulsive disorders
- Eating disorders
- Personality disorder
- Alcohol and drug dependency
- General observations and recording: assessment tools for mental health
  - General observations and recording
  - Mood
  - Sleep charts
  - Weight charts
  - ABC charts
- Mental State Examination (MSE)
  - Appearance
  - Behaviour
  - Cognition
  - Experiences
  - Mood and affect
  - Speech
  - Thought content
- Specific mental health assessment tools
  - Assessment of dual diagnosis (ADD)
  - Learning disability version of the cardinal needs schedule (LDCNS)
  - Psychiatric Assessment Schedules for Adults with Developmental Disabilities (PAS-ADD)
  - The Hamilton Rating Scale for Depression (HRSD)
  - Beck Anxiety Inventory (BAI)
  - Schedule for Affective Disorders and Schizophrenia (SADS)
- Treatments
  - Medication
  - Talking therapies
  - Electroconvulsive therapy (ECT)
  - Other approaches
- The Care Programme Approach
- The Mental Health Act 1983
  - Involuntary admission: Assessment

- Part II of the Mental Health Act

- Part III of the Mental Health Act

- Assessment or treatment

- Admission for assessment under MHA 1983

- Part II: Compulsory admission to hospital and guardianship

- Part X: Miscellaneous and supplementary

- Part III: Patients concerned in criminal proceedings or under sentence

- Admission for Treatment MHA 1983

- Part II: Compulsory admission to hospital and guardianship

- Part III: Patients concerned in criminal proceedings or under sentence

- Appropriate treatment test

- Assessment of mental capacity: IMCAs and DOLS

Competences

NMC Competences and Competencies

Domain 1: Professional values - Field standard competence and competencies – 1.1; 2.1; 3.1; 4.1.

Domain 2: Communication and interpersonal skills - Field standard competence and competencies – 1.1; 2.1; 3.1; 4.1.

Domain 3: Nursing practice and decision making - Field standard competence and competencies – 1.1; 3.1; 5.1; 8.1.

Domain 4: Leadership, management and team working - Field standard competence and competencies – 1.1; 1.2; 2.1; 6.1; 6.2.

An Bord Altranais Competences and Indicators

Domain 1: Professional/ethical practice – 1.1.2; 1.1.3; 1; 1.1.5; 1.1.6; 1.1.7; 1.1.8; 1.2.4; 1.2.6.

Domain 2: Holistic approaches to care and the integration of knowledge – 2.1.1; 2.1.2; 2.1.3; 2.1.4; 2.2.1; 2.2.3; 2.2.4; 2.3.3; 2.3.4; 2.4.1; 2.4.2.

Domain 3: Interpersonal relationships – 3.1.1; 3.1.2; 3.1.3; 3.2.1; 3.2.2.

Domain 4: Organisation and management of care – 4.1.3.

Domain 5: Personal and professional development – 5.1.1; 5.1.2; 5.1.3.

THE NATURE OF MENTAL HEALTH AND WELL-BEING

Whereas all people are prone to mental health difficulties (Singleton et al., 2001), prevalence studies suggest that people with learning disabilities present with significantly higher rates mental ill-health than does that of the general population; 25% to 40% (Mental Health Foundation, 2007;

Cooper et al., 2007; Raghavan and Waseem et al., 2005; Department of Health, 2001), and are more prone to developing mental ill health than the rest of the population. Health services, at least in the United Kingdom, for people with learning disabilities, until relatively recently, had developed over many years into a separate medical speciality. That speciality resided within psychiatry (Royal Society of Psychiatrists, 1996), and this has given rise to separate services for people with learning disabilities. This is still in part the case, particularly around their mental health needs. Until the 1970s this was not challenged, but the growth of the concept of normalisation, in conjunction with the development of the social model of disability, has led to philosophical changes in clinical commissioning of learning disabilities services away from 'separateness' and toward 'inclusion'. This has resulted in the almost complete closure of all long-stay learning disability hospitals during the 1980s and 1990s, and a move to so-called community-based services. These services strive for integration and inclusion into mainstream activities that range from employment to health, as outlined in the government's white paper *Valuing People* (DH, 2001), and the subsequent 'refresh' *Valuing People Now* (DH, 2009).* Other more general mental health policy temporally is in keeping with this shift, and can be seen, for example, in the National Service Framework (NSF) for Mental Health (DH, 1999), which seeks to ensure that mental health services are accessible and available to all.

There is much more to good health than simply being physically healthy; any notion of health must also incorporate a healthy mind (see Chapter 4). Someone who has a healthy mind should be able to think (relatively) clearly and respond to and be able to deal with the everyday challenges of living. Additionally, that person should be able to make and sustain good relationships with his or her friends and the colleagues with whom he or she works, as well as his or her own immediate family. Finally, he or she should feel some sense of inner peace, and be able to enjoy life and share a feeling of well-being with others in the community. When these things are present, that is when we might consider someone to have good mental health.

Achieving good mental health is every bit as challenging as achieving good physical health. Every year, about one in four people in the United Kingdom may experience some kind of mental health problem (Mental Health Foundation, 2007). Of these problems, mixed anxiety and depression are probably the most common manifestations of mental ill health, with approximately 9% of people meeting the criteria for diagnosis (Singleton, 2001), although most of these presentations will not be severe enough to require specific treatment. Mental health problems include eating disorders, obsessive compulsive disorder, dependency on drugs and alcohol, personality disorder, bipolar disorder, and schizophrenia. There are a good and wide range of treatment options for mental ill health and psychological disorders, and these include medication, psychotherapy, or other treatments (Mental Health Foundation, 2007). It must be borne in mind that a mental illness is a medical condition where a person's thinking, feeling, mood, ability to relate to others, and daily functioning can all be disrupted. In just the same way as physical illnesses can affect someone's life, mental illnesses are medical conditions that often result in a diminished capacity for coping with the ordinary demands of life. In general terms, mental illness is a complex condition of altered mental health, but one where recovery is possible.

---

* This policy shift refers primarily to England—see Chapter 1 for relevant policy for Wales, Scotland and Northern Ireland, as well as Ireland, but the trajectory for specialist services, and a move to 'community care' away from congregated forms of living is similar in all countries.

Mental illnesses can affect anyone, regardless of age, race, religion, or income (although these factors may have a predisposing influence), and it must also be borne in mind that mental illness is not the result of some personal weakness. Nor is it a reflection of some flaw in an individual's persona, nor an indication of the way in which someone has been brought up, although significant childhood events can lead to a lack of resilience in adulthood. Most importantly, it should be remembered that mental illnesses are treatable (Mental Health Foundation, 2007). In other words, mental ill health is something that could, and does, affect all kinds of people and from all walks of life. This is an important thing for any nurse or health and social care professional to try and help others understand, and could do much to reduce or positively inform the negative stereotyping and ignorance that has surrounded mental ill health for centuries. Most people who are diagnosed with a serious mental illness can experience relief from their symptoms by actively participating in some kind of a treatment plan, and this includes people with learning disabilities.

MANIFESTATIONS OF MENTAL ILL HEALTH

In the past, presentation of psychiatric disorder was broadly divided into two major types of mental illness, and these types were broadly based upon manifestation of symptomology.

Neuroses was a term historically used to refer to a range of mental illnesses that encompassed symptoms that were extreme manifestations of the normal range of emotional experiences, and they typically included disorders such as depression, anxiety, or panic attacks. Generally, neuroses tend to be more amenable to treatment, and were often said to be characterised by 'insight' by the person experiencing the illness into both their condition and the presenting symptoms. These illnesses are now more frequently called common mental health problems. However, it should be remembered that this will not necessarily mean the illnesses are less severe conditions than those with psychotic symptoms.

Psychoses was a term historically used to describe a range of mental illnesses with symptoms that interfered with a person's perception of reality and typically included hallucinations, delusions, or paranoia, with the person seeing, hearing, smelling, feeling, or believing things that no one else does is able to perceive or understand. In the past this group was further subdivided into organic disorders (for example, vascular dementia), metabolic disorders (for example, porphyria), functional disorders (for example, schizophrenia), and affective disorders (for example, manic depressive psychosis, which is now referred to as bipolar disorder). Generally, they tend to be more challenging to treat than neuroses, and were often said to be characterised by a lack of 'insight' by the person experiencing the illness both about their condition and symptoms, that to a lesser or greater extent are characterised by thought disorder/s, hallucinations, and delusions. These illnesses are now more generally referred to as severe mental health problems.

This following section identifies a range of common and severe mental health problems that adults and children with learning disabilities may experience. Such problems include affective disorders, anxiety, suicide and deliberate self-harm (DSH), schizophrenia, obsessive compulsive disorders, eating disorders, personality disorder, and, finally, alcohol and drug dependency.

Affective disorders

Affective disorders refer to a wide range of mental disorders that are all characterised by dramatic changes or extremes of mood. Affective disorders can include manic (elevated, expansive, or irritable mood with hyperactivity, pressured speech, and inflated self-esteem) or depressed (dejected mood with little interest in life, sleep disturbance, agitation, and feelings of worthlessness or guilt) episodes, and often the two are combined. People with an affective disorder may or may not have psychotic symptoms such as delusions, hallucinations, or a loss of contact with reality. The reported prevalence rate of affective disorders in people with learning disabilities is known to vary considerably, and in a relatively recent study overall prevalence of these disorders was thought to be 6.6% (Cooper et al., 2007). How affective disorders vary between people with mild and severe learning disabilities is poorly understood.

Depression

Depression is a disorder, primarily of emotion, and is typically characterised by an all-pervasive lowering of mood (Katona and Robertson, 2000). In psychiatry, two main types of depression are proposed. These are *'endogenous'* and *'exogenous'*. The former is more severe and perhaps explained by biological factors, and often not associated with external triggers to the depression. The latter, sometimes referred to as reactive depression, is less severe, milder, can sometimes be explained by external 'triggers' of significant life events such as loss, and will sometimes manifest itself with an overlapping anxiety. In the population of people with mild learning disabilities people who, perhaps, present with well-developed communication skills, rather than those with moderate, severe, or profound learning disabilities with complex needs, have the ability not only to recognise but also to articulate their emotions. This means that assessing their level of mood can be undertaken using a standard assessment method. Where an individual is unable to report or articulate his or her emotions, one often has to rely on reports from carers and supporters of overt changes in behaviour to arrive at a diagnosis. It is worth noting that depression is one of the most frequently diagnosed psychiatric disorders in people with learning disabilities (Benson, 1985), and this is especially so for those with Down syndrome (Burt et al., 1992; Collacott et al., 1992; Myers and Pueschel, 1995; Szymanski, 1988). Weight loss is a common symptom of depression, but people with learning disabilities may also atypically present with an increased appetite, and therefore significant weight gain (RCN, 2010). As a learning disability nurse you should be acutely aware of other signs or symptoms, such as social withdrawal, because they could well be indicative of a depression. Also important is to directly look for or indirectly seek carers' reports about changes in other aspects of someone's behaviour. For example, behavioural changes to look out for include changes in personal hygiene and appearance; of particular note is diurnal mood variation, where the mood is worse on waking but improves as the day proceeds. Again, all of these can be indicative of a depression.

Bipolar disorder

Bipolar disorder was known in the past as manic-depressive psychosis, and it is a condition that is characterised principally by its affect on mood and which in classical presentation swings from the extreme of mania to that of depression. Bipolar disorder is actually relatively common, with

John is in his late 30s, and until fairly recently had a good appetite and was described by support staff as being very happy and content. He is known to his local community team for people with learning disabilities (CTPLD), because a number of years ago he was diagnosed by his general practitioner with depression following the traumatic death of his father from a cerebral vascular accident (stroke). John lives in supported living, and since the recent closure of his day service that he had been attending for many years, it has been noticed that he has become somewhat withdrawn. John now works for two days a week at a local Mencap charity shop. He has a very close relationship with his brother, who calls round every week to take John out to a local pub on a Wednesday evening, where they are both members of a local darts team. He receives little help where he lives, with only a support worker calling in once a day, twice a week, in the mornings, just to make sure he is up, washed, and ready to go to work part-time in a charity shop, where he works from 9:30 a.m. until 3:30 p.m. John's brother has noticed that he havs recently lost a lot of weight, and reports *'that his clothes just hang off him'*. John's brother has called the charity shop to see how John is getting on there, and they say that he seems very quiet and that almost as soon as he arrives he spends most of the day asking if it is time to go home. John's brother has also left a letter for the support worker asking her to phone him because he is a little worried about his brother. The support worker says she does not know John very well, because she has only been supporting him for a few weeks, but that she has noticed when she calls round at 8:00 a.m. John is nearly always asleep; he is very difficult to rouse, saying that he has been awake since very early and he is now tired. He often says he doesn't want breakfast because he feels sick. John's brother decides to ask John if he thinks he should go to the doctor to check that all is well. Initially, John said no, because he was frightened of his doctor. This was surprising to John's brother, who knows that John's GP is very supportive of John; eventually he agrees.

Learning Activity 5.1

John and his brother visit the GP. The GP diagnoses depression. He prescribes Citalopram (Cipramil) 20 mg in the morning, and suggests that the CTLD might be able to offer John some help, as they did before, including looking for more things to do during the week, and he subsequently makes a referral. The GP has asked John's brother to come along with John in three weeks' time just to see how things are, and in the meantime makes a referral to your CTLD. You are asked to visit John at home where his brother will be present.

What kinds of things are you, as a community learning disability nurse, able to offer John?

John and his brother tell you that he has been on the tablets for a week now and that he does not feel better. What explanation might you offer him?

John says that he has real problems with a dry mouth, and that he feels very sleepy all of the time. What explanation and advice might you offer him?

How do you think the GP made his diagnosis? What things would he have been looking for? Would he have used any tools to help him in his assessment? Why has he prescribed this particular type of medicine?

something like one person in 100 in the general population being diagnosed with this condition. It can occur at any age, though it tends to develop more commonly between 18 and 24 years of age, and rarely after the age of 40, and it affects men and women equally. There are different types of bipolar disorder (see Table 5.1).

The pattern of mood swings in bipolar disorder is known to vary widely between people. For example, some will only have only a few bipolar episodes in their lifetimes, and will be stable in between, whereas others may experience many episodes. During an episode, depression is typically experienced where the person feels very low and lethargic, and then mania where they will feel very high and overactive. This may manifest in a lesser nature and is then referred to as hypomania. The symptoms of bipolar disorder will, therefore, depend on the presenting mood being experienced. And, unlike normal mood swings, which we all may experience at some time in our lives—for example, elation at winning a competition or great sadness at losing a family pet—the mood swings in bipolar disorder are extreme, and some episodes of disorder may last for many weeks or even months. Some people may report that they do not experience a 'normal' mood very often, and that the changes in their moods may not be associated with any particular life event or experience that may account for such a mood swing. During the manic phase of this disorder, symptoms commonly reported include elevated mood, delusions (characteristically some of these can be grandiose), being overly talkative (pressure of speech), ideas that seem to jump (flight of ideas), the use of rhyming language (clang association), and possibly overactive, and at times uninhibited, behaviour.

Table 5.1 Typology of bipoltar disorders

Bipolar I
Here there has been at least one 'high' or manic episode lasting longer than one week. Some people with bipolar I will have only manic episodes—most will also have periods of depression. Untreated, manic episodes generally last between three and six months. Depressive episodes last longer: 6 to 12 months without treatment.
Bipolar II
Here there has been more than one episode of severe depression, but only mild manic episodes. These are called 'hypomania'.
Rapid cycling
This is characterised by more than four mood swings in a 12-month period. This affects around 1 in 10 people with bipolar disorder, happens with both types I and II, and is more common in people with learning disabilities.
Cyclothymia
Here, mood swings are not as severe as those in full bipolar disorder but can last longer and develop into full bipolar disorder.

Source: Royal College of Psychiatrists, 2014. Available at http://www.rcpsych.ac.uk/healthadvice/problemsdisorders/bipolardisorder.aspx.

This type of disorder is estimated to occur more frequently in people with learning disabilities than in the general population. A tendency to cyclical changes in behaviour has been observed in ~4% of people with learning disabilities (Deb and Hunter, 1991). It is also thought that the gender ratio of bipolar disorder is similar in people with learning disabilities as that observed in the general population. Typically, changes in levels of activity, appetite, and sleep can be observed in people with learning disabilities, but grandiose delusions, which can often be characteristic of mania, are said to be less capacious in people with learning disabilities. It is also suggested that 'rapid cycling' bipolar disorder is more common in people with learning disabilities (moving from depression to mania and vice versa), and that this is associated with brain injury and abnormal electroencephalogram (EEG) readings (RCN, 2010).

Anxiety

This disorder is characterised by an at time almost unbearable emotional state that combines fear, a sense of impending doom, and a range of accompanying physical symptoms such as palpitations, tachycardia, sweating, dizziness, derealisation, dyspnoea, and generalised discomfort. It should be noted that anxiety is a normal phenomenon often experienced as a response to a range of external stressors in most, if not all, people. However, some people will experience this without an external stressor being present, and when this happens, and it becomes debilitating, it is known as a disorder. It can be experienced as part of a phobic disorder such as agoraphobia or depression, or as a generalised anxiety disorder (GAD).

There is considerable variation in the reported prevalence rates of anxiety disorders, although some claim that the rate is higher in the population of people with learning disabilities when compared with the general population. A recent study reported a rate of 3.8% (Cooper et al., 2007), although Raghavan (1998) has in the past suggested that it is poorly researched. It is also suggested that anxiety disorders manifest themselves equally in males and females with learning disabilities as compared with the general population, where incidence is said to be higher in women (RCN, 2010).

It is suggested that the presentation of anxiety disorders might differ within the population of people with learning disabilities from that of the general population (RCN, 2010). Some people with learning disabilities are unable to describe their internal thinking as possible symptoms of anything other than some kind of physical discomfort, and this may result in them describing experiences of mental distress as manifestations of physical illness. So, for example, an acute anxiety attack may be reported as a stomachache or as a headache or as feeling sick. So, as is the case with depression in people with learning disabilities, where no accurate self-report is likely to be forthcoming, the learning disability nurse must directly, or indirectly through carers or supporters, seek evidence of behavioural signs of acute anxiety and/or sleep disturbance.

Suicide and deliberate self-harm (DSH)

Suicide refers to intentional self-inflicted death, and deliberate self-harm to nonfatal self-inflicted harm. Episodes of self-harm tend to be less severe and suicidal attempts less frequent in people with learning disabilities than is the case in the general population. Nevertheless, where any attempts are made at either suicide or DSH they should be treated seriously. In years gone by, such behaviour/s were frequently referred to as 'attention seeking'; this is an outdated response, and certainly lacks the compassion needed to try to understand people's distress, and what it might mean (Heslop and Macaulay, 2009). Learning disability nurses need to ensure that they, as well as others, treat people with dignity, respect, and compassion:

> **People who have self-harmed should be offered the same quality of care and range of treatments as any other patient.... Staff should not behave in a punitive, threatening, dismissive or judgmental manner towards people who self-harm**
>
> *(Royal College of Psychiatrists' Centre for Quality Improvement, 2006, p. 7)*

Some forms of DSH can be very distressing not only for the person with a learning disability but also for those caring or supporting the person, and the learning disability nurse needs to be aware of this. Suicides are said to occur rarely in the population of people with learning disabilities, but we need to be mindful that this may be in part be accounted for as an artefact of lack of or under-reporting (Priest and Gibbs, 2004). All suicidal threats or attempts must be taken very seriously, regardless of the level of sophistication in constructing and/or executing them.

Schizophrenia

Schizophrenia is a serious mental illness that affects thinking, emotion, and behaviour, and it is the most common form of psychosis. It is estimated that approximately 1 in 100 people in the general population will develop schizophrenia. It most commonly commences between the ages of 15 and 35 years, but it is also known to manifest in young children. Generally the course of this illness can last for a long period of time, and it is widely described as incapacitating. The prevalence of schizophrenia in the population of people with learning disabilities is thought to be three times that of the wider population. For example, Deb et al. (2001) have suggested a prevalence of between 1.3% and 3.7%. Schizophrenia seemingly has an earlier onset of 22.5 years in people with learning disabilities as compared with 26.6 years in the general population (Meadows et al., 1991).

As is the case in other mental illnesses, in people with severe or profound learning disabilities with complex needs, diagnosing this condition can be difficult. Also, in the population of people with learning disabilities, some of the cardinal symptoms such as delusions are suggested to be more simplistic than those that might ordinarily be found in the wider population, perhaps because delusions in people with learning disabilities are a construct of their potentially limited life experiences. So, for example, a delusion found in someone from the general population believing that the police and secret service are regularly screening all of their telephone calls and mail might manifest itself in someone with learning disabilities as all people are talking about them. Notwithstanding, a note of caution, it is important to exclude such a belief from perceived reality, as it is known that people with learning disabilities are now the subject of both 'hate' and 'mate' crimes (Mencap, 2010).

It has also been suggested that hallucinations tend to be uncomplicated, even simple (RCN, 2010). It is also said that people with learning disabilities are less likely to have thought echo, second-person hallucinations, and running commentary; essentially this involves someone hearing their own thoughts, as opposed to them being externally located.

It should be remembered that any potential decline in social functioning or self-help skills may be masked by the support a person with learning disabilities receives from support workers or carers. Conversely, another form of masking can occur when poor social functioning or self-help skills are attributed to their learning disabilities, as opposed to being symptomatic of a major mental illness such as schizophrenia.

It should also be remembered that some behaviours seen in people on the spectrum of autistic conditions might be similar to those seen in schizophrenia. For example, neologisms (the making of new words) are also commonly seen in autism as well as bizarre motor mannerisms. It has been suggested that many people with learning disabilities do not demonstrate a sufficient range of symptoms to meet the standard criteria (ICD-10) for schizophrenia, so often a diagnosis of 'psychotic episode' is reported.

Obsessive-compulsive disorders

It is suggested that obsessive-compulsive disorder (OCD) is a relatively common form of anxiety that is characterised by obsessive thinking concomitant with compulsive behaviour. These obsessions can be very distressing, and those with this condition typically present with repetitive thoughts, which they may freely articulate as completely irrational but state that they cannot be disregarded. Compulsions are ritual actions that people feel compelled to repeat to relieve concomitant anxiety, or, alternatively, to prevent obsessive thoughts. It is as if the rituals have some magical property. For example, a very common compulsion is someone believing his or her hands are dirty, so he or she will wash them over and over again, often resulting in dry and cracked skin that may become sore and infected. This is a symbolic ritual that has significant meaning, and many instances can be found in literature and history: Pontius Pilate and Jesus of Nazareth and Jaggers the solicitor in *Great Expectations* by Charles Dickens. It has been calculated that 2% to 3% of people will experience some form of obsessive compulsive disorder at some time during their lives (Mental Health Foundation, 2007). The prevalence of OCD in people with learning disabilities is thought to be 3.5% (Vitello et al., 1989). It is difficult to give a clear diagnosis of OCD without being clear that a patient is able to articulate how they fight not to engage in compulsive behaviour. It is also difficult in some circumstances to differentiate between true compulsions, and some stereotypical movements, mannerisms, or even complex spasms. Finally, it is also the case that compulsions and stereotypic behaviour are not uncommon in people with autistic spectrum conditions, and this may make diagnosis difficult.

Eating disorders

Eating disorders are typically characterised by an abnormal attitude toward food that causes someone to significantly change his or her eating habits and behaviour. It is common for someone with an eating disorder to focus his or her thinking disproportionately on his or her weight and bodily appearance, and this can lead to making unhealthy choices about food, with subsequent damage to his or her health and well-being. Common eating disorders include anorexia nervosa and bulimia and binge eating. Anorexia nervosa and bulimia are said to be less common in people with learning disabilities than is the case in the general population, but hyperphagia (excessive hunger or increased appetite) and pica (persistent ingestion of non-nutritive substances) are more prevalent. However, in people with mild learning disabilities, prevalence rates of eating disorders may be similar to those seen in the wider population. Weight loss may not always be indicative of an eating disorder, and may be symptomatic of another mental health problem, such as depression, or a physical health problem. It is important to note that any diagnosis of bulimia or anorexia nervosa will need to be based upon an individual being able to report his or her thinking of distorted body image, which will require relatively well-developed and sophisticated verbal skills. Of particular relevance to eating disorders is overeating, and this is particularly associated with Prader–Willi syndrome.

Research Prader–Willi syndrome and identify how the constant desire to eat food, driven by a permanent feeling of hunger, which can lead to dangerous weight gains, can best be managed.

Personality disorder

Personality disorder is now, and within an historical context has always been seen as, a highly contentious diagnostic label. Currently, there are nine categories of personality disorder, which are arranged into three clusters. These have collectively replaced the now old and unused single term: psychopathic disorder. It has often been thought that using personality as a basis for diagnosis, where presenting symptoms fail to fit neatly into a recognised cluster for any other diagnosis to be made, is problematic. Notwithstanding, the diagnostic term of personality disorder is reserved for people who have difficulty in coping with life and whose behaviour persistently causes distress to themselves as well as others. Personality disorders tend to be characterised by long-lasting rigid patterns of thought and behaviour (Mental Health Foundation, 2007). The International Classification of Mental and Behavioural Disorders (ICD-10) (World Health Organisation, 1992) has defined a personality disorder as

a severe disturbance in the characterological condition and behavioural tendencies of the individual, usually involving several areas of the personality and nearly always associated with considerable personal and social disruption.

(World Health Organisation, 1992)

The behaviours of people with such a disorder usually seem to exaggerate part/s of their personality, and subsequently their behaviours seem increasingly at odds with what is generally regarded as normal behaviour. In the field of learning disability, it is suggested that some clinicians believe it is *'unfair or improper to use this diagnosis in this population'*, and this is especially so for those with severe learning disabilities (RCN, 2010). It is argued that personality disorders are more prevalent in people with learning disabilities than in the general population. However, caution must be exercised, and before a diagnosis of personality disorder is made a full assessment of an individual's circumstances, as well other known conditions such as autism, because these may offer alternative explanations for presenting personality characteristics has to be undertaken.

Alcohol and drug dependency

The level of drug and alcohol misuse evidenced from research would suggest that what little that is known is equivocal, with mostresearch suggesting that substance misuse, and problematic use, is not common among this group of people (Cooper et al., 2004). There is limited evidence that alcohol and cannabis tend to be the drugs of choice for people with learning disabilities (Burgard et al., 2000). A factor accounting for this kind of dependency being lower in this group of people, even amongst those who lead more independent lifestyles, is a lack of disposable income, along with a lack of social skills that is required for obtaining such substances. Perhaps unsurprisingly, it is suggested that drug and alcohol misuse will be less commonly found in environments where support staff are involved in an individual's life and where, for example, the use of money is under the supervision of carers. Manthorpe (1996) has pointed to the social significance of people with learning disabilities having such choices. She has argued that if normalisation and integration into community life are the true goals of deinstitutionalisation and empowerment, then social activities such as *'drinking in the pub'* should be accessible to people regardless of their disability. However, it must be remembered that people without learning disabilities, quite correctly, are living much more independent and self-directed lifestyles. With this comes the attendant risk/s of being exposed and becoming vulnerable to developing substance misuse (Huxley et al., 2007).

GENERAL OBSERVATIONS AND RECORDING: ASSESSMENT TOOLS FOR MENTAL HEALTH

There are numerous approaches and tools that can be used to assess mental health or mental ill health. Some of these approaches or tools have been designed specifically for people with learning disabilities, whereas the general population has designed others for use. And of the latter, some of these are less helpful for people with learning disabilities. No matter which approach or tool is used to identify a mental health disorder, a diagnosis can be made more easily if the assessment is supported with good observational skills to corroborate any diagnosis. These observations are of particular use in people with learning disabilities who may not report changes to their mental well-being, and this could be for a number of reasons. For example, they may not be able to recognise the significance of changes in their thoughts and feelings or their symptoms may be cloaked by the kinds of support they may be in receipt of. When this is the case then either through the direct and/or indirect input from the learning disability nurse they should seek to elicit observations from family and/or care staff. This makes it of critical importance for the learning disability nurse to make sure that he or she directs carers and support staff on what to record, as well as how to document their observations in a range of areas such as changes to mood or sleep disturbance/s or sudden and unexplained changes in weight or behaviour.

General observations and recording

As a precursor to undertaking a MSE or using a specific mental health assessment tool, general observations and recording can be used to establish the likelihood of an underlying mental health problem. This process of titration of approach and tools used is helpful and can prevent unnecessary distress or wasting valuable resources—of which time tends to be the most important. The following observations are useful.

Mood

Whereas mood is variable in all people, sustained changes to someone's 'normal' mood might be indicative of an underlying psychopathology. The learning disability nurse can help carers develop an easy-to–use record that captures an individual's mood over a pre-determined period of time. One way to do this might be to divide the day up into sections and use a series of visual keys to record mood, such as smiley or sad faces.

Sleep charts

If an individual presents with significant changes in his or her sleeping patterns, this may be symptomatic of a range of mental health disorders. For example, waking up early in the morning or even sleeping in very late may be signs of depression. Alternatively, lack of sleep may be a sign of hypomania. Once again, maintaining a record, where possible, can be helpful.

Weight charts

Given that weight gain, or loss, is classically associated with evidence about how people are looking after themselves, careful observations of weight could elicit useful information; lack of, or increased appetite, may be a sign of an underlying mental health problem. This is simply recorded by maintaining weight charts that can be completed on a weekly or monthly basis and making ongoing judgments.

ABC charts

The use of antecedent/behaviour/consequence (ABC) charts is well established in the field of learning disabilities (see Chapter 9). Their use is to provide a structured record of behaviours that might be described as distressed or challenging. They offer an opportunity to identify why particular behaviour/s might occur, by recording behaviour/s before, during, and after a particular behavioural incident. As well as potentially identifying triggers to, and functions of, that behaviour, they also enable us to hypothesise or predict how an incident/s might best be managed or resolved in the future.

MENTAL STATE EXAMINATION (MSE)

The Mental State Examination (MSE) is much more thorough than a general overview of how someone appears to be functioning. MSEs are an incredibly helpful and fundamental component of mental health assessment and one that learning disability nurses should be well versed in. The structure of an MSE should be similar to that used within the general population, but practitioners need to be cognisant of an individual's level of communication and cognitive capacity, and this may determine how questions are framed or reframed. It is important that a full history, including, where possible, that of family, is made before conducting the MSE proper; this can assist in making sense of presenting behaviour and comparing this with that of their 'normal' behaviour. When an MSE is undertaken by a learning disability nurse, the nurse will need to be informed by the following areas, which are of central importance to assessing someone's mental state. (Remember the acronym for a MSE: [ABC – EMST] A boy called early morning [a] silly teenager).

Appearance

Here, the learning disability nurse should focus on general health, manner, presenting persona, cleanliness, facial expression/s, or general demeanour. These may be helpful, but the observations need to be made within the context of someone having a learning disability. And, conversely, it must be remembered that the label of learning disability can sometimes result in 'masking' or overshadowing a diagnosis of mental illness, with 'learning disability' being the only thing a clinician sees or hears.

Behaviour

Here, an overall impression needs to be formed as to the parameters of the person with the learning disability and his or her presenting behaviour/s, and whether this can be described broadly as normal. For some people with learning disabilities, this may be more difficult to do than imagined. Some people with learning disabilities can present as childish, or be over-familiar, particularly to those perceived to be in authority. The issue here is one of making a judgment based on relative 'norms', so, for example, a distinction will need to be made between behaviour that seems depressed, whereas that person is normally very quiet and subdued. What is being looked for in this assessment are significant deviations of behaviour that materially and substantially move away from how the person normally behaves. Another important issue here is that of 'dual diagnosis', which refers to an individual with learning disabilities' concomitant mental health needs (Wallace, 2002). This group of people tends to be marginalised and is sometimes exposed to prejudices, abuse, and social isolation, compounding the integrity of the group's mental health. Finally, a note of caution, sharp distinctions need to be drawn between perceived behaviour and behaviour that might be explained by other, already known and diagnosed conditions such as autism. But this should not stop the clinician from looking for signs of restlessness or agitation or its opposite psycho-motor retardation, and also observe for level of eye contact, and level of engagement—cooperative or otherwise.

Cognition

Cognition refers to the mental actions or process of acquiring knowledge and understanding through thought, experience, and the senses. It includes perception, discernment, awareness, apprehension, learning, understanding, comprehension, enlightenment, insight, intelligence, reason, reasoning, thinking, and (conscious) thought. Clearly any assessment of cognitive processes will vary as a subsequence of someone's level of ability and his or her concentration, orientation, and memory may all be compromised. This component of the MSE may be particularly compromised where dementia is suspected, which may be the case particularly in people with Down syndrome. Any questions asked to assess cognition must be constructed in an accessible and meaningful way that is cognisant with someone's developmental level. So, questions need to be relevant and straightforward, such as 'What is your brother's name?', 'Where do you live?', and 'When do you go to the pub?' These questions can be used to expand your assessment and to come to a decision, if possible, about a person's cognitive state.

Experiences

Hallucinations occur when someone sees, hears, smells, tastes, or feels things that don't exist outside of their mind; they can involve any of the senses. Hallucinations tend to be fairly common in people with schizophrenia and are often experienced as hearing voices. They can be frightening, because they may be unexpected or unwanted. More frequently than not, an identifiable cause can be isolated. They can, for example, occur as a result of taking drugs or alcohol, or, as already stated, as part of a mental illness. Hallucinations can also occur as a result of extreme tiredness or recent bereavement. However, these are rare occurrences. It should be borne in mind that hallucinations can be very difficult to isolate in people with learning disabilities. One area of potential confusion may occur in olfactory, gustatory, or visual hallucinations, where their manifestation is commonly accounted for by the aura of a seizure (refer to Chapter 6).

Mood and affect

It is helpful to seek an individual's subjective experiences, or mood, before making a judgment about his or her observed manifestation of emotion/s, or affect. This should be surfaced through careful and sensitive questioning and prompts. Pictures can help people with learning disabilities locate their feelings, and images such as those from the *Books Beyond Words* series—for example, *Ron's Feeling Blue* (Hollins et al., 2011) or *Sonia's Feeling Sad* (Hollins et al., 2011)—are useful in identifying the different emotions they might be experiencing. Some individuals may have problems in reporting their emotional state for a number of reasons (for example, difficulty in understanding emotions). In these instances, the learning disability nurses' observations will play a greater role in helping to diagnose a mood disorder. As before, in the general observations, seek input from person's carer if they have one, or alternatively family and/or friends.

Speech

This can be extremely helpful, but clearly only if the person is able to speak at a level of sophistication where a judgment can be made as to whether speech is disordered. Things to look for include rate, quantity, pressure (flight of ideas), poverty (an absence of ideas), and tone (expressiveness or otherwise); sometimes the use of neologisms, or clang association, is also observed.

Thought content

It is important that any individual's presentation is placed within the context of his or her normal range of functioning. That said, changes in thinking might be one of the strongest indications of a mental health problem. The range of thought disorders include *flight of ideas*, which refers to language that may be difficult to understand when it jumps from one seemingly unrelated idea to another; *circumstantiality*, which refers to language that may be difficult to understand or is long-winded and convoluted; *word salad*, which to words that are strung together, resulting in gibberish; *neologisms*, which means *new word*, and, whereas it is common in children, is considered indicative of brain damage or a thought disorder (such as schizophrenia) when present in adults; *thought insertion*, which is a delusional thought that things are being placed into a person's mind by someone or an external source, and is often a symptom of schizophrenia; and, finally, *Knight's move* thinking, which is a phenomenon that is similar to derailment of thought or loosening of associations, and is characterised by strange associations and directions between ideas—the name for this disorder derives from the move used by the knight in the game of chess. Given the complexity and sometimes subtle nature of thought disorder, it is important in people with learning disabilities to be sure that thinking is really disordered and not merely an artefact of their development level. It would be relatively easy to interpret someone's thought content as delusional if he or she is not able to articulate a rational explanation for something he or she may say.

SPECIFIC MENTAL HEALTH ASSESSMENT TOOLS

For some people with learning disabilities, using standard mental health assessment tools may not be appropriate. Some instruments have been designed specifically for people with learning disabilities. The person who is being assessed will require adequate preparation, and the information and support will be necessary for any additional investigations that may be required. In the following, three learning disability–specific and three standard assessment tools for assessing mental health are provided; in the resources section others are given.

Assessment of dual diagnosis (ADD)

This assessment tool has been the subject of preliminary evaluation of inter-rater, as well as test-re-test, reliability. The authors found that the tool had high stability across raters and over time. In addition, the good internal consistency provides information on diagnosis, developing treatment plans, and evaluating outcomes (Matson and Bamburg, 1998).

Learning Disability version of the Cardinal Needs Schedule (LDCNS)

The LDCNS is based on the systematic assessment of needs using the Cardinal Needs Schedule (CNS) (Marshall et al., 1995). This provides a model of needs assessment that includes assessment of functioning of the individual's symptoms, behaviour problems, and personal and social skills in a number of areas of functioning, determining whether problems exist in any of these areas of functioning, applying a set of criteria to establish the appropriateness of addressing an identified problem, and, finally, determining the need for appropriate intervention in the areas of functioning where problems have been identified (Raghavan et al., 2004).

Psychiatric Assessment Schedules for Adults with Developmental Disabilities (PAS-ADD)

This is the generic name for a series of mental health assessment tools originally developed for people with learning disabilities. Most recently, this system has incorporated children and adolescents (including those with and without intellectual disability), making child mental health assessments more reliable and valid throughout generic children's services. Whereas the PAS-ADD system maximises the contribution of the individual, and, where possible, the individual's family carers, frontline staff, and a range of professionals, its clinical emphasis provides a structured frameworks for assessment. PAS-ADD is presented in different formats; there is a semi-structured interview for professional staff that assesses mental state and a checklist version for carers and support staff of potential indicators of mental health problems (Moss, 2002).

The Hamilton Rating Scale for Depression (HRSD)

This is a multiple-item questionnaire and is used to assess for depression and as a guide to evaluate recovery. The questionnaire is designed specifically for adults and is used to rate severity of depression by exploring mood, feelings of guilt, suicide ideation, insomnia, agitation or retardation, anxiety, weight loss, and somatic symptoms. The questionnaire is scored on each item, and the total score is then compared. It takes approximately 20 minutes to complete. A score of 0–7 is considered to in the normal range of mood, whereas scores of 20 or higher indicate moderate, severe, or very severe depression (Maier et al., 1988)

Beck Anxiety Inventory (BAI)

The Beck Anxiety Inventory (BAI) comprises 21 questions about how an individual has been feeling in the last week, as expressed symptomatically of anxiety, and includes numbness and tingling, sweating not due to heat, and fear of the worst thing happening. It has been designed for use in adults within the age range of 17–80. Each question has the same set of four possible answer choices, which are answered by making a mark with a cross with the answer most accurately describing how the respondent has felt. These include not at all (0 points), mildly (1 point), moderately (2 points), and severely (3 points). The BAI has a maximum score of 63; 0–7 is indicative of minimal level of anxiety, 8–15 of mild anxiety, 16–25 of moderate anxiety, and 26–63 of severe anxiety (Beck et al., 1988).

Schedule for Affective Disorders and Schizophrenia (SADS)

The SADS was developed in the 1970s and provides health practitioners with a clinical schedule to assist them in the diagnosis, as well as providing descriptive evaluations, of possible affective disorder or schizophrenia. The schedule enables the construction of a detailed description of the features of the current episode of illness when the episode is at its most severe, along with a description of the major features during the week prior to an evaluation, a detailed description of past psychopathology and level of functioning, and, finally, a series of questions and criteria that enable a diagnosis to be made (Endicott and Spitzer, 1978).

TREATMENTS

Broadly speaking, there are a wide range of treatments available to treat and ameliorate mental ill health, and these typically include medication, talking therapies, and physical treatments such as electroconvulsive therapy, as well as personal management strategies for mental ill health and the maintenance of well-being.

Medication

Antipsychotics

Antipsychotics are used to treat symptoms of acute psychosis or to prevent further episodes. Antipsychotics are generally divided into two classes: the older 'typical' agents, the neuroleptics, and the newer 'atypical' agents, these have been developed since the 1990s.

Typical agents include Chlorpromazine (Largactil), usual dosage 75–300 mg in a daily divided dose; haloperidol (Haldol), usual dosage 3–15 mg in a daily divided dose; and trifluoperazine (Stelazine), usual dosage 5-20 mg in a daily divided dose. Problems with the typical agents include extensive side effects that include stiffness and shakiness (extrapyramidal side effects), often called pseudo-Parkinson's disease, sluggish and slow thinking, restlessness (akathisia), lowering of blood pressure (postural hypotension), and sexual dysfunction. The pseudo-Parkinson's condition can be controlled with anticholinergic drugs—orphenadrine (Disipal) and procyclidine (Kemadrin) are the two most commonly used anticholinergics. There is a longer-term problem, tardive dyskinesia (TD), that is all too often found. TD is difficult to treat, and, more often, an incurable form of dyskinesia, where involuntary, repetitive body movements of the mouth, tongue, and jaw occurs. This is thought to affect about 1 in 20 people every year who are taking such medicines.

Atypicals are usually described as having less-distressing side effects. Examples include amisulpride (Solian), usual dosage 50–800 mg in a daily divided dose; aripiprazole (Abilify), usual dosage 10–30 mg in a daily divided dose, and clozapine (Clozaril), usual dosage 200–450 mg in a daily divided dose. Side effects of atypical antipsychotics are not homogenous but can include weight gain, diabetes mellitus, hyperlipidemia, myocarditis, sexual dysfunction, extrapyramidal side effects, and cataract (Üçok and Wolfgang, 2008).

Depot injections

This medication is normally administered into the upper outer aspect of the buttock or lateral mid aspect of the thigh, by an intramuscular injection, where a delivered 'reservoir' of medicine slowly releases itself into the bloodstream. This is useful for patients who may not remember to take their medicine. The injection is given every one to four weeks, depending on the dose required. The medication is slowly released into the body over a number of weeks. The benefits and side effects of the depot injection are much the same as is if it were taken orally. Examples include Modecate (fluphenazine decanoate), up to 100 mg by one injection every two to five weeks, according to response and severity of condition; Depixol (flupenthixol decanoate), up to 400 mg by one injection every two to four weeks, according to response and severity of condition; and Clopixol (zuclopenthixol decanoate), up to 600 mg by one injection every 1 to 4 weeks.

Antidepressants

Antidepressants are very commonly prescribed for depression. Generally, modern management of depression indicates that antidepressants are not recommended for the initial treatment of mild depression; it is the case that risks may outweigh the benefits. Current practice is based upon using self-guided cognitive behaviour therapy (CBT), or short courses of cognitive therapy with a therapist. Whereas for severe depression, a combination of antidepressants along with individual CBT should be considered, this combination is thought to be more cost effective than either treatment approach on its own.

Selective serotonin reuptake inhibitors (SSRIs)

Fluoxetine (Prozac), usual dosage 20 mg per day, usually in the morning; citalopram (Cipramil), usual dosage 20 mg per day, usually in the morning; paroxetine (Seroxat), usual dosage initially 20 mg, then up to 60 mg per day, usually in the morning; and sertraline (Lustral), usual dosage initially 25 mg per day, after one week increase to 50 mg every morning or evening.

Serotonin-adrenaline reuptake inhibitors (SNRIs)

Duloxetine (Cymbalta and Yentreve), usual dosage 60 mg once a day; venlafaxine (Efexor), usual dosage initially 37.5 mg orally twice a day, or 25 mg orally three times a day.

Tricyclic antidepressants (TCAs)

Amitriptyline (Tryptizol), usual dosage 50–75 mg per day, either in divided doses or as a single nighttime dose increasing to 150–200 mg per day; clomipramine (Anafranil), usual dosage 25 mg orally once per day at bedtime, may be increased to 100 mg per day during the first two weeks; and imipramine (Tofranil), an initial dose of 100 mg per day given in three to four divided doses, this dose may be gradually increased to 300 mg per day.

Monoamine oxidase inhibitors (MAOIs)

Moclobemide (Manerix), initial dose is 300 mg daily, this can be increased to 600 mg daily, usually administered in two to three divided doses, tablets should be taken immediately after a meal; and phenelzine (Nardil), usual dosage 15 mg orally three times daily, dosage should be increased to at least 60 mg daily, and in some cases 90 mg daily.

Learning Activity 5.4

Patients on monoamine oxidase inhibitors (MAOIs) are routinely told to avoid a range of foods and medications during phenelzine therapy, and for two weeks after discontinuing use. Why is this?

Sleeping and anxiety medication

Minor tranquillisers and hypnotics, primarily benzodiazepines, are used to treat anxiety and sleep problems. They are usually prescribed only on a short-term basis because of their addictive nature. These include benzodiazepines such as diazepam (Rimapam), withj a usual dosage 2 mg three times daily, which can be increased, if necessary, to 15–30 mg daily in divided doses, and hypnotics. Other examples include nitrazepam (Mogadon), usual dosage 5 mg at night; and zopiclone (Imovane), usual dosage 3.75 mg, which may be increased to 7.5 mg.

Mood stabilisers

Mood-stabilising medications are used to treat bipolar disorder. They are usually taken long term, even when a person is not experiencing an episode of mania, hypomania, or depression. The oldest mood stabiliser is lithium; anticonvulsant drugs developed to treat epilepsy are now often used as mood stabilisers. Additionally, some antipsychotic medications also appear to be effective as mood stabilisers. Examples of medicines used as mood stabilisers include lithium (Lithane), usual dosage 1800 mg per day in divided doses; sodium valproate (Epilim), usual dosage 400–600 mg per day in daily divided doses; carbamazapine (Tegretol), usual dosage 200 mg orally in tablet or capsule form every 12 hours, a maintenance dose of up to 1200 mg per day in three or four divided doses may be necessary; and lamotrigine (Lamictal), where dosage is introduced based on concurrent medication, which can be very complicated. It is advisable to refer to the latest edition of the British National Formulary.

Talking therapies

Talking therapies, also known as psychological therapies, are frequently used to help people better understand their thoughts and feelings, and to assist them in making connections to their behaviours, moods, and psychological well-being. Talking therapies are best understood when organised under the general heading of psychotherapy and include

- Supportive therapies, such as occupational and music therapy
- Re-educative therapies, such as behaviour therapy or cognitive behaviour therapy (CBT)
- Reconstructive therapies, such as psychoanalysis with the Jungian or Kleinian approaches

Talking therapies can help people find important ways to change their lives by encouraging them to act and think in a more positive way. It should be noted that such therapies are not always suitable for all people with learning disabilities, and as a general rule such therapies are more suited to those with mild learning disabilities.

Electroconvulsive therapy (ECT)

The National Institute for Health and Clinical Excellence recommends that electroconvulsive therapy (ECT) should be used only for the treatment of severe depressive illness, or a prolonged or severe episode of mania or catatonia, to gain fast and short-term improvement of severe symptoms. As with any significant treatment in medicine or surgery, all potential patients must give their informed consent, or permission, for the ECT to be done. There is a general consensus that ECT should be used only after all other treatment options have failed, or when the situation is thought to be life threatening (refer to the Resources section for further information).

Other Approaches

Other important factors to consider in the overall management of mental ill health, and for the maintenance of good mental health and well-being, include

- *Support from family and friends*—To be connected with others is really important to one's mental health and well-being. Helping people stay in touch with family and friends is something that the learning disability nurse can do for a patient

- *Undertaking something worthwhile to do during the day*—Since the demise of most day services in England, many people with learning disabilities have little meaningful daytime occupation. This means it is really important to assist people in accessing, for example, part-time work, voluntary work, interest groups, reading groups at libraries, and walking groups.

- *Peer support*—When our mental health is compromised, it is sometimes helpful to be able to speak with others who have had similar experiences. This can be achieved through support groups. Learning disability nurses must be cognisant of all resources in their locality that they can help people with learning disabilities access. Community learning disability nurses might consider setting up small groups for people if such groups do not already exist.

- *Alternative therapies*—Consider, for example, relaxation exercises, reflexology, massage, meditation, and yoga. These all have the potential to bring about a sense of well-being and relaxation.

- *Hobbies*—Having a hobby is a good way to maintain an interest in something that may have nothing to do with jobs or our normal routines; we undertake hobbies solely because we enjoy the activity. It is also a way of meeting like-minded people. Hobbies include car booting, model building, needlework, and knitting. Most people enjoy being able to spend time on a favourite hobby, and people with learning disabilities are no different.

- *Physical exercise*—Maintaining a good level of physical activity is known to increase a sense of well-being, and this is something to be particularly aware of as people with learning disabilities can lead very sedentary lives.

- *Spirituality and religion*—This has the potential to bring peace and a sense of order and meaning to people's lives. It is really important that learning disability nurses ensure that attention is given to the religious and spiritual needs of all those with whom they work.

Finally, a straightforward way of explaining how to maintain good mental health to people with learning disabilities is to use the example five a day (see Figure 5.1). **Walk.** Get outside and get

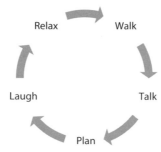

Figure 5.1 The five-a-day way to good mental health.

the sun on your face—walking and getting out in the sunlight, even if it's cloudy, is good for you. **Talk.** Spend time talking and listening to others. It's good to spend time making friends; it's good to say and hear kind things. **Plan.** Plan your day. It's good to have a structure to your day, so that you have some routine, and have things to look forward to. Make plans for the weekend, like meeting up with a friend or going to the park or for a swim—whatever it is you enjoy. **Laugh.** There's an old saying: *'Laughter is the best medicine'.* It's always good to have a laugh and it's even better if it's with other people or friends. Remember to have a sense of humour! **Relax.** Do things that help you to relax: listen to music, read a book, go for a walk, have a nice hot bath, or do yoga! Whatever works for you! The most important thing is to find the five a day that works for you and keep at it every day, if you can!

THE CARE PROGRAMME APPROACH

The Care Programme Approach (CPA) is addressed comprehensively in Chapter 7; therefore, its inclusion here is simply to place it into a context of supporting someone with learning disabilities with mental ill health needs. CPA is a particular way of assessing, planning, and reviewing someone's mental health care needs and represents a comprehensive, person-centred, systematic and integrated approach to multiagency care planning that simultaneously involves managing risk. It provides a way of supervising people known to mental health services, and who have been previously sectioned under the Mental Health Act. To receive CPA an individual must be assessed against a list of criteria, and the following is a list of the criteria that will be of relevance to someone with learning disabilities and a severe mental illness who has been discharged into the community

- Severe mental disorder (including personality disorder) with a high degree of clinical complexity
- Current or potential risk(s) of suicide, self-harm, harm to others, relapse history requiring urgent response, disinhibition, physical/emotional abuse, cognitive impairment, child protection issues
- Current or significant history of severe distress/instability or disengagement
- Presence of learning disabilities
- Current/recent detention under the Mental Health Act
- Multiple service provision from different agencies including criminal justice

THE MENTAL HEALTH ACT 1983

Background

The Mental Health Act seeks, where necessary, to compel people with mental disorder to be assessed and treated for that disorder. The Mental Health Act of 1983 was amended in 2007. The amendments to the Act were intended to limit the impact of mental disorder on the individual and society, including safeguards against the abuse of process, and access to independent review. The nature and scope of these amendments are comprehensively dealt with in Chapter 7. It should also be noted that the act's principle scope is limited to England and Wales; Scotland, Northern Ireland and the Republic of Ireland all have different, but nonetheless similar, mental health legislation.

Involuntary admission for assessment

Involuntary admission to hospital must take place only if a person is suffering from a mental disorder within the meaning of the Mental Health Act (MHA), and where detention in a hospital is deemed necessary for a person's health and safety or the protection of others. Within the Act, mental disorder refers to any disorder or disability of the mind. Of particular importance is that a person with learning disabilities cannot be considered to be suffering from a mental disorder, within the meaning of the Act, unless his or her disability is associated with abnormally aggressive or seriously irresponsible conduct. There are 10 parts to the Act. In the 10th part there are supplemental provisions that include its application to Scotland, Northern Ireland, and the Isles of Scilly; there are also six schedules. For the purposes of this chapter, parts II and iii are possibly the most significant in relation to mental ill health in people with learning disabilities, but other parts are also referred to.

Part II of the Mental Health Act

Part II of the MHA makes civil provision as well as arrangements for compulsory admission to hospital and guardianship. The vast majority of people who are admitted involuntarily to hospital for assessment or treatment of mental disorders are admitted under Part II of the Act.

Part III of the Mental Health Act

Part III of the Act makes provision and arrangements for patients who are concerned with criminal proceedings, or under sentence to be detained to hospital for assessment or treatment of a mental disorder.

Assessment or treatment

Sometimes it can be unclear whether a patient who needs to be detained should be admitted for assessment or treatment. People with learning disabilities who are admitted for assessment will often need to receive treatment, and the same is true of patients who are admitted for treatment; they will need to be assessed as part of the treatment process.

Admission for assessment MHA 1983

The primary reason for assessment for most people with learning disabilities will be to obtain an understanding of problematic or offending behaviour, as well as any relationship between their learning disabilities and their behaviour that might result in harm to themselves or harm to others.

Indications for assessment

- The person with learning disabilities has never previously been admitted to hospital or has not been in regular contact with specialist services.

- The diagnosis or cause of the patient's problems is unclear. Previously established treatment or interventions may need to be re-formulated and this may include an assessment of need for informal treatment.

- The presenting needs or condition are judged to have changed since an earlier involuntary admission.

Part II: Compulsory admission to hospital and guardianship

Section 2: Admission for assessment. This is for up to 28 days and requires evidence of mental disorder, and that this cannot be achieved without detention.

Section 4: Admission for assessment in an emergency. This is for up to 72 hours and is used out of urgent necessity, and with a view to admission for assessment under Section 2.

Section 5: (2) This is commonly referred to as a doctor's holding power, which is for up to 72 hours. The patient should already be receiving treatment for a mental disorder as inpatient, and there should be a view to admission for assessment under Section 2.

Section 5: (4) This is commonly referred to as a nurse's holding power; this is for a period of up to six hours. There must be evidence of immediate risk of harm. The use of this section requires a need to secure attendance of a responsible approved clinician as soon as possible.

Part X: Miscellaneous and supplementary

Section 135: This permits a warrant for the police to search for, and remove, a patient to place of safety for a mental health assessment; this is for a period of up to 72 hours. The use of this section requires evidence to suggest mental disorder, as well as a need for a mental health assessment.

Section 136: This provides for police power to remove a person from a public place to a place of safety for a mental health assessment; this is for a period of up to 72 hours. The use of this section requires evidence to suggest a mental disorder, as well as a need for a mental health assessment.

Part III: Patients concerned in criminal proceedings or under sentence

Section 35: Remand to hospital for report on an accused's mental condition. This is for up to three periods of 28 days, but this must not to exceed 12 weeks in total. It requires evidence to suggest that an accused person, who is to be remanded awaiting trial or sentence, is suffering from a mental disorder and requires assessment in hospital.

Admission for treatment under MHA 1983

Treatment for many people with learning disabilities who are involuntarily admitted to a hospital will be focused on addressing the 'abnormally aggressive' and 'seriously irresponsible conduct' that resulted in their detention. In the context of forensic nursing treatment, treatment measures may include

- Behavioural interventions, such as the development or implementation of effective behavioural support and management plans that can be generalised to other settings or manage risk

- Offence-specific treatment, such as sex offender treatment programmes, treatment of arson behaviour, or treatment of violent offending

- Related treatment, such as anger management, anxiety management, problem solving, and cognitive skills programmes

- Interventions to improve day-to-day functioning, such as social skills programmes, activities for daily living skills programmes, and interpersonal skills training.

Some people who are admitted involuntarily for treatment will also require specific treatments for mental illnesses, such as schizophrenia or a bipolar disorder.

Part II: Compulsory admission to hospital and guardianship

Section 3: Admission for treatment. This is for periods of six months and then renewable annually. This requires evidence of suffering from a mental disorder that needs treatment in hospital, and cannot be treated without detention.

Part III: Patients concerned in criminal proceedings or under sentence

Section 36: Remand of accused person to hospital for treatment. This is for up to three periods of 28 days, not exceeding 12 weeks in total. This requires evidence that the accused person who is to be remanded awaiting trial or sentence is suffering from mental disorder that requires treatment in hospital.

Section 37: This can be with or without a restriction order (Section 41). It is also known as a hospital order; this gives courts the power to order hospital admission for treatment. This may include Ministry of Justice restrictions in discharge (Section 41). This is for two periods of six months and then renewable annually. This is used where a conviction for an imprisonment offence requires treatment in a hospital for mental disorder; the hospital order replaces the sentence.

Section 38: This is known as an interim hospital order. This is for periods of 28 days; it is renewable by the court for a total period not exceeding one year. This is used where a conviction for an imprisonment offence requires a period of treatment in a hospital to allow assessment regarding the appropriateness of Section 37.

Section 47 with or without a restriction order (S.49): This section covers the transfer to a hospital of a person serving a prison sentence. This may include Ministry of Justice restrictions in discharge (Section 49) until the restriction order expires. This is used when the person serving a sentence of imprisonment requires treatment for a mental disorder in hospital.

Appropriate treatment test

Finally, the availability of appropriate treatment is a requirement of detention in a hospital for treatment of a mental disorder. Treatment must be appropriate, taking into account the nature and degree of the person's mental disorder and all the other circumstances of the person's case. The MHA revised code of practice (2008) now provides extensive guidance regarding this appropriate treatment test.

Assessment of mental capacity: IMCAs and DOLS

Under the Mental Capacity Act 2005, people are presumed to be able to make their own decisions *'unless all practical steps to help him (or her) to make a decision have been taken without success'*. Thus, all people, and that includes those with learning disabilities, are presumed to be able to make their own decisions. Decisions can only be made for others if all practical steps to help them to make a decision have been taken and without success. It must be remembered that incapacity is not based on the ability to make wise or sensible decisions; if that were the case, most of us would be deemed to be lacking capacity (well certainly I would). To assess for incapacity, you will need to consider whether the person you're looking after is able to understand the particular issue that he or she is making a decision about. Due consideration needs to be given to whether there is

- An impairment or disturbance in the functioning of the mind or brain
- An inability to make decisions

A person is only deemed unable to make a decision if he or she cannot

- Understand the information relevant to the decision
- Retain that information
- Use or weigh that information as part of the process of making the decision
- Communicate the decision

If an individual is unable to make a decision, and therefore give his or her consent, and in this context we are looking at decisions around treatment for mental health, then what is known as a 'best interests' decision will need to be made. When this is the case, all involved should be mindful that they should

- Not make assumptions on the basis of the person's age, appearance, condition or behaviour
- Ensure that they consider all the relevant circumstances
- Make sure that they have assessed and considered whether or when the person has capacity to make the decision
- Ensure that the person's participation is supported in any acts or decisions made for him or her
- Ensure that they do not make a decision about life-sustaining treatment
- Make sure that they considered the person's expressed wishes and feelings, beliefs, and values
- Take care to account for the views of others with an interest in the person's welfare, his or her carers, and those appointed to act on the person's behalf

Most organisations provide policies governing how this should be managed. You are strongly advised to refer, and adhere, to all requirements.

Also under the Mental Capacity Act 2005 a new service was created: the Independent Mental Capacity Advocate (IMCA) service. The purpose of this service was to help vulnerable people who lack capacity and have no one to appropriately consult regarding certain important decisions that will affect these people. Such decisions include medical treatment where a local authority is proposing to arrange accommodation for someone for longer than eight weeks, or where the NHS is proposing to arrange accommodation for someone for longer than 28 days. More recently, local authorities and the NHS are now required to instruct an IMCA in certain cases that involve care reviews and adult protection cases. The NHS and local authorities have a duty to consult an IMCA about decisions that involve people who have no family or friends, or when it is not appropriate to consult these parties. For example, it could be that a family member or friend is unwilling to be consulted about a best interests decision. It is the case that family members or friends may be unwell or elderly and therefore not able to contribute to any consultation. Also, there may be other reasons that make it impractical to consult with the family member or friend; for example, he or she lives some distance away, or sometimes a family member may refuse to be consulted. Additionally there may be issues of known abuse by the family member or friend. There are a number of benefits of the IMCA Service for someone who lacks capacity, including having an independent person to review significant decisions being proposed, and having someone who is articulate and knowledgeable about legislation and an individual's rights, as well as health and social care systems. It is also important to have someone skilled in supporting people who may have difficulties in communicating their views. Having an independent person who can support someone and represent them when serious decisions are being made, and when they have nobody else who can be consulted, is critical. There are also enormous benefits for statutory bodies making or proposing such life-changing decisions. This can be particularly so for practitioners working in such organisations and agencies who may find that IMCAs may assist them in making decisions. Complex decisions can be made with somewhat more confidence, and in many cases more quickly, because of the involvement of an IMCA.

This leads to a consideration of deprivation of liberty, an issue that has contemporaneously risen to the top off the learning disability agenda again. As from 2009, new procedural safeguards, known as 'Deprivation of Liberty Safeguards' (2005) (or DOLS) were introduced to protect individuals from unlawful deprivation of their liberty. These new procedures were introduced by the Mental Health Act 2007 as an amendment to the Mental Capacity Act 2005. They were developed as a long-needed response to what has become known as *'the Bournewood gap'*, an apparent 'gap' in the law that relates to deprivation of liberty that was identified in a case involving Bournewood Hospital, England.* This gap arose because it was found that restraining or restricting an individual's liberty was lawful under the Mental Capacity Act 2005. Whereas, depriving an individual of his or her liberty was not lawful under the Mental Capacity Act 2005. It is possible to justify restraint or restrictions on someone's liberty under the Mental Capacity Act 2005 provided that

- Reasonable steps are taken to establish that the individual lacks capacity in relation to the matter in question.
- It is reasonably believed that the individual does lack capacity in relation to the matter in question.
- It is in the best interests of that individual for the act to be done.
- It is reasonably believed that it is necessary to do the act to prevent harm to that individual.
- The act in question is a proportionate response to the likelihood of the individual suffering harm.
- The act in question is a proportionate response to the seriousness of that harm.

---

* This case concerned a young man who was taken to Bournewood hospital, and detained there. Originally, he had been admitted informally in his 'best interests'—solicitors were engaged to pursue a case of unlawful detention.

However, making a distinction between restraining, restricting, and depriving of liberty can be problematic. It should be remembered that it is possible to *'deprive someone of their liberty'* not only through physical confinement but also by levels of control that are applied to an individual's movements. Such deprivations of liberty are also possible by using other high levels of control over an individual, such as who can visit them, and controlling when they can undertake particular activities, the cumulative effect being that someone is being deprived of his or her liberty. By way of contrast, an individual who, for example, resides in a locked unit during the night for his or her own safety is unlikely to be thought of as being deprived of his or her liberty, because broader contextual issues need to be taken into any assessment. Therefore, concepts of restraint, restriction, and deprivation of liberty are probably best understood as existing on a 'spectrum of control', with deprivation of liberty involving a higher degree or intensity of control over an individual. Ultimately, the concept is one to be interpreted in view of the specific circumstances of that individual. That is why DOLS procedures were introduced: to 'safeguard' the liberty of the individuals by ensuring that rigorous and transparent procedures were followed prior to any deprivation of liberty. The DOLS procedure aims to ensure that those caring for, or involved with, individuals are able to engage with the decision-making process whenever questions about the liberty of an individual are being explored. The DOLS procedure also aims to ensure that such decision making is conducted carefully and is subject to independent scrutiny. The procedure designates two types of bodies—the managing authorities and supervisory bodies. The hospital or care home that is, or will become, responsible for an individual's care is referred to as the 'managing authority'. When the Primary Care Trusts (PCTs) ceased to exist in 2013, their supervisory body responsibilities under the Deprivation of Liberty Safeguards relating to hospitals passed to local authorities, so it is they who are the 'supervisory body'. It should be noted that the Regulations in England and Wales that govern the application and assessment procedure are different, so it is important that the correct regulations are followed.

CONCLUSION

In this chapter, it has been established that there is high prevalence of mental health problems in the population of people with learning disabilities when compared with the general population. It has been advocated that there is need to prepare learning disability nurses to promote good mental health and well-being or its maintenance in this group of people, whose mental health is particularly vulnerable. In this chapter, the nature and manifestations of good mental health, as well as manifestations of mental ill health, assessment tools used in nursing practice and how to conduct a mental state examination have all been outlined in detail. Additionally, a range of approaches to treatments has been outlined as well as the Care Programme Approach. This chapter has accounted for important aspects of relevant mental health legislation, assessment of mental capacity, Independent Mental Capacity Advocates (IMCAs), and Deprivation of Liberty Safeguards (DOLS).

ACKNOWLEDGEMENT

Grateful thanks to Briege Gates, Clinical Group Manager, Luton CAMHS, South Essex Partnership NHS Trust for the use of the five-a-day model for the maintenance of good mental health.

REFERENCES

An Bord Altranais 2005. *Requirements and Standards for Nurse Registration Education Programmes* (3rd ed.). Dublin: An Bord Altranis.

Beck, A.T., Epstein, N., Brown, G., and Steer, R.A. 1988. An inventory for measuring clinical anxiety: Psychometric properties. *Journal of Consulting and Clinical Psychology*, 56(6):893–897.

Benson, B. 1985. Behavioral disorders and mental retardation. *Applied Research in Mental Retardation*, 84:465–469.

Burgard, J.F., Donohue, B., Azrin, N., and Teichner, G. 2000. Prevalence and treatment of substance abuse in the mentally retarded population: An empirical review. *Journal of Psychoactive Drugs*, 32(3):293–298.

Burt, D.B., Loveland, K.A., and Lewis, K.R. 1992. Depression and the onset of dementia in adults with mental retardation. *American Journal on Mental Retardation*, 96:502–511.

Collacott, R.A., Cooper, S.A., and McGrother, C. 1992. Differential rates of psychiatric disorders in adults with Down syndrome compared with other mentally handicapped adults. *The British Journal of Psychiatry*, 161:671–674.

Cooper, S.A., Melville, C., and Morrison, J. 2004. People with intellectual disabilities. *British Medical Journal*, 329:414.

Cooper, S.A., Smiley, E., Morrison, J., Williamson, A., and Allan, L. 2007. Mental ill-health in adults with intellectual disabilities: Prevalence and associated factors. *The British Journal of Psychiatry*, 190:27–35.

Deb, S. and Hunter, D. 1991. Psychopathology of people with mental handicap and epilepsy: I Maladaptive behaviour. *British Journal of Psychiatry*, 159:822–834.

Deb, S., Matthews, T., Holt, G., and Bouras, N. 2001. *Practice Guidelines for the Assessment and Diagnosis of Mental Health Problems in Adults with Intellectual Disability.* Brighton: Pavilion Publishing.

Department of Health. 1999. *The National Service Framework (NSF) for Mental Health.* London. DH.

Department of Health. 2001. *Valuing People: A New Strategy for Learning Disability for the 21st Century.* London: DH

Department of Health. 2009. *Valuing People: Now.* London: The Stationery Office.

Department of Health. 2011. *No Health without Mental health.* UK: Department of Health.

Deprivation of liberty safeguards. 2005. Code of practice to supplement the main Mental Capacity Act 2005 code of practice. London: TSO.

Endicott, J. and Spitzer, R.L. 1978. A diagnostic interview: The schedule for affective disorders and schizophrenia. *Arch Gen Psychiatry*, 35(7):837–844.

Ferguson, D. 2009. Mental health and learning disability. In: Jukes, M. (Ed.), *Learning Disability Nursing Practice.* London: Quay Books, pp. 309–326.

Heslop, P. and Macaulay, F. 2009. *Hidden Pain? Self-injury and People with Learning Disabilities.* Bristol: Bristol Crisis Service for Women.

Hollins, S. and Kopper, L. 2011. *Sonia's Feeling Sad.* London: Books Beyond Words and Royal College of Psychiatrists.

Hollins, S., Banks, R., and Curran, J. 2011. *Ron's Feeling Blue.* London: Books Beyond Words and Royal College of Psychiatrists.

Huxley, A., Adam, Taggart, L., Baker, G., Castillo, L., and Barnes, D. (2007) Substance misuse amongst people with learning disabilities. *Learning Disability Today*, 7(3):34–38.

Huxley, A., Copello, A., and Day, E. 2005. Substance misuse and the need for integrated services. *Learning Disability Practice*, 8(6):14–17.

Katona, C. and Robertson, M. 2001. *Psychiatry at a Glance* (2nd ed.). Oxford: Blackwell Science.

Maier, W., Buller, R., Philipp, M., and Heuser, I. 1988. The Hamilton Anxiety Scale: Reliability, validity and sensitivity to change in anxiety and depressive disorders. *Journal of Affective Disorders*, 14(1):61–68.

Manthorpe, J. 1996 People with learning difficulties: Alcohol and ordinary lives. In: Harrison, L. (Ed.), *Alcohol Problems in the Community*. London: Routledge

Marshall, M., Hogg, L., Gath, D. 1995. The cardinal needs schedule—a modified version of the MRC needs for care assessment schedule. *Psychological Medicine*, 25:605–617.

Matson, J.L. and Bamburg, J.W. 1998. Reliability of the assessment of dual diagnosis (ADD). *Research in Developmental Disabilities*, 19(1):89–95.

Mencap 2010. *Don't Stand By: Ending Disability Hate Crime Together.* London: Mencap.

Mental Health Act 1983. London: HMSO.

Mental Capacity Act 2005. London: HMSO.

Mental Health Foundation. 2007. *The Fundamental Facts: The latest facts and figures on mental health.* London: The Mental Health Foundation.

Meadows, G., Turner, T., Campbell, L., Lewis, S., Roueley, M., and Murray, R. 1991. Assessing schizophrenia in adults with mental retardation: A comparative study. *British Journal of Psychiatry*, 158:103–105.

Moss, S. 2002. *The Mini PAS-ADD Interview Pack.* Brighton: Pavilion Publishing.

Myers, B.A. and Pueschel, S.M. 1995. Major depression in a small group of adults with Down syndrome. *Research in Developmental Disabilities*, 16(4):285–299.

Nursing and Midwifery Council. 2010. *Standards for Pre-Registration Nursing Education*, London: NMC.

Pueschel, S.M. 1991. Psychiatric disorder in person with Down syndrome. *J Nerv Ment Dis.*, 179:609–613.

Priest, H., and Gibbs, M. 2004. *Mental Health Care for People with Learning Disabilities.* Edinburgh: Churchill Livingstone.

Raghavan, R. 1998. Anxiety disorders in people with learning disabilities: Review of the Literature. *Journal of Learning Disabilities for Nursing Health and Social Care*, 2(1):3–9.

Raghavan, R., Marshall, M., Lockwood, L., and Duggan, L. 2004. Assessing the needs of people with learning disabilities and mental illness: Development of the learning disability version of the cardinal needs schedule. *Journal of Intellectual Disability Research*, 48:25–37.

Raghavan R. and Waseem F. 2007. Services for young people with learning disabilities and mental health needs from South Asian communities. *Advances in Mental Health and Learning Disabilities*, 1(3):27–31.

Royal College of Nursing. 2010. *Mental Health Nursing of Adults with Learning Disabilities*. London: Royal College of Nursing.

Royal College of Psychiatrists. 1996. *Meeting the Mental Health Needs of People with Learning Disability Part 1: Adults with Mild Learning Disability*. London: Royal College of Psychiatrists.

Royal College of Psychiatrists. 2014. Typology of bipolar disorders. (Online) Available at http://www.rcpsych.ac.uk/healthadvice/problemsdisorders/bipolardisorder.aspx (accessed May 5, 2014). Royal College of Psychiatrists, London.

Royal College of Psychiatrists' Centre for Quality Improvement. 2006. *Better Services for People Who Self-Harm: Quality Standards for Healthcare Professionals*. London: Royal College of Psychiatrists.

Royal College of Psychiatrists. 1997. Meeting the mental health needs of people with learning disability. Council Report CR 56. London: RCP

Szymanski L.S. 1988. Diagnosis of mental disorders in retarded persons. In: Stark J.A., Menolascino, F.J., Albarelli, M.H., Grey, V.C. (Eds), *Mental Retardation and Mental Health: Classification, Diagnosis, Treatment Services*. New York: Springer Verlag.

Singleton, N., Bumpstead, R., O'Brien, M., Lee, A., Meltzer, H. 2001. *Psychiatric Morbidity among Adults Living in Private Households, 2000: Summary Report*. London: Office for National Statistics.

Üçok, A. and Wolfgang, G. 2008. Side effects of atypical antipsychotics: A brief overview. *World Psychiatry*, 7(1):58–62.

Vitiello, B., Spreat, S., and Behar, D. 1989. Obsessive compulsive disorder in mentally retarded patients. *Journal of Mental and Nervous Disease*, 177:232–235.

Wallace, B. 2002. Boxed In: The challenge of dual diagnosis. *Learning Disability Practice*, 5(4):24–26.

WHO. 1992. *ICD-10 Classification of Mental and Behavioural Disorders. Clinical Descriptions and Diagnostic Guidelines*. Geneva: World Health Organisation.

FURTHER READING

Katona, C. and Robertson, M. 2001 *Psychiatry at a Glance* (2nd ed.). Oxford: Blackwell Science.

Priest, H. and Gibbs, M. 2004. *Mental Health Care for People with Learning Disabilities.* Edinburgh: Elsevier.

Raghavan, R. and Patel, P.R. 2005 *Learning Disabilities and Mental Health: A Nursing Perspective*. Oxford: Blackwell.

USEFUL RESOURCES

National Association for the Dually Diagnosed the DM-ID: A Clinical Guide for the Diagnosis of Mental Disorders in Persons with Intellectual Disabilities, available from The National Association for the Dually Diagnosed. www.thenadd.org

Royal College of Psychiatrists DC-LD: Diagnostic criteria for psychiatric disorders for use with adults with learning disabilities/mental retardation, available from the Royal College of Psychiatrists/Gaskell Publishing. www.rcpsych.ac.uk

World Health Organisation ICD-10: Guide for Mental Retardation. www.who.int

Down Syndrome and Dementia Resource: Dodd, K., Turk, V., and Christmas, M. 2002.

British Institute of Learning Disabilities: www.bild.org.uk

Mental Health in Learning Disabilities: A training resource: Holt, G., Hardy, S., and Bouras, N. 2005. www.pavpub.com

Understanding Depression in People with Learning Disabilities: Hollins, S. and Curran, J. 1997. www.pavpub.com

IMCA - Wales: http://mhmbcb.com/imca/imca_web.htm

ECT: http://www.rcpsych.ac.uk/healthadvice/treatmentswellbeing/ect.aspx

6 Learning disability nursing and people with profound learning disabilities and complex needs

Bob Gates

INTRODUCTION

People with profound learning disabilities and complex needs are one of the most marginalised and potentially vulnerable groups of people in any society. They are at continuing risk of social exclusion, and simultaneously experience poorer health than does the rest of the population (Mansell, 2010). Therefore, arguably, the role of the learning disability nurse in supporting, and where necessary providing, direct care for this group of people is particularly relevant because of the high levels of dependence they may have on others throughout their lives. Nursing, or directed social care, should be regarded as a way of systematically planning and documenting interventions to meet the needs of and to support this group of people in all aspects of their lives. This chapter will examine the learning disability nurse's direct and indirect role in supporting or caring for this group of people. As in previous chapters, this will be contextualised within the Nursing and Midwifery Council for the United Kingdom (2010) and An Bord Altranais (2005) standards for competence.

This chapter will focus on the following issues:

- Understanding profound learning disabilities and complex needs
- How many people have profound learning disabilities and complex needs?
- Attitudes toward people with profound intellectual disabilities and complex needs
- The nature of learning disability nursing interventions for people with profound learning disabilities and complex needs
- Care planning for people with profound learning disabilities and complex needs
- Maintaining a safe environment

- Communication
- Breathing
- Eating and drinking
- Eliminating
- Washing and dressing
- Maintaining body temperature
- Mobilising
- Working and playing
- Expressing sexuality
- Sleeping
- Dying
- Spirituality
- Relationships
- The implementation of Care Plans
- Evaluating Care Plans

Competences

NMC Competences and Competencies

Domain 1: Professional values - Field standard competence and competencies – 1.1; 2.1; 3.1; 4.1.

Domain 2: Communication and interpersonal skills - Field standard competence and competencies – 1.1; 2.1; 3.1; 4.1.

Domain 3: Nursing practice and decision making - Field standard competence and competencies – 1.1; 3.1; 5.1.

Domain 4: Leadership, management and team working - Field standard competence and competencies – 1.1; 1.2; 2.1.

An Bord Altranais Competences and Indicators

Domain 1: Professional/ethical practice – 1.1.3; 1.1.5; 1.1.6; 1.1.7; 1.1.8; 1.2.4.

Domain 2: Holistic approaches to care and the integration of knowledge – 2.1.1; 2.1.2; 2.1.3; 2.1.4; 2.2.1; 2.2.3; 2.3.3; 2.3.4; 2.4.1; 2.4.2.

Domain 3: Interpersonal relationships – 3.1.3; 3.2.1; 3.2.2; 5.1.1.

Domain 4: Organisation and management of care – 4.1.3.

Domain 5: Personal and professional development – 5.1.1; 5.1.2; 5.1.3.

UNDERSTANDING PROFOUND LEARNING DISABILITIES AND COMPLEX NEEDS

Lacey (1998) has defined profound and multiple learning disabilities as comprising the following characteristics:

- Profound intellectual impairment (which refers to people who score below 20 on an Intelligence Quotient [IQ] test)
- Additional disabilities, which may include sensory disabilities, physical disabilities, autism or mental illness

More recently, the Profound and Multiple Learning Disability (PMLD) Network (2013) has defined profound and multiple learning disabilities as

> **Children and adults with profound and multiple learning disabilities have more than one disability, the most significant of which is a profound learning disability. All people who have profound and multiple learning disabilities will have great difficulty communicating. Many people will have additional sensory or physical disabilities, complex health needs or mental health difficulties. The combination of these needs and/or the lack of the right support may also affect behaviour. Some other people, such as those with Autism and Down's syndrome may also have profound and multiple learning disabilities. All children and adults with profound and multiple learning disabilities will need high levels of support with most aspects of daily life.**

(http://www.pmldnetwork.org/, accessed August 27, 2014)

Regardless of definition, Mencap (2014) have rightly reminded us that people with profound learning disabilities and complex needs are all different and should be treated as individuals. It is important that people with profound learning disabilities and complex needs not be perceived as a list of ailments (Carnaby, 2001), but as people first, capable of experiencing the same range of human experience as their fellow citizens (Davies and Evans, 2001).

Historically, a number of labels have been used to refer to this group of people and these have included '*severe disabilities and complex needs*', '*profound learning disabilities*', and '*the most severely disabled*' (PMLD Network, 2002). This can lead to confusion, not least for parents and carers, and difficulties with accessing appropriate services. Problematic with the many terms used to refer to this group of people is that such terms are associated with the 'medical model' (Ho, 2004), which is now seen by many to have become outdated. Paradoxically, however, this group of people often present with complex health problems. Notwithstanding this and for the purposes of this chapter, the term '*profound learning disabilities and complex needs*' will be used throughout, and its use is grounded in the definitions already provided by Lacey (1998) and the PMLD Network (2013).

HOW MANY PEOPLE HAVE PROFOUND LEARNING DISABILITIES AND COMPLEX NEEDS?

As outlined in Chapter 1, in the United Kingdom it has been calculated that of the three to four persons per 1000 population with learning disabilities, approximately 30% will present with severe or profound learning disabilities. Within this group it is common to find multiple disabilities that include physical or sensory impairments or disability, as well as behavioural difficulties. Based on these estimates, one can assume that there are some 2,30,000 to 3,50,000 persons with severe learning disabilities in the United Kingdom. And of this number, Emerson (2009) has calculated that there are somewhere in the region of 16,000 adults with profound learning disabilities and complex needs in England. Interestingly it has also been calculated and predicted that there will be a significant rise in this number, with an estimation that it will increase by something of the order of 1.8% per year until to 2026. This will result in an increase in the total number of adults with profound learning disabilities and complex needs being in the region of some 22,000 people. To put this in context, given a geographical area that has a population of 2,50,000, we would see a rise from 78 adults in 2009, to 105 in 2026, which is a rise of over 30%. The PMLD Network concurs with this prediction suggesting that it may be accounted for as a result of ongoing developments in medical technology, better control of epilepsy, and an increase in the use of tube feeding (PMLD Network, 2001).

Whereas people with profound learning disabilities and complex needs clearly represent a small section of society, it is nonetheless a highly significant and vulnerable section. This group of people generally requires lifelong support to carry out activities of daily living, and, like other citizens, they are entitled to access the resources that enable them to meet their health and social care needs as and when required. It must be emphasised, as in Chapter 1, learning disability is a lifelong condition—therefore, when we talk about people with people with profound learning disabilities and complex needs we are talking about children and adults, as well as older people. As has been described in Chapter 3, learning disability nursing contributes to the health and well-being of people with learning disabilities across the entire age spectrum (U.K. Chief Nursing Officers, 2012).

ATTITUDES TOWARD PEOPLE WITH PROFOUND INTELLECTUAL DISABILITIES AND COMPLEX NEEDS

There remains considerable lack of knowledge not only in the general public, but also more worryingly in health and social care professions about people with profound learning disabilities and complex needs. Consider the following statements from parents of people with learning disabilities:

> **'You shouldn't have to look after someone like that. He should be in an institution', 'If you will keep her at home what do you expect?' and, 'At the end of the day people thought my sons were worthless, utterly worthless, and we were too. I thought they were very special'.**

> *(Mencap, 2001, p. 5)*

And in relation to health care professionals, parents report on equally disturbing attitudes expressed:

> **'I overheard the doctor say: that's not coming in my room. It will destroy the equipment—we had to stay with Anthony from 10am to 10pm because no one was feeding him'**

> *(Mencap, 2004)*

> **'Victoria was rushed to hospital after a series of seizures. She needed to be put on a ventilator. The Doctor came up and spoke to us. He was suggesting that it wasn't worth trying to save her'**

> *(Mencap, 2004)*

'To be told that your child is a cabbage and that you will lose all your friends if you don't place them in institutional care is inhuman. To be told without empathy for your situation reinforces the damage—and it still happens. Fortunately we have learned to ignore experts.'

(Mansell, 2010)

Mansell (2010) has supported such concerns over attitudes, and questions why this still persists. He has noted:

Why is it that people with profound intellectual and multiple disabilities have such difficulty in getting help? The evidence from families themselves is that prejudice, discrimination and low expectations underlie their plight.

(Mansell, 2010, p. 5)

To evidence Mansell's assertion, consider a relatively recent publication from Mencap England, *Death by Indifference* (Mencap, 2007). In this harrowing report, Mencap asserted that people with learning disabilities had died unnecessarily due to institutional discrimination while in NHS care. This prompted the then Secretary of State for Health, Patricia Hewitt, to establish an independent inquiry, chaired by Sir Jonathan Michael, into access to health care for people with learning disabilities. It was clear from his report that this group of people had been failed (Michael, 2008). It stated that people with learning disabilities were facing suffering and sometimes even death because current legislation designed to give them access to health care was not being adhered to. The report also concluded that there was not a case for new legislation as it was already in place—so the challenge was to make effective use of existing legislation. The report identified examples of good practice but noted that these were 'patchy', and often the result of committed individuals. The report took evidence from the public, people with learning disabilities, carers, and professionals in the fields of health and social care. All of this ultimately led the report to make 10 recommendations, which were:

1. That all undergraduate and postgraduate clinical training must ensure that curricula include training in learning disabilities.
2. That all health care organisations collect data to allow people with learning disabilities to be identified by the health service so their pathways of care can be tracked.
3. That family and other carers should be involved in the provision of treatment and care, unless good reason is given, and that Trust Boards should ensure reasonable adjustments are made to enable them to do this effectively.
4. That Primary Care Trusts should identify and assess the needs of people with learning disabilities and their carers as part of their Joint Strategic Needs Assessment.
5. That awareness training is needed in the health service of the risk of premature avoidable death, and the Department of Health should establish a learning disabilities Public Health Observatory.
6. That the government directs the Department of Health to immediately amend Core Standards for Better Health, to include an explicit reference to the requirement to make 'reasonable adjustments'.
7. That inspectors and regulators of the health service develop and extend their monitoring of the standard of general health services provided for people with learning disabilities.

8. That the Department of Health should direct Primary Care Trusts (PCTs) to commission enhanced primary care services, which include regular health checks provided by general practitioners (GP) practices, and improve data, communication, and cross-boundary partnership working. This should include liaison staff that work with primary care services to improve the overall quality of health care for people with learning disabilities across the spectrum of care.

9. That all Trust Boards should ensure that the views and interests of people with learning disabilities and their carers are included.

10. That all Trust Boards should demonstrate in routine public reports that they have effective systems in place to deliver effective, 'reasonably adjusted' health services, including advocacy services, for those people who happen to have a learning disability (see Box 6.2 as to progress since the Michael Report) (Michael 2008, pp. 54–56).

And yet even more recently, in the Confidential Inquiry into the premature deaths of people with learning disabilities (CIPOLD), Heslop et al., (2013) have identified that the mean age of death of people with learning disabilities (65 years for men; 63 years for women) is significantly less than that for the U.K population (78 years for men and 83 for women). Subsequently men with learning disabilities are dying, on average, 13 years sooner than do men in the general population and women with learning disabilities are dying, on average, 20 years younger than do women in the general population. The CIPOLD (Heslop et al., 2013) found the most frequent reasons

---

Box 6.1 Progress since the Michael Report

Following a period of five years, what has changed? On the 3rd of January 2013, the Guardian newspaper in the United Kingdom reported on the avoidable deaths of 74 more people with learning disabilities who had died while in the care of the NHS (Bawden and Campbell, 2012); it also highlighted a further 17 serious incidents. Families were continuing to allege that hospital blunders, poorly trained staff, and indifference were to blame. This newspaper, in collaboration with Mencap, had been continuing to campaign to stop people with learning disabilities from receiving unequal health care. Of the cases highlighted in the report, 59 took place within the last five years. And more recently in the Times newspaper, Barrow (2012) has reported on an interview with Sir Jonathan Michael, who said that, four years later, he still doubted *'that all lives were seen to be equally valuable'* across the health service. This article reports how Sir Jonathan recalled being shocked by what he found in 2008, saying that there are still concerns about attitudes toward the lives of patients with severe mental illness. Hospitals and GPs were failing to make essential adjustments to ensure that vulnerable patients received the highest standard of care. Sir Jonathan said:

> **The number of patients with learning disabilities is relatively small in number but we felt then, as I do now, that if the NHS can't look after the most vulnerable, there is something fundamentally wrong**

> *(Barrow, 2012)*

for premature deaths were delays or problems with diagnosis or treatment and difficulties with identifying needs and providing appropriate care in response to changing needs. In addition, the CIPOLD highlighted a lack of reasonable adjustments made to facilitate health care of people with learning disabilities, in particular when accessing clinics for appointments and investigations. These were found to be a contributory factor in a number of the deaths investigated (Heslop et al., 2013). Also known is that this vulnerability is of particular relevance and concern for those with profound learning disabilities and complex needs using General Hospitals (Garrard, 2010).

It is not unusual to hear people say that they have never seen or met a person with profound learning disabilities and complex needs (PMLD Network, 2002). One explanation for this in the past might have been that many of these people were historically *'shut away'* from the communities in which they had previously lived. Even today, many children with profound learning disabilities and complex needs attend special schools resulting in fewer opportunities to interact with the wider community (Foreman et al., 2004). In the past, many people with profound learning disabilities and complex needs lived as *'inpatients'* in long-stay hospitals for the mentally handicapped, as they were known then, where they were cared for predominantly by nursing and medical staff. Most of these hospitals have now closed, and the 'patients' now live in community-based settings where they are rightly regarded as *'clients'* or *'service users'* or *'citizens'*. Because of these hospital closures many children and adults now live in their family home or in a small residential home or supported living, where they are often supported by relatives or unqualified social care staff (Ward, 1999). Therefore, to advise or assist them in recognising the many health care needs of such individuals, learning disability nurses must be able to work in collaboration with a wide variety of people, including family members, paid carers, and professionals from other disciplines and in a number of environmental settings.

Since the almost universal closure of the old long-stay hospitals, and the impact of the white paper *Valuing People* (DH, 2001), and *Valuing People Now* (DH, 2009), significant progress has been made toward the social inclusion of people with profound learning disabilities and complex needs, but there is still a long way to go (McNally, 2004; Gooding, 2004, Mansell, 2010). The PMLD Network (2002) has argued that this group of people still needs to be made more visible in society.

Carnaby (2001) has suggested that this group have been perceived as *'difficult to engage'*, *'passive'*, and an *'expensive'* demand on resources. Such negative perceptions can be damaging and must be challenged if attitudes are to improve. Klotz (2004) has argued that people with profound learning disabilities and complex needs can, and do, live socially meaningful lives, and furthermore within the United Kingdom, the Human Rights Act 1998 has enshrined in law that everyone has a fundamental right to life. Additionally, nurses are bound by a professional code of conduct, which has explicitly stated that all patients and clients must be treated with respect and dignity (NMC, 2004; An Bord Altranais, 2005). These values are also central to the policies set out by the learning disabilities white paper *Valuing People* (DH, 2001, 2009), and more recently a national drive in the United Kingdom to ensure that health care service, particularly that of nursing care, is delivered to all with compassion and care respecting the rights and dignity of all (DH, 2012).

Respect and dignity are relatively abstract concepts that can be interpreted in many different ways. For the purposes of this chapter, respect is being defined as

A feeling of deep admiration for someone elicited by their qualities or achievements or due regard for the feelings or rights of other.

(Oxford English Dictionary, 2002)

Dignity has been defined as

The state or quality of being worthy of honour or respect.

(Oxford English Dictionary, 2002)

In the field of learning disabilities some interpretations of respect have led to ideological fanaticism that in order to treat people with profound learning disabilities and complex needs with respect, they must be treated in a way that is appropriate to their chronological age; age appropriateness. However, dictionary definitions of the terms 'respect' and 'dignity' arguably lend support to Carnaby's view that the most respectful and dignified approach to interaction with this group of people is to be cognisant of an individual's specific abilities and disabilities (Carnaby, 2001). Notwithstanding treating an adult as an *'eternal child'* could be equally disrespectful, and could also hinder an individual's development (Wolverson, 2003). Therefore, all approaches to support or care must balance the necessity for developmental appropriateness on the one hand, with that of securing socially acceptable age-appropriate interactions on the other. And in nursing, more generally, a contemporary vision based around six values—care, compassion, courage, communication, competence, and commitment—has been articulated. This vision seeks to embed these values, known as the so-called Six Cs, in all nursing, midwifery, and care-giving settings throughout the NHS and social care to improve care for patients. The action to achieve this includes:

- Recruiting, appraising, and training staff according to values as well as technical skill
- Regularly reviewing organisational culture and evidence for staffing levels
- Doing more to assess patients' experience
- Helping staff make every contact count for improving health and well-being (DH, 2012)

THE NATURE OF LEARNING DISABILITY NURSING INTERVENTIONS FOR PEOPLE WITH PROFOUND LEARNING DISABILITIES AND COMPLEX NEEDS

Nurses have a duty of care to patients, which means that clients are entitled to receive safe and competent care that should be informed by evidence-based practice (NMC, 2010; An Bord Altranais, 2005). In the context of this chapter, evidence-based practice refers to a way of managing nursing interventions by making clinical decisions that use the best available research evidence, clinical expertise, including professional judgment, and an understanding of patient preferences (Craig and Smyth, 2002). However, it has to be said that little evidence has been established concerning an evidence-based practice for people with profound learning disabilities and complex needs, and therefore good practice is sometimes based on research that has been undertaken with people with mild and moderate intellectual disabilities (Carnaby, 2001; Klotz, 2004). This should necessarily cause us to question both the validity and reliability of 'evidence' gathered from one population and then applied to another (Gates and Wray, 2000; Gates and Atherton, 2001). This issue of referring to and treating people with learning disabilities as one homogenous group is commonplace but problematic.

Even the relatively recent white paper, *Valuing People* (DH, 2001), in England made little reference to the needs of people with profound learning disabilities and complex needs (Aylott, 2001; Cooper and Ward, 2011). The policies set out by *Valuing People* were based on the principles of rights, independence, choice, and inclusion. Putting these values into practice for people with profound learning disabilities and complex needs poses specific challenges. For example, some people are extremely limited in their abilities to make and communicate choices, and the ways in which these people require support will therefore be different from their peers. The PMLD Network (2001) has argued that the policies set out in *Valuing People* are of little use for this group, and in conjunction with Mencap has published their own report that made recommendations that the government needed to make to address the needs of this group a priority (Mencap, 2001). This was partially addressed in the *Valuing People Now* (DH, 2009). More recently Mansell (2010) has challenged us all to raise our sights and the level of our expectations of this group of people. In particular, he advocated extending good services that could be found in individualised and person-centred care, treating families as experts, focusing on the quality of relationship between staff and the disabled person, and sustaining cost-effective packages of care; this could be done by *'raising our sights'* (Mansell, 2010). He identified a number of obstacles that acted as barriers to improvement that include housing, community facilities, health, wheelchairs, communication aids and assistive technology, further education, employment and day-time activity, short breaks, training clinical procedure, and funding. With some 33 recommendations, his report provides a blueprint for improving services for this group of people, along with their families and carers.

When developing care plans for people, whose contribution to its construction is potentially limited, it is critically important to include family members, people who know and care for the person, and all relevant professionals. Carnaby (2001) and more recently Mansell (2010) have both stressed the importance of joint working between professionals for providing comprehensive and

Case History 6.1

Clara has profound intellectual disabilities and complex needs. She is 16 years old and lives in her family home with her parents and two younger brothers. Clara has cerebral palsy and is unable to walk, sit up unaided, or control the movements of her limbs and hands. Clara spends her days in a wheelchair, which she reilies on others to manoeuvre. She also relies on others to wash, dress, and feed her. Clara is unable to speak and she seemingly communicates through eye contact, facial expressions, and vocalisations. Clara is considered to be significantly underweight for her age.

Clara experiences a number of health problems, including:

- Epilepsy – poorly controlled tonic–clonic seizures
- Being underweight
- Constipation
- Frequent chest infections
- Repeatedly developing pressure sores on her ankles, elbows, and sacral area
- Poor eyesight
- Frequently experiences menorrhagia

Clara attends a local school for young people with special educational needs. She has respite care for two nights per month at a unit for young people with profound learning disabilities and complex health needs.

Learning Activity 6.1

Take some time to think about some of the people who might be involved directly or indirectly in Clara's care. Construct a realistic list, and then compare your list with items identified in Box 6.2.

Box 6.2 *People who might be involved in Clara's care*

1. Close family
2. Consultant
3. GP
4. Neurologist
5. Community nurse - learning disabilities
6. Speech and language therapist
7. Physiotherapist
8. Occupational therapist
9. Continence nurse
10. Dietician
11. Advocate
12. School teacher
13. School nurse
14. Transition worker
15. Respite care staff

seamless care. The appointment of a key worker is thought to be essential for joint working to be effective (Mencap, 2001; Wake, 2007; Mansell, 2010).

In Case History 6.1, Clara is presented as someone with profound learning disabilities and complex needs. Clara is a young woman who presents with potential threats and challenges to her health, which include epilepsy, nutritional problems, chest infections, constipation, pressure areas, and visual impairments.

Are there any people, professionals, or other informal carers listed in Box 6.2 that you have not thought of? Or have you listed people that we have not identified? Either way, it might be worth spending some time thinking about this list, and accounting for any differences with a colleague.

CARE PLANNING FOR PEOPLE WITH PROFOUND LEARNING DISABILITIES AND COMPLEX NEEDS

First, as with all care plans, these must be constructed in a person-centred way, and this is especially important for those with profound learning disabilities and complex needs. This is because in many instances this group of people can be almost entirely dependent on a range of people offering care and support, and this can extend to nearly all aspects of someone's life. This dependency can include, for example, having to be fed, toileted, moved, positioned, washed, bathed, dressed, and even assisted with body elimination. With this in mind, the PMLD Network (2001) has argued that person-centred planning can be used effectively with people who have limited communication abilities if a *'circle of support'* is in place to support the planning process. A circle of support has been described as a group of people who know and care about the person and are committed to spending time developing a deep understanding about the person to plan for and advocate services that might improve the person's life (Tomlinson, 2012). Care plans must be written in such a way that all people providing direct care can understand and follow them; this is contemporarily referred to as co-production. In the field of learning disabilities, it has been estimated that approximately 75% of the workforce is unqualified (Ward, 1999). It is also important that care plans are constructed in such a way that they can be readily understood by care staff that originate from a variety of backgrounds, and bring various prior experiences and knowledge with them. Consistency of care is important in terms of effective outcomes, but so too is fostering a sense of security and predictability for the person with profound learning disabilities and complex needs. Ideally, day or education services, residential care, and family carers should all be following the same care plans. To maintain confidentiality, care plans must contain information and be shared on a professional basis with those who need to know to ensure that patients are supported by the wider health and social care team supporting someone with learning disabilities. As the NMC (2010) and An Bord Altranais (2005) have said:

Learning disabilities nurses must use a structured, person-centred approach to assess, interpret and respond therapeutically to people with learning disabilities, and their often complex, pre-existing physical and psychological health needs. They must work in partnership with service users, carers and other professionals, services and agencies to agree and implement individual care plans and ensure continuity of care

(NMC, 2010)

Plans care in consultation with the client taking into consideration the therapeutic regimes of all members of the health care team

(An Bord Altranais, 2005)

People with profound learning disabilities and complex needs present with a wide range of needs. Focusing on one particular area of need can potentially result in the neglect of other areas of care. For example, Male (1996) found that at a special school for people with profound learning disabilities and complex needs, high levels of personal and health care support reduced opportunities for social and educational activities; care plans must therefore ensure that the full range of needs is addressed.

There is also a risk of needs being neglected when all aspects of life take place in one location (Goffman, 1961; Mansell, 2010). Most people experience work, leisure, and relaxation activities in very different places. For people with profound learning disabilities and complex needs, it is possible that all these activities could all take place within the person's home. This inevitably is likely to lead to a risk of social exclusion, whereas access to a number and variety of environments might provide wider social, leisure, and educational opportunities, and therefore a more inclusive lifestyle (Mansell, 2010).

Arguably, neither a medical nor social model of care can adequately meet the care needs of this group. Current ideas about nursing emphasise the importance of holistic care. Narayanasamy et al. (2002) have argued that there is a need for a holistic approach to care that includes, for example, attention to mind, body, and spirit. The challenge for nurses who are planning care for people with profound learning disabilities and complex needs is to balance a high level of need related to the 'body' with needs related to the 'mind' and 'spirit'. It is generally accepted that all three areas have an impact on quality of life (Swinton, 2001; Narayanasamy et al., 2002; Shalock, 2004) but psychological and spiritual needs tend to be lower in the order of priorities.

One way of ensuring the provision of holistic learning disability nursing care is to adopt a nursing model. These have been devised to help organise both the planning and provision of care. The remainder of this chapter discusses care planning through the use of the Roper, Logan, and Tierney model of nursing, which is applied to the case history of Clara (See Case History 6.1). This model was chosen because it is well known and still widely used within the nursing profession. Nurses might find other models that are equally useful and also find that with experience they rely less on a model for care planning and more on their own knowledge, skills, and understanding.

Tierney (1998) has argued that the strength of the Roper, Logan, and Tierney model is that it focuses on holistic care and is based on the concept of health rather than illness and disease. Arguably, these factors make it an appropriate model for learning disability nursing, and it is particularly useful when working with people with profound learning disabilities and complex needs. The model also has practical utility because it focuses on understanding the needs of people in terms of the activities they perform. The model embraces the idea that independence and dependence operate along a continuum relating to each activity of living separately. This is consistent with the generally accepted idea that the level of skills of people with learning disabilities can and do vary across different domains (American Association of Intellectual and Developmental Disability, 2010).

The model can be put into practice in a systematic way using the four stages of the nursing process: assessment, planning, implementation, and evaluation (Yura and Walsh, 1978). The first stage, assessment, involves determining an individual's ability to carry out each of the 12 activities

---

Box 6.3 Some of the people who might be involved in the direct implementation of Clara's care plan

1. Family
2. School teacher
3. Respite care staff
4. Physiotherapist (some aspects)
5. Neurologist/consultant psychiatrist (learning disabilities)/paediatrician
6. Speech and language therapist
7. Certain aspects of the care plan such as communication should be used by all those who come into contact with Clara
8. Community nurse – learning disabilities – indirectly

Factors Influencing Activities of Living	Activities of Living	Dependence/ Independence Continuum
	Maintaining a safe environment	←——————————→
Biological	Communicating	←——————————→
	Breathing	←——————————→
Psychological	Eating and drinking	←——————————→
	Eliminating	←——————————→
Sociocultural	Personal cleansing and dressing	←——————————→
	Controlling body temperature	←——————————→
Environmental	Mobilising	←——————————→
	Working and playing	←——————————→
Politico-economic	Expressing sexuality	←——————————→
	Sleeping	←——————————→
	Dying	←——————————→

Figure 6.1 The Model of living. (from Holland, K. et al., *Applying the roper logan tierney model in practice.* London: Churchill Livingstone, 2003.)

of living listed in Box 6.3 along with his or her health care needs and challenges. In the planning stage problems are identified and documented, along with the goals that aim to address these problems. In relation to people with profound learning disabilities and complex needs, improvements are likely to be small and goals identified should reflect this. Care plans can include specific and direct nursing interventions or indirect actions and supports recommended by the nurse, but the emphasis must always be on the person and the nurse, carer, or supporter working together toward the goals. The nursing process advocates that care plans should be implemented within normal daily routines as much as possible (Holland et al., 2003).

The final stage of the nursing process, evaluation, is an ongoing process in which the individual's ability to carry out the activities of daily living and health challenges should be re-examined to see if the goals have been met. Due to the severity and enduring nature of profound learning disabilities and complex needs, an appropriate goal, for example, might be to maintain a condition or prevent its deterioration. Care plans should be adjusted according to the outcome of evaluation, and this can be performed by using the nursing process in a problem-solving oriented way.

In order to use the Roper, Logan, and Tierney model effectively, nurses must have an understanding of the five factors (biological, psychological, sociocultural, environmental, and politico-economic) that influence the activities of living (Holland et al., 2003). Figure 6.1 provides some examples of how the model and the factors that influence the activities of living might be used to develop a care plan for Clara.

Having considered how these factors may influence the activities of daily living, the following sections discuss each of these activities of living in turn. The case illustration of Clara is used throughout to consider how care planning might be carried out. Some of the more general issues that may arise when applying this model to the care and support more generally to people with profound learning disabilities and complex needs are also considered.

MAINTAINING A SAFE ENVIRONMENT

A large number of people with profound learning disabilities and complex needs have epilepsy, and it is thought that 30% of people (nearly 1 in 3) who have a mild to moderate learning disability has epilepsy, and approximately 50% of people with severe learning disabilities have some form of epilepsy (The Epilepsy Society, 2014). Maintaining a safe environment in its widest sense is an important issue to consider for people with epilepsy. Reflect on the risks associated with bathing, falls, swimming, medicines compliance, and climbing ladders, and consider the need for a medic alert bracelet or perhaps using plastic glasses.

Carers play a vital role in monitoring and managing epilepsy and ensuring that these people receive appropriate care from specialist health services and that they maintain a safe environment is critical. Carers are the most likely people to witness seizures, and it is vital that they are able to record a thorough description of seizures, because this can help medical professionals to make an accurate diagnosis as well as help manage the environment around them to reduce possible harm. A thorough knowledge of the person's medication is also essential to monitor its use and be alert to possible side effects.

Clara has been diagnosed with generalised, tonic–clonic seizures. This type of seizure is characterised by a stiffening of the muscles, followed by rhythmical relaxing and tightening of the muscles, which causes the body to jerk and shake. During a seizure Clara's breathing becomes more difficult, and her skin turns a blue-grey colour. When the jerking stops, her breathing and colour go back to normal and she usually sleeps for a few hours. There are other types of epilepsy, and a range of medications is routinely used to treat epilepsy (see Box 6.4). Witnessing a seizure can be frightening. However, along with training and comprehensive care plans, this should enable carers to know how to respond in the event of a seizure; all of these aspects related to the care management of epilepsy are things which the learning disability nurse should do (see Box 6.5).

Additionally in relation to maintaining a safe environment, another thing the learning disability nurse must be mindful of is the possibility of abuse. Although Clara lives at home, the potential for abuse must always be an issue that learning disability nurses are sensitised to, and the potential for this to happen to people with learning disabilities from those caring for them is well known. This has been reported consistently, and for some considerable time, in the research literature, in both the United Kingdom (Martin, 1984; Brown and Craft, 1989; Allington, 1992; Williams, 1995; ARC/NAPSAC, 1996; Brown, 1999; Cambridge, 1999; Moore, 2001) and internationally (for example, Endicott, 1992; Herr et al., 2003), and it may be institutionalised within configurations of human service delivery systems (Buckinghamshire County Council, 1981; Flynn, 2012). We also know that there are a number of factors connected with abuse toward people with intellectual disabilities and these include age and degree of disability (Brown et al., 1995; Williams, 1995). However, whereas we know about such lamentable practice, less well understood is the extent to which people with learning disabilities are abused, and this is for a number of reasons that include inconsistent and

---

Learning Activity 6.2

Go back to the list of people who might be involved in Clara's care. From this list, identify who is likely to be involved in the **direct** implementation of her care plans.

Box 6.4 Types of epilepsy and examples of chemotherapy used in treatment

Partial seizures (Focal)*: Altered state of consciousness

Simple partial seizures—Usually originates from one area of the brain, electrical activity tends not to spread, common sensations include déjà vu; if the seizure does progress this may be referred to as an aura.

May be treated with carbamazepine (Tegretol), lamotrigine (Lamictal), sodium valproate (Epilim), levetiracetam (Keppra).

Complex partial seizures—Usually originates from one area of the brain, person loses awareness of surroundings, may follow on from a simple partial seizure, may experience automatisms (lip smacking, chewing, messing with buttons or clothes); the person may wander around and may be confused for some time, and as the seizure subsides the person becomes more aware of their environment.

May be treated with Carbamazepine (Tegretol), Lamotrigine (Lamictal), Sodium valproate (Epilim), Levetiracetam (Keppra).

Primary generalised seizures (non-focal): Complete loss of consciousness

Absence seizures—The commonest type of primary generalised seizure, usually found in children (rare in adults); may stare blankly, sometimes blink, person unaware they are having a seizure, may experience repeated episodes in any one day, distinguished from complex partial because there is no aura or automatisms.

May be treated with sodium valproate (Epilim), ethosuximide (Zarontin).

Myoclonic seizures—Most common type (juvenile myoclonic epilepsy) presents often in adolescence, commences with sudden, brief muscle jerking of the limbs which occur singly or in a cluster, often early in the morning.

May be treated with sodium valproate (Epilim), levetiracetam (Keppra), clonazepam (Rivotril).

Tonic–clonic seizures—Represents a convulsive seizure; the person will lose consciousness and collapse to the ground. They may cry out and their body stiffens followed by rhythmical jerking (convulsion); tongue or cheek may be bitten. The seizure normally terminates after a short while, followed by drowsiness.

May be treated with carbamazepine (Tegretol), lamotrigine (Lamictal), sodium valproate (Epilim), clobazam (Frisium).

Tonic seizures—Sudden stiffening of the muscles, the person falls to the ground and there is a loss of consciousness.

May be treated with sodium valproate (Epilim), lamotrigine (Lamictal).

Atonic seizures—Sudden loss of muscle tone with instantaneous collapse/person falls to the ground. Drop attack (often causing facial injuries).

May be treated with sodium valproate (Epilim), lamotrigine (Lamictal).

---

* Partial seizures may progress if electrical activity spreads across the brain, and therefore does remain focal, resulting in a generalised tonic–clonic seizure.

Box 6.5 *Example of one aspect of Clara's care plan that focuses on maintaining a safe environment*

Name

Clara

Activity concerned

Maintaining a safe environment

Problem

Uncontrolled, tonic-clonic epileptic seizures

Goals

To ensure that Clara does not suffer injury whilst having a seizure

To respond appropriately when Clara has a seizure

To provide appropriate emotional support

To monitor and record Clara's seizures

To monitor Clara's medication

To access appropriate health and medical care

To liaise with epilepsy specialists

To be achieved by

Ongoing, to be reviewed at regular intervals

Nursing Intervention (This should be based on a consideration of the five factors that affect the activities of living.)

Physical	Physical effects of a seizure
	History of seizures
	Type of seizures
	Medication
Psychological	Behavioural signs of seizure activity
	Mood and behaviour following a seizure
	Psychological effects of epilepsy
	Emotional support needed to cope with epilepsy
Sociological	Restrictions of epilepsy on daily life
	Reactions of others who may witness a seizure
	Disruption of routines
	Concerns of others, information for carers and relatives
Environmental	Seizure triggers
	Risks of injury from the environment
Politico-economic	Ability of carers to manage epilepsy (training)
	Access to services
	Availability and access to an epilepsy nurse and neurologist

inadequate operationalisation of the term abuse, difficulty in ensuring such abuse is reported, and suggestions of unreliability of persons with intellectual disabilities as witnesses for any potential criminal proceeding against the perpetrator/s. This further compounds difficulties in estimating prevalence. More recently Northway et al. (2013) have advocated amongst other things for people with learning disabilities to have greater access to personal safety and abuse awareness courses. They articulated that when people with learning disabilities disclose abuse, then others people must listen to them, but in relation to people with profound learning disabilities and complex needs this will prove problematic.

COMMUNICATION

It has been estimated that 50% to 90% of people with learning disabilities have difficulties with communication, and that some 20% of people with learning disabilities have no verbal communication at all (BILD, 2002).

People with profound learning disabilities and complex needs are often unable to use formal methods of communication and may subsequently rely on others to interpret their facial expressions, and their non-verbal behaviours. However, Hogg (1998) has found that carers often believed that they were able to interpret needs and emotions through facial expressions, vocalisations, eye contact, and posture, but that these were not always reliable and valid interpretations (Hogg, 1998). Improving communication with people who have profound learning disabilities and complex needs is therefore an important part of the carer's role; particular attention should be given to this aspect of care within the care planning process, and the learning disability nurse must be mindful of directing carers.

Clara should be, if she has not already, referred to a speech and language therapist to conduct a communication assessment, as they have the necessary skills to recommend appropriate communication strategies for an individual (Bradshaw, 2001). One strategy thought to improve communication with people who have profound intellectual disabilities and complex needs is the use of a 'communication passport'. A communication passport aims to help carers understand and interpret choices, preferences, likes, and dislikes, and provides specific information about how to communicate with an individual based on his or her level of (dis)abilities. If the communication passport is produced in a user-friendly, accessible format it is much more likely to be used. It can also provide the individual with more opportunities to communicate effectively with a larger number of people who he or she may come into contact with, both within his or her own home, along with the services he or she may use in the community.

Another communication strategy that is beneficial for some people who are at a very early stage of development is 'Intensive Interaction' (Nind and Hewett, 1994). Intensive Interaction involves developing the repetitive, pre-linguistic behaviours that are used routinely by the individual into a shared 'language', which is thought to enable others to gain access to the person's world (Caldwell, 1997). In this way, it is thought that meaningful communication sequences can be experienced that are mutually enjoyable and relaxing (Hewett, 2005; Hewett et al., 2012).

To perceive and understand the world, people with profound learning disabilities and complex needs are thought to rely more heavily on multiple sources of sensory stimulation (Ayer, 1998). However, it is common for this group to experience sensory impairments that might further disadvantage their ability to communicate and experience the world (Bradshaw, 2001).

Regular hearing and sight assessments are therefore vital to pick up and respond to problems as early as possible. Appointment details should be recorded, and strategies should be in place to ensure that the results of assessments are disseminated to everyone involved in the person's direct care.

It is thought that by documenting responses to a range of choices offered, over time patterns may emerge that suggest that consistent, valid choices are being made. Aylott (2001) has used the term 'choices inventory' to refer to this strategy. Belfiore and Toro-Zambrana (1994) have developed a protocol that aims to achieve this. They drew a distinction between choice and preference—whereas choice is essentially a selection of one option from a number of options offered, preference refers to a relatively predictable behaviour. This can be applied in a systematic way by observing and recording how an individual responds to various environmental stimuli. For example, if it is observed that someone becomes distressed when there is a lot of noise and relaxed when it is quiet, then it could be inferred that the individual is demonstrating a preference for quietness. This information can help carers to support people to make choices and exercise some degree of control over their environment. This kind of approach to careful monitoring and reporting on preference has been more recently reported by the Joseph Rowntree Foundation, which identified that control of decisions could be enabled by

a rigorous approach to building evidence of the process, including careful and creative recording and monitoring

(Values into Action, 2001)

Therefore, over a period of time, it would be possible to establish a range of preferences for Clara, and incorporate these into her care plan.

BREATHING

Respiratory problems are common in people with profound intellectual disabilities and complex needs, and this group is particularly susceptible to chest infections (Wake, 2003). Recent studies and reports have found that respiratory disorders were a leading cause of death for people with intellectual disabilities (Hollins et al., 1998; Glover and Ayub, 2010; Heslop et al., 2013).

For people like Clara, who experience difficulties with breathing, a care plan might need to address methods of enhancing respiratory function. This could include instructions on

- Appropriate positioning
- Postural drainage to remove excess sputum
- Oral and nasal suction
- Minimising the risks of aspiration
- Methods of promoting awareness amongst carers of the signs to look for to identify chest infections promptly

Carers also need to be alert to signs and symptoms of asthma, and hay fever, which can further exacerbate breathing difficulties.

EATING AND DRINKING

Some people with profound intellectual disabilities and complex needs experience 'dysphagia'. This refers to difficulties with swallowing. Dysphagia is a condition that affects approximately 1 in 3 people with a learning disability (Howesman, 2013). Some 99% of children with severe cerebral palsy will have dysphagia (Calis et al., 2008). Dysphagia is not limited to people with learning disabilities; the general population is also affected. It is thought that as many as 68% of people with dementia living in care homes (Steele et al., 1997) and significant numbers of nursing home residents will have dysphagia.

Dysphagia is defined as a disorder of swallowing usually resulting from physical impairment or neurological disorder (Royal College of Speech and Language Therapists [RCSLT], 2009). It is often associated with stroke, dementia, multiple sclerosis, Parkinson's disease, head and neck cancers, acquired brain injury, and respiratory conditions (Terrado et al., 2001; RCSLT, 2009).

Poor management of dysphagia can lead to avoidable fatalities, and there is a clear need for the enhancement of knowledge in our health care staff in this condition (Mencap, 2007; Heslop et al., 2013). Particularly problematic is that people with learning disabilities are at great risk of developing respiratory infections caused by aspiration or reflux if they have difficulties with swallowing (RCN, 2007).

This condition is common in people with cerebral palsy, who may have poor muscle tone in the mouth area, poor reflexes, and immature feeding skills (Harding and Wright, 2010). Difficulties with eating and drinking can lead to malnourishment and potential dehydration, which can be prevented by monitoring food and fluid intake and weight and responding promptly if problems arise.

Clara is underweight and is continuing to lose weight. She does not eat very much and is frequently constipated. This is concerning, and indicates an urgent need for a thorough multidisciplinary assessment (Harding and Wright, 2010). A speech and language therapist, who has been specially trained in feeding difficulties and management, should be asked to assess Clara's specific difficulties and recommend a strategy to ensure that she receives adequate nutrition, safely. A dietitian could also be involved to assess the nutritional content of Clara's diet, and make recommendations for how her diet might be improved.

In addition to the difficulties Clara has with eating and drinking, she also encounters frequent chest infections, and both of these problems are signs of aspiration problems. Aspiration is potentially life threatening and needs to be addressed as a matter of urgency. A referral must be made to the speech and language therapist who specialises in this area (Harding and Wright, 2010).

If Clara is able to eat orally, the care plan would need to include details about the appropriate consistency of food, how often and how much she should be fed, the appropriate utensils to use, and how to ensure that she maintains a posture that maximises her ability to eat safely. A high risk of aspiration can indicate the need for non-oral feeding by gastrostomy. There are a number of excellent texts that provide more comprehensive coverage of feeding for people with profound learning disabilities and complex needs (Wake, 2007).

Even if Clara is unable to eat orally, it is important that she should not miss out on the shared mealtime experience with her family. This can be an important social time when families get together not only to eat, but also to share one another's company and conversation; her inclusion in all family events is important.

ELIMINATING

Constipation is relatively common among people with profound learning disabilities and complex needs, and it can be caused by lack of fibre in the diet and lack of mobility. Improving this condition can be achieved by increasing the amount high-fibre foods such as vegetables, pulses, and fruits in the diet. This is a natural way of increasing bulk and fibre. For people who have difficulties chewing or swallowing, the use of *'smoothies'* can be an alternative and pleasurable way to increase the fibre content of the diet. If this does not solve the problem, Clara's GP could prescribe medication, but this should be used as a last resort. The use of all medications should be closely monitored and regularly reviewed. Swimming (hydrotherapy) can be a useful and enjoyable physical exercise, and can assist in making the abdominal wall 'work' and thereby encourage bowel movement. Alternative therapies such as bowel massage have also been shown to improve the condition for some people (Emly et al., 2001). However, the availability of these therapies is variable across different geographical areas of the United Kingdom and Ireland.

WASHING AND DRESSING

Personal and intimate care is a significant and time-consuming part of life for many people with profound learning disabilities and complex needs. When developing a care plan for Clara, safety is of paramount importance for both carers and Clara. Moving and handling guidelines must be adhered to, as well as the policies in place to protect vulnerable people from abuse (Cambridge and Carnaby, 2000a). The family will need support to ensure they have the correct equipment and training to enable them to carry out care tasks safely. When providing personal care, consideration should be given to individual preferences and cultural customs.

Personal care provides a valuable opportunity for sensory experiences and one-to-one interaction (Cambridge and Carnaby, 2000b). It should not be rushed but used as a time for social interaction and the development of skills.

Due to the nature of their disabilities, many people with profound learning disabilities and complex needs are incontinent. Continence care involves invading a person's intimacy and must be attended to with sensitivity. Privacy and respect are vital when carrying out all aspects of personal and intimate care. This means more than simply closing the door when providing care. It means being careful not to make insensitive comments in front of other people and giving undivided attention whilst carrying out care activities. Carers should try to avoid becoming blasé about continence care—even though it can become a routine part of their work.

People with incontinence are particularly susceptible to perineal dermatitis (Gray et al., 2002). Protecting the skin is therefore a prime consideration when carrying out continence care. The care plan should detail routine preventive measures, the signs of skin breakdown, and a treatment plan to follow if skin breakdown does occur (Smith and Carey, 2013). Preventive measures include the use of appropriate continence pads, keeping the skin clean and dry without scrubbing, and using appropriate cleaning and moisturising products (Gray et al., 2002). Some people with sensitive skin have allergies to certain products, and in these cases the use of detergents, biological washing agents, talcum powder, and products containing lanolin or perfume should be avoided (Gibbons, 1996). Alternatives such as emollients, non-biological washing agents, and perfume-free products are readily available. The pharmacist or GP can give advice about the choice and use of these products to suit an individual's needs.

People with profound learning disabilities and complex needs are often reliant on others to ensure that their teeth are cleaned, and this should be done at least twice a day and checked by the dentist every six months. However, some people with learning disabilities do not like having their teeth cleaned, and this can cause difficulties. If this is the case, it is worth checking with a dentist to find out whether the person has a dental problem that makes brushing painful. Using a small, soft toothbrush, and trying flavoured toothpastes may also be preferred. In some areas, specialist services give advice on dental care for people with learning disabilities. Dental care is necessary for maintaining good health and for preventing halitosis, which is important for social acceptability.

One particularly important consideration with respect to medication in the management of epilepsy concerns the use of phenytoin (Epanutin), but it is not routinely used today. This particular medicine is responsible for causing gingival hyperplasia and hypertrophy that makes the management of oral hygiene even more critical, and the advice of a dentist and oral hygienist should be sought if this medicine is used.

MAINTAINING BODY TEMPERATURE

It may be more difficult for people with profound learning disabilities and complex needs to maintain their body temperature due to poor circulation caused by restricted mobility. Regular monitoring of Clara's temperature is important to enable carers to respond promptly and appropriately if she develops a high or low temperature as this could indicate an underlying health problem, and a raised temperature is usually a sign of an underlying infection.

Clara would be unable to communicate whether she was too hot or cold, and carers must therefore be mindful about weather conditions and ensure that she wears appropriate clothing. Such clothing might include gloves, hats, and scarves in the winter, and cool, cotton clothing in the summer. Clothing should also be comfortable and suitable for Clara's age and culture.

Sunburn and heatstroke should be prevented by applying high-factor sun cream and ensuring that Clara avoids the sun around mid-day and at particularly hot times. Carers should remember that dark skins, as well as fair skins, are susceptible to sunburn. Fluid intake should be increased when the weather is hot, to avoid dehydration.

MOBILISING

Issues of mobility are highly relevant for people who have physical disabilities, and this is often the case for those people with profound learning disabilities and complex needs where therapeutic positioning is of the utmost importance (Hill and Goldsmith, 2010). Clara is completely reliant on others for her comfort and to ensure that the correct measures are taken to improve and maintain her posture. The role of a physiotherapist would be to assess Clara's needs for orthotics, wheelchairs, seating, and special footwear, and to carry out a review at prescribed intervals to determine any changes in need. This is particularly important at Clara's stage in life, as she is going through puberty and is likely to require larger equipment to account for her growth.

Clara's care plan should describe the correct use of equipment such as hoists, splints, and body braces and give instructions about how to carry out interventions as recommended by the physiotherapist. Her care plan might include a series of passive exercises and the correct use of equipment, such as a standing frame, to improve or maintain her posture.

When considering issues of mobility for people with very restricted movement, carers should be mindful of the effects this might have on an individual. Located in one plane of orientation for prolonged periods of time can make sudden or extreme movements seem unpleasant and even frightening. Carers should remember that some people with profound learning disabilities and complex needs can, in a sense, be physically locked into their own bodies, and this may result in a lack of self-determination on their part and total reliance on others for movement.

Also problematic for some people with profound learning disabilities and complex needs are destructive changes in body shape as a consequence of poorly aligned posture when lying for prolonged periods in a supine position. It is critically important to maintain good posture by keeping the body in a symmetrical position (Hill and Goldsmith, 2010). Hydrotherapy is thought to be a particularly valuable way of increasing mobility and maintaining posture and also offers the individual an opportunity to experience weightlessness for the period of time that he or she is in the water; this can be particularly helpful for the management of pressure areas.

WORKING AND PLAYING

Providing meaningful activities to people with profound learning disabilities and complex needs can be challenging. This group is reliant on others to initiate activities, and their involvement may largely be passive. It is also difficult to assess how meaningful the activity is for someone who has limited communication abilities. Choice of activities should therefore be based on understanding the individual's abilities and preferences, which can be developed through the use of a communication profile and choices inventory as discussed previously in this chapter.

Studies have shown that people with profound learning disabilities and complex needs often spend large periods of time unengaged (Bradshaw, 2001). This is likely to reduce their capacity and motivation to learn and practice communication skills. It is conceivable that the development of communication strategies could be achieved alongside the provision of meaningful activities.

Multi-sensory rooms or 'snoezelens' are often found in special schools, day centres, and larger residential homes. The literature suggests that multi-sensory rooms can be used for relaxation, sensory stimulation, leisure, and entertainment (Ayer, 1998; Patterson, 2004). Their purpose is therefore not entirely clear and will probably depend on how they are used. If multi-sensory rooms are to be used effectively and meaningfully, their use should therefore be based on individual assessment and observation. Hirstwood and Gray (1995) have suggested that these rooms can be used as *'dumping grounds'* whilst staff conduct activities in other areas. This is unacceptable; someone with profound learning disabilities and complex requires the support of other people to benefit from the environment and to have a meaningful experience. It would also be dangerous for Clara, due to the risk of her having an epileptic seizure. Care plans should specify the precise aims of the use of multi-sensory room and be accompanied by risk assessments that detail how the room should be used safely.

Carers should not forget that the world is full of natural and man-made environments that could provide stimulation, enjoyment, and opportunities for social interaction for this group. Including people with profound intellectual disabilities and complex needs in everyday activities, such as cooking, is important, and an individual's preferences for such activities can be monitored by developing a choices inventory.

Occupational therapists in particular and local Mencap (England, Northern Ireland, and Wales), Enable, or PAMIS (Scotland) or Inclusion Ireland are all possible sources of ideas for providing suitable activities.

EXPRESSING SEXUALITY

The sexuality of people with learning disabilities is poorly understood and has often been neglected by health and social services (Oakes, 2007). Over recent years, a move away from the medical model of care toward a holistic model of health care has lead to greater recognition of the sexuality of people with learning disabilities (Oakes, 2007).

The law in relation to sex is fairly clear for people with profound intellectual disabilities and complex needs. It is unlawful for a person to have sex with someone who is unable to give consent (The Home Office, 2003). Holland et al. (2003) have argued that expressing sexuality is essential for well-being. It has been argued that to encompass the wide range of sexual needs and experiences that people have, sexuality should be viewed in a broad way (Batcup and Thomas, 1994). For people with profound intellectual disabilities and complex needs, care plans might include activities to encourage bodily awareness, opportunity and support with masturbation, information about how clothing and appearance can be used as an expression of sexuality and sexual identity, and how people should be supported through developmental changes such as puberty, menstruation, and menopause, the first two of these being particularly relevant to Clara.

SLEEPING

People with profound intellectual disabilities and complex needs are dependent on others to ensure they have a safe and comfortable place to sleep. Clara is known to be at risk of developing pressure sores on her ankles, elbows, and sacral areas, and this is thought to be caused by her positioning in bed. The physiotherapist might recommend the use of a 'sleep system' to enable carers to position Clara in such a way that removes pressure from the areas prone to sores.

The time at which a person goes to bed and gets up should be determined by the individual's own sleep pattern. The amount of time people need to sleep varies. Lying in bed when not asleep may be boring and become uncomfortable, and not having enough sleep is thought to be detrimental to physical and psychological health and quality of life (Dogan et al., 2005; Brostrom et al., 2004). To aid restful sleep, carers should ensure that the bedroom is quiet, neither too hot nor cold, and free from draughts.

DYING

Although life expectancy for people with intellectual disabilities is increasing, this group has an increased risk of early death (Hollins et al., 1998; Heslop et al., 2013)

Problems recognising and assessing symptoms of illness mean that diagnoses, and therefore access to appropriate treatment, are often delayed in this group (RCN, 2013). Pain is often the earliest indicator of illness, but Donovan (2002) has found that carers can have difficulties recognising that a person with profound intellectual disabilities and complex needs is in pain, suggesting that illnesses could therefore be easily missed.

People with profound learning disabilities and complex needs are at greater risk of pain as a result of associated physical conditions such as cerebral palsy and gastro-oesophageal reflux (Davies and Evans, 2001). Pain management strategies, which might include the administration of analgesics and correct positioning, should be detailed in the care plan.

The Royal College of Nursing (2013) has pointed out that an increase in life expectancy has resulted in conditions such as cardiovascular cancer becoming more common in people with intellectual disabilities. When required to provide palliative care, carers should seek the support of specialist services (see Chapter 3). Some of the issues that might need to be considered at this stage of life include pain and symptom control, consent, ways of communicating about illness and death with the individual and his or her family, and how relatives can be supported through this difficult time (RCN, 2013). Consideration should also be given to how carers will be supported to cope with the effects of their own experience of loss and bereavement.

In any kind of congregated living arrangement, people with profound learning disabilities and complex needs are also likely to be affected by the loss of a resident. Research on bereavement and people with intellectual disabilities has suggested that the experience of grief can be prolonged and its effects can include anxiety, depression, and irritability (Oswin, 1991; Hollins, 1997; Blackman, 2003).

These findings have challenged the widespread belief that people with learning disabilities are incapable of experiencing grief; the reader might care to refer back to Chapter 3.

One limitation of the Roper, Logan, and Tierney model is that it does not include spirituality or relationships as activities of daily living. As both of these are thought to be equally as important to the human experience, they should be considered as an integral part of the care planning process for people with profound learning disabilities and complex needs.

SPIRITUALITY

Spirituality has been considered a significant dimension of well-being (Narayanasamy et al., 2002). Hatton et al., (2004) have argued that meeting people's religious and spiritual needs is an essential role for services to fulfil. However, spiritual needs are probably one of the most challenging and neglected areas of care for people with profound intellectual disabilities and complex needs.

Care planning and decision making can be problematic in this area, as differences in values and beliefs between different members of care staff and family members can cause tensions. Person-centred approaches offer a solution to some of these problems. By encouraging open discussion and prioritising the individual's needs above the aspirations of family and staff, decisions can be made about how to meet religious and spiritual needs.

Narayanasamy et al., (2002) have argued that a distinction must be made between religion and spirituality. They have found that services largely failed to address spiritual needs but were better at meeting religious needs, which might have involved supporting individuals with religious activities and practices. Legere (1984) has defined spirituality as 'to give meaning and purpose', which might be a helpful way for carers to start to think about how to meet this area of human need.

There are some resources that might be useful for developing care plans to address religious and spiritual needs (see Hatton et al., 2004). However, these do tend to concentrate on the needs of people with mild to moderate intellectual disabilities, and our understanding about how these needs might best be met for people with profound learning disabilities and complex needs is a long way off.

RELATIONSHIPS

Carers play a vital role in supporting people with profound intellectual disabilities and complex needs to maintain and develop relationships throughout their lives. Parents will have had varying experiences of parenting a child with profound learning disabilities and complex needs. Some may have had difficulties coming to terms with their son or daughter's disability, and carers should be sensitive to the worries and concerns parents may have about their son or daughter's care.

The need for human touch has been well established (Montagu, 1971; Dobson et al., 2002). However, policies in human services are sometimes interpreted in a way that restricts the use of touch. This is regrettable, as touch might be a person's only, or most meaningful, way of communicating and connecting with the social world. Touch can also be used to provide sensory stimulation and to offer comfort. The need for touch could be addressed through the use of massage and communication strategies.

THE IMPLEMENTATION OF CARE PLANS

Ultimately, the success of care planning is dependent on its implementation. Care plans should not be paper exercises whereby forms are filled out and filed away in a cabinet and retrieved only at the next date for review. They should be active documents that should be updated on a regular basis and used by all those involved in providing care.

There is a very high turnover of staff in learning disabilities services, and this can have serious consequences for service quality (Felce et al., 1993; Hatton et al., 1995; Hatton et al., 2001). Care plans can be pivotal in ensuring that information is passed on to new carers when staff leave and therefore attempt to bring about some form of continuity in someone's life.

The majority of staff who provide direct 'hands-on' care may not have relevant care-related qualifications. The white paper *Valuing People* and its follow-up policy document *Valuing People Now* (DH, 2001; DH, 2009) suggested that the lack of trained staff in learning disabilities services should be addressed by the introduction of a Learning Disabilities Awards Framework (LDAF) (Gates and Statham, 2013). Service providers were charged with the responsibility of establishing and maintaining a competent workforce, and were to ensure that all new staff members were enrolled onto the LDAF schemes; this did not happen. This makes it imperative for specialist professionals such as learning disability nurses, speech and language therapists, physiotherapists, clinical psychologists, consultant psychiatrists in learning disabilities, and occupational therapists to be able to offer valuable training to paid social carer staff as well as family carers.

Hogg (1998) has acknowledged that whereas people might use especially trained staff to support people with profound learning disabilities and complex needs, this does not mean that they always have to use special services.

EVALUATING CARE PLANS

As previously stated, care plans must be seen as active documents that should constantly evolve in response to the evaluation of current and past interventions, changes in the individual's needs, and development of new knowledge and ideas.

A lack of consensus on what constitutes quality of life (Petry et al., 2001) poses a challenge for the evaluation of care plans, as what may be a desirable outcome for one person could be entirely different for someone else. Physical outcomes are probably easier to evaluate because a comparison can be made about objective measurements (such as blood pressure or the frequency of seizures) that are taken before and after the intervention. Measuring abstract concepts, such as spiritual well-being, is more problematic. The use of communication profiles was discussed previously in this chapter. These could help carers to develop an understanding of the success of the care plan from the individual's perspective. However, for the most part, evaluation will be based on the reports and opinions of other people. Reflective practice provides an opportunity for staff to consider these different perspectives and their own contribution to care planning. The use of adopting multiple perspectives has been advocated in the context of learning disability research (Gates and Atherton, 2001; Mafuba and Gates, 2012).

> **Autobiographical, participatory, oral and life history research provides evidence of a different nature that represents authentic accounts from people with learning disabilities concerning their experiences of disability and having to cope with professionals and caring agencies. While the reliability of such accounts may be problematic in some cases, they are clearly some of the most valid types of evidence professionals in learning disabilities presently have at their disposal. This is because the reliability of such methods is, in a sense, held ransom to the vagaries nature of human memory. Whereas human memory can be unreliable, the authenticity of such accounts represents highly valid data.**

(Gates and Atherton, 2001, p. 519)

Establishing long-term relationships and building and maintaining family relationships and community links are extremely valuable. Family members might be the only consistent presence in a person's life, as carers tend to come and go. Professionals should remember that a family carer is usually *'the expert'* when it comes to the care of their loved one.

CONCLUSION

This chapter has attempted to demonstrate how learning disability nursing care can be planned and delivered for people with profound learning disabilities and complex needs, both through direct interventions and indirectly through prescribed care plans for social care staff and support workers. It has been argued that this group represents one of the most marginalised groups of people in society. They are at risk from social exclusion and experience poorer health than the rest of the population. Care plans in this chapter have been presented as one way of ensuring that this group of people receives systematic planning and documentation of interventions by their paid carers. Such an approach should be adopted to meet an individual's daily needs for support in all aspect's of his or her life, and it has been suggested in this chapter that the use of a specific model of nursing might assist in this being undertaken in a more organised and guided way. Further, it has been suggested that care planning is particularly relevant for this group of people because of the high level of dependence they may have on others throughout their whole lives. In particular, this chapter has considered the role of the intellectual disability nurse in care planning and delivery for some of the most vulnerable people in our society.

REFERENCES

American Association of Intellectual and Developmental Disability. 2010. *Intellectual Disability: Definition, Classification, and Systems of Supports* (11th ed.). AAIDD: Washington.

Allington, C.L.J. 1992. Sexual abuse within services for people with learning disabilities. *Mental Handicap,* 20:59–63.

An Bord Altranais. 2005. *Requirements and Standards for Nurse Registration Education Programmes* (3rd ed.). Dublin: An Bord Altranis.

ARC/NAPSAC. 1996. *It Could Never Happen Here! The Prevention and Treatment of Sexual Abuse of Adults with Learning Disabilities in Residential Settings.* Chesterfield and Nottingham, ARC/NAPSAC.

Ayer, S. 1998. Use of multi-sensory rooms for children with profound and multiple intellectual disabilities. *Journal of Intellectual disabilities for Nursing, Health and Social Care,* 2(2):89–97.

Aylott, J. 2001. The new intellectual disabilities white paper: Did it forget something? *British Journal of Intellectual disabilities,* 10(8):512.

Barrow, M. (January 27, 2012) NHS gives 'second-rate care' to mentally disabled patients. London. *The Times*

Bawden, A. and Campbell, D. (January 3, 2012) NHS accused over deaths of disabled patients: Mencap inquiry finds institutional discrimination against people with learning disabilities led to at least 74 deaths. Manchester. *The Guardian*

Batcup, D. and Thomas, B. 1994. Mixing the genders, an ethical dilemma: How nursing theory has dealt with sexuality and gender. *Nursing Ethics,* 1(1):43–52.

Belifore, P.J., Toro-Zambrana, W. 1994. *Recognising Choices in Community Settings by People with Significant Disabilities.* Washington: American Association on Mental Retardation.

BILD. 2002. *Factsheet: Communication.* Birmingham: BILD.

Blackman, N. 2003. *Loss and Learning Disabilities*. London: Worth Publishing.

Bradshaw, J. 2001. Communication partnerships with people with profound and multiple intellectual disabilities. *Tizard Intellectual Disability Review,* 6(2):6–15.

Brostrom, A., Stromberg, A., Dahlstrom, U., and Fridlund, B. 2004. Sleep difficulties, daytime sleepiness, and health-related quality of life in patients with chronic heart failure. *Journal of Cardiovascular Nursing,* 19(4):234–242

Brown, H. 1999. Abuse of people with learning disabilities: Layers of concern and analysis. In: Stanley, N., Manthorpe, J., and Penhale, B. (Eds.), *Institutional Abuse: Perspectives Across the Lifecourse*. London: Routledge, pp. 89–109.

Brown, H. and Craft, A. 1989. *Thinking the Unthinkable: Papers on Sexual Abuse and People with Learning Disabilities*. London: FPA Education Unit.

Brown, H., Stein, J., and Turk, V. 1995. The sexual abuse of adults with learning disabilities: Report of a second two-year incidence survey. *Mental Handicap Research,* 8(1):3–24.

Buckinghamshire County Council. 1998. *Independent Longcare Inquiry. Buckinghamshire County Council,* Buckingham.

Caldwell, P. 1997. 'Getting in touch' with people with severe learning disabilities. *British Journal of Nursing,* 6(13):751–756.

Calis, E., Veugelers, R., Sheppard, J., Tibboel, D., Evenhuis, H., and Penning, C. 2008. Dysphagia in children with severe generalized cerebral palsy and intellectual disability. *Developmental Medicine & Child Neurology*, 50(8):625–630.

Cambridge, P. 1999. The first hit: A case study of the physical abuse of people with learning disabilities and challenging behaviours in residential services. *Disability and Society,* 14:285–308.

Cambridge, P. and Carnaby, S. (2000a) A personal touch: Managing the risks of abuse during intimate and personal care. *The Journal of Adult Protection*, 2(4):4–16.

Cambridge, P. and Carnaby, S. (2000b) *Making it Personal: Providing Intimate and Personal Care for People with Intellectual Disabilities*. Brighton: Pavillion.

Carnaby, S. 2001. Editorial. *Tizard Intellectual Disability Review*, 6(2):2–5.

Carnaby, S. 2004. *People with profound and multiple learning disabilities: A review of research about their lives.* London: Mencap.

Cooper, V. and Ward, C. 2011. Valuing people now and people with complex needs. *Tizard Learning Disability Review*, 16(2):39–43.

Craig, J. and Smyth, R. 2002. *The Evidence Based Practice Manual for Nurses.* London: Churchill Livingstone.

Davies, J. 2012. *An ordinary life: Supporting families whose child is dependent on medical technology or has complex health needs.* London: Foundation for People with Learning Disabilities.

Davies, D. and Evans, L. 2001 Assessing pain in people with profound intellectual disabilities. *British Journal of Nursing,* 10(8):513–516.

Department of Health. 2001. *Valuing People: A New Strategy for Intellectual Disability for the 21st Century.* London: The Stationary Office.

Department of Health. 2009 *Valuing People Now.* Leeds: Department of Health.

Department of Health. 2012. *Compassion in Practice, Nursing, Midwifery and Care Staff: Our Vision and Strategy.* Leeds: DH.

Dobson, S., Upadhyaya, S., Conyers, I., and Raghavan, R. 2002. Touch in the care of people with profound and complex needs. *Journal of Learning Disabilities,* 6(4):351–362.

Dogan, O., Ertekin, S., and Dogan, S. 2005. Sleep quality in hospitalized patients. *Journal of Clinical Nursing,* 14(1):107–113.

Donovan, J. 2002. Learning disability nurses' experiences of being with clients who may be in pain. *Journal of Advanced Nursing,* 38(5):458–466.

Emerson, E. 2009. *Estimating Future Numbers of Adults with Profound Multiple Learning Disabilities in England.* Lancaster: Centre for Disability Research.

Emly, M., Wilson, L., and Darby, J. 2001. Abdominal massage for adults with learning disabilities. *Nursing Times,* 97(30):61–62.

Endicott, O. 1992. How does Canada measure up against international human rights standards? *Entourage,* (7)1:5–9.

Felce, D., Lowe, K., and Beswick, J. 1993. Staff turnover in ordinary housing services for people with severe or profound mental handicaps. *Journal of Intellectual Disability Research,* 37(Pt 2):143–152.

Flynn, M. 2012. *Winterbourne View Hospital: A Serious Case Review.* Gloucester: Gloucestershire Safeguarding Adults Board.

Foreman, P., Arthur-Kelly, M., Pascoe, S., and King, B.S. 2004. Evaluating the educational experiences of students with profound and multiple disabilities in inclusive and segregated classroom settings: An Australian perspective. *Research and Practice for Persons with Severe Disabilities,* 29(3):183–193.

Garrard, B., Lambe, L., and Hogg, J. 2010. *Invasive Procedures: Minimising Risks and Maximising Rights. Improving Practice in the Delivery of Invasive Procedures for People with Profound and Multiple Learning Disabilties.* Dundee: PAMIS and White Top research unit.

Gates, B. and Atherton, H. 2001. The challenge of evidence-based practice for learning disability professionals in health and social care. *British Journal of Nursing.* 10(8):173–178.

Gates, B. and Statham, M. 2013. Lecturers and students as stakeholders for education commissioning for learning disability nursing: Focus group findings from a multiple method study. *Nurse Education Today,* 33(10):1119–1123.

Gates, B. and Wray, J. The problematic nature of evidence. In: Gates, B., Gear, J., and Wray, J. (Eds). 2000. *Behavioural Distress: Concepts and Strategies.* London: Bailliere Tindall.

Gibbons, G. 1996. Nurse prescriber supplement: Skin care and incontinence. *Community Nurse,* 2(7):37.

Glover, G. and Ayub, M. 2010. *How People with Learning Disabilities Die.* Durham: Improving Health and Lives Learning Disabilities Observatory.

Goffman, E. 1961. *Asylums: Essays on the Social Situation of Mental Patients and Other Inmates.* Harmondsworth: Penguin.

Gooding, L. 2004 Valuing People has yet to make a real impact. *Learning Disability Practice,* 7(3):6.

Gray, M., Ratliff, C., and Donovan, A. (2002) Tender mercies: Providing skin care for an incontinent patient. *Nursing,* 32(7):51–54.

Harding, C. and Wright, J. 2010. Dysphagia the challenge of managing eating and drinking difficulties in children and adults who have learning disabilities. *Tizard Learning Disability Review,* 15(1):4–13.

Hatton, C., Brown, R., Caine, A., and Emerson, E. 1995. Stressors, coping strategies and stress-related outcomes among direct care staff in staffed houses for people with learning disabilities. *Mental Handicap Research,* 8:252–271.

Hatton, C., Emerson, E., Rivers, M., Mason, H., Swarbrick, R., Mason, L., Kiernan, C., Reeves, D., and Alborz, A. 2001. Factors associated with intended staff turnover and job search behaviour in services for people with intellectual disability. *Journal of Intellectual Disability Research,* 45(3):258–270.

Hatton, C., Turner, S., Shah, R., Rahim, N., and Stansfield, J. 2004. *Religious Expression, a Fundamental Human Right: The Report of an Action Research Project on Meeting the Needs of People with Learning Disabilities.* London: The Mental Health Foundation.

Herr, S.S., Gostin, L.O., and Koh, H. H. 2003. *The Human Rights of Persons with Intellectual Disabilities. Different But Equal.* New York: Oxford University Press.

Hewett, D. 2005. How Does Intensive Interaction Work? (Online.) Available at http://www.intensiveinteraction.co.uk/about/how-does-intensive-interaction-work/ (accessed on October 10, 2013).

Hewett, D., Barber, M., Firth, G., and Harrison, T. 2012. *The Intensive Interaction Handbook.* London: SAGE.

Heslop, P., Blair, P., Fleming, P., Hoghton, M., and Marriott A. 2013. *Confidential Inquiry into Premature Deaths of People with Learning Disabilities, Final Report.* Bristol: Norah Fry Research Centre.

Hill, S. and Goldsmith, J. 2010. Biomechanics and prevention of body shape distortion. *Tizard Learning Disability Review,* 15(2):15–29.

Hirstwood, R., Gray, M. 1995. *A Practical Guide to the Issue of Multiple Sensory Rooms.* Stourport on Seven: Toys for the handicapped 1995.

Ho, A. 2004. To be labeled, or not to be labeled: That is the question. *British Journal of Learning Disabilities,* 32(2):86–92.

Hogg, J. 1998. Competence and quality in the lives of people with profound and multiple intellectual disabilities: Some recent research. *Tizard Intellectual Disability Review,* 3(1):6–17.

Holland, K., Jenkins, J., Solomon, J., and Whittma, S. 2003. *Applying the Roper Logan Tierney Model in Practice.* London: Churchill Livingstone.

Hollins, S. and Esterhuyzen, A. 1997. Bereavement and grief in adults with learning disabilities. *British Journal of Psychiatry,* 170:497–501.

Hollins, S. Attard, M.T., von Fraunhofer, N., McGuigan, S., and Sedgwick, P. 1998. Mortality in people with learning disability: Risks, causes and death certification findings in London. *Developmental Medicine and Child Neurology,* 40(1):50–56.

Howeseman, T. 2013. Dysphagia in people with learning disabilities. *Learning Disability Practice,* 16(9).

Human Rights Act. 1998. London: HMSO.

Klotz, J. 2004. Sociocultural study of intellectual disability: Moving beyond labeling and social constructionist perspectives. *British Journal of Learning Disabilities*, 32:93–94.

Lacey, P. 1998 In: Lacey, P. and Ouvry, C. (Eds.), *People with Profound and Multiple Intellectual disabilities: A collaborative Approach to Meeting Complex Needs*. London: David Foulton.

Legere, T. 1984. A spirituality for today. *Studies in Formative Spirituality*, 5(3):375–385.

Mafuba, K. and Gates, B. 2012. Sequential multiple methods as a contemporary method in learning disability nursing practice research. *Journal of Intellectual Disabilities*, 16(4):1–10.

Male, D. 1996. Who goes to SLD schools? *Journal of Applied Research in Intellectual Disabilities,* 9(4):307–323.

Mansell, J. 2010 *Raising Our Sights: Services for Adults with Profound Intellectual and Multiple Disabilities.* Kent: Tizard Centre.

Martin, J.P. 1984. *Hospitals in Trouble.* Oxford: Basil Blackwell.

McNally, S. 2004. Plus ça change? Progress achieved in services for people with an intellectual disability in England since the publication of Valuing People. *Journal of Learning Disabilities,* 8(4):323–329.

Mencap. 2001. *No Ordinary Life: The Support Needs of Families Caring for Children and Adults with Profound and Multiple Intellectual Disabilities.* London: Mencap.

Mencap. 2004. *Treat Me Right! Better Healthcare for People with a Learning Disability.* London: Mencap.

Mencap. 2007. *Death by Indifference: Following the Treat Me Right!* Report. London: Mencap.

Mencap. 2014. PMLD (profound and multiple learning disabilities) Information for professionals who work with or support people with PMLD (Online). Available at http://www.mencap.org.uk /all-about-learning-disability/information-professionals/pmld (accessed March 28, 2014).

Michael, J. 2008. *Healthcare for All: A Report of the Independent Inquiry into Access to Healthcare for People with Learning Disabilities.* London: HMSO.

Montagu, A. 1971. *Touching, the Human Significance of the Skin.* New York: Harper and Row.

Moore, D. 2001 Friend or foe? A selective review of literature concerning abuse of adults with learning disabilities by those employed to care for them. *Journal of Learning Disabilities for Nursing, Health and Social Care,* 3:245–258.

Narayanasamy, A., Gates, B., and Swinton, J. 2002. Spirituality and Intellectual disabilities: A qualitative study. *British Journal of Nursing,* 11(14):948–957.

Nind, M. and Hewett, D. 2001. *A Practical Guide to Intensive Interaction*. Kidderminster: BILD Publications.

Northway, R., Jenkins, R., Jones, V., Howarth, J., and Hodges, Z. 2013. Researching policy and practice to safeguard people with intellectual disabilities from abuse: Some methodological challenges. *Journal of Policy and Practice in Intellectual Disabilities,* 10(3):188–195.

Nursing and Midwifery Council. 2004. *The NMC Code of Professional Conduct: Standards for Conduct, Performance and Ethics.* London: NMC.

Nursing and Midwifery Council. 2010. *Standards for Pre-Registration Nursing Education.* London: NMC.

Oakes, P. 2003. Sexual and personal relationships. In: Gates, B. (Ed.), *Learning Disabilities: Toward Inclusion.* London: Churchill Livingstone.

Oswin, M. 1991. *Am I Allowed to Cry? A Study of Bereavement amongst People Who Have Learning Difficulties.* London: Human Horizons.

Oxford English Dictionary. 2002. 10th ed. Revised. Oxford: Oxford University Press.

Patterson, I. 2004. Snoezelen as a casual leisure activity for people with a developmental disability. *Therapeutic Recreation Journal,* 38(3):289–300.

Petry, K., Maes, B., and Vlaskamp, C. 2001. Developing a procedure for evaluating quality of life for people with profound and multiple disabilities. *Tizard Learning Disability Review,* 6(2):45–48.

PMLD Network. 2001. *No Ordinary Life: The Support Needs of Families Caring for Children and Adults with Profound and Multiple Learning Disabilities.* London: Mencap.

PMLD Network. 2002. *Valuing People with Profound and Multiple Intellectual Disabilities (PMLD).* London: Mencap.

PMLD Network. 2013. About profound and multiple learning disabilities. (Online) Available at https://www.mencap.org.uk/about-learning-disability/information-professionals/pmld/about-pmld (accessed August 27, 2014).

Royal College of Nursing. 2007. *Meeting the Health Needs of People with Learning Disabilities.* London: Royal College of Nursing.

Royal College of Nursing. 2013. *Meeting the Health Needs of People with Learning Disabilities: RCN Guidance for Nursing Staff.* London: RCN.

Royal College of Speech and Language Therapists. 2009. *Resource Manual for Commissioning and Planning Services for SLCN.* London: RCSLT.

Shalock, R.L. 2004, The concept of quality of life: What we know and do not know. *Journal of Intellectual Disability Research,* 48(3):203–216.

Smith, D. and Carey, E. 2013. Person-centred care planning for clients with complex needs. *Learning Disability Practice,* 16(10):20–23.

Steele, C., Greenwood, C., Ens, I., Robertson, C., and Seidman-Carlson, C. 1997. Mealtime difficulties in a home for the aged: Not just dysphagia. *Dysphagia,* 12:43–50.

Swinton, J. 2001. *A Space to Listen: Meeting the Spiritual Needs for People with Learning Disabilities.* London: The Mental Health Foundation.

Terrado, M., Russell, C., and Bowman, J.B. 2001. Dysphagia: An overview. *MEDSURG Nursing,* 10(5).

The Home Office. 2003. *The Sexual Offences Act.* London: The Home Office.

The Epilepsy Society. 2014. Learning Disability and Epilepsy. Available at http://www.epilepsynse
.org.uk/pages/info/leaflets/learning.cfm (accessed March 20, 2014).

Tierney, A. 1998. Nursing models: Extant or extinct? *Journal of Advanced Nursing,* 28(1):77–85.

Tomlinson, C. 2012. Love is simply not enough. *Tizard Learning Disability Review,* 17(1):26–31.

U.K. Chief Nursing Officers. 2012. *Strengthening the Commitment. The Report of the UK Modernising Learning Disabilities Nursing Review.* Edinburgh: Scottish Government.

Values into Action. 2001. *Demonstrating Control of Decisions by Adults with Learning Difficulties Who Have High Support Needs.* York: Joseph Rowntree Foundation.

Wake, E. 2003. Profound and multiple disability. In: Gates, B. (Ed.), *Learning Disabilities: Toward Inclusion.* London: Churchill Livingstone.

Ward, F. 1999. *Modernising the Social Care Workforce: The First National Strategy for England. Supplementary Report on Learning Disability.* Leeds: Training Organisation for the Personal Social Services.

Williams, C. 1995. *Invisible Victims: Crime and Abuse Against People with Learning Difficulties.* London: Jessica Kingsley.

Wolverson, M. 2003. Challenging behaviour. In: Gates, B. (Ed.), *Learning Disabilities: Toward Inclusion.* London: Churchill Livingstone.

Yura, H. and Walsh, M.B. 1978. *The Nursing Process.* New York: Appleton-Century-Crofts.

FURTHER READING

Chadwick, D.D., Jolliffe, J., and Goldbart, J. 2002 Carer knowledge of dysphagia management strategies. *International Journal of Language and Communication Disorders,* 27(3):135–144.

Lacey, P. and Ouvry, C. (Eds.). 1998. *People with Profound and Multiple Learning Disabilities: A Collaborative Approach to Meeting Complex Needs.* London: David Fulton.

Pawyln, J. and Caranaby S. 2008. *Profound Intellectual and Multiple Disabilities: Nursing Complex Needs.* Oxford: Wiley Blackwell.

USEFUL RESOURCES

Epilepsy: www.epilepsynse.org.uk

Cerebral palsy: www.scope.org.uk

Eating and swallowing difficulties: www.dysphagiaonline.com (free registration)

Intensive interaction: www.intensiveinteraction.co.uk

General information: www.learningdisabilties.org.uk

PAMIS: www.dundee.ac.uk/pamis

PMLD: www.pmldnetwork.org/

7 Learning disability nursing in forensic settings

*Mick Wolverson**

INTRODUCTION

This chapter explores key competencies, skills, and the knowledge base required for learning disability nurses working in forensic settings. Explicit links will be made to the NMC (2010) standards for competence, and the An Bord Altranais (2005) domains of competence that demonstrate how these prepare nurses for working in forensic settings. Forensic is an adjective, which, when used with other terms, has come to mean an activity that is linked to courts and criminal investigation. In relation to learning disabilities the term forensic is usually applied, although not always, to people who have offended and been dealt with by the courts. In relation to those who have not offended, the term forensic is often applied to people with learning disabilities who present a significant risk to others and who *may* commit an offence and those who have a significant history of self-injurious behaviour.

It therefore follows that forensic nursing involves assessing and planning the care of people who have usually offended and have had contact with the criminal justice system. This is a relatively new and expanding specialist area of learning disability nursing practice (Kingdon, 2010). Learning disability nursing in forensic settings is a highly complex area of practice that involves balancing the

---

This chapter will focus on the following issues:

- Case study
- Epidemiology/prevalence
- Service development and configuration
- Inappropriate sexual behaviour
  - Assessment
  - Formulation
  - Treatment
- Arson
  - Causation
  - Assessment
  - Interventions

---

* Michael Wolverson, Lecturer in Learning Disabilities, York University, UK

- Risk assessment and risk management
- The Mental Health Act
  - Section 17: Supervised community treatment—compulsory treatment orders (CTOs)
  - Section 37: Hospital order
  - The Mental Capacity Act (MCA) 2005 Deprivation of Liberty Safeguards (DOLS)
- De-escalation and control and restraint

tensions between offering person-centred and therapeutic care within the framework of a contemporary rights culture, and the need to manage risk within controlling systems and environments.

People with a learning disability and with forensic histories have a diverse range of complex needs. Their behaviours constitute a risk, and often result in offending, and include arson, sexually inappropriate behaviour, physical aggression, destruction of property, and self-injurious behaviours. The causation of these behaviours is often extremely complex with a multifactorial range of contributory factors, including a dual diagnosis of mental disorder and learning disabilities, the presence of autism or Asperger syndrome, acquired brain injury, and psychosocial issues such as dysfunctional family dynamics, abuse, and institutionalisation. People with learning disabilities and a forensic history will often have had involvement with a wide range of clinical professionals and agencies, including psychiatry, psychology, education, the police, and criminal justice system.

It is evident that this complex area of practice requires learning disability nurses who specialise in this area to acquire an evidence-based body of knowledge, and the requisite skills and competencies to deliver effective nursing care within a multidisciplinary and multiagency context. Mason and Phipps (2010) have commented that there can be a lack of clarity in relation to the core nursing competencies expected of the forensic learning disability nurse. Mason and Phipps (2010) and Kingdon (2010) have suggested that there is some degree of consensus about the required knowledge base and core competencies of the forensic learning disability nurse.

This chapter will explore this core knowledge base and the core competencies by specifically focusing on sexually inappropriate behaviour, arson, managing risk, and the Mental Health Act 1983. The case illustration provided by 'Jason' will be used to illustrate key points throughout.

NMC Competences and Competencies

Domain 1: Professional values - Field standard competence and competencies – 1.1; 2.1; 3.1; 4.1

Domain 2: Communication and interpersonal skills - Field standard competence and competencies – 1.1; 2.1; 3.1; 4.1.

Domain 3: Nursing practice and decision making - Field standard competence and competencies – 1.1; 3.1; 5.1.

Domain 4: Leadership, management and team working - Field standard competence and competencies – 1.1; 1.2; 2.1; 6.1.

Competences

An Bord Altranais Competences and Indicators

Domain 1: Professional/ethical practice – 1.1.1; 1.1. 5; 1.1.6; 1.1.7; 1.2.2; 1.2.3.

Domain 2: Holistic approaches to care and the integration of knowledge – 2.1.1; 2.1.3; 2.1.4; 2.2.1; 2.2.3; 2.2.4; 2.3.1; 2.3.2; 2.3.4; 2.4.1; 2.4.2.

Domain 3: Interpersonal relationships – 3.1.1; 3.2.1; 3.2.2.

Domain 4: Organisation and management of care– 4.1.2; 4.1.3; 4.3.

Domain 5: Personal and professional development – 5.1.1; 5.1.2; 5.1.3.

Case Study 7.1

Jason, who is 19 years of age, is currently detained under section 37/41 of the Mental Health Act 1983 in a medium-secure unit operated by a private company. He is accommodated in a 12-bedded unit within a large forensic hospital campus, which has six other units that provide treatment for specific groups of people requiring treatment in a forensic setting. The campus, which is eight miles from the town centre and 130 miles from Jason's hometown, is on the site of a pre-existing psychiatric hospital and some of the older buildings have been retained and modernised. The specific purpose of Jason's unit (which is referred to as a ward) is to assess and treat men with learning disabilities who have offended in law. It is predominantly staffed by learning disability nurses and unqualified support staff, although there are two registered mental nurses and one registered general nurse. The hospital also employs an extensive multidisciplinary team, including two psychiatrists, psychologists, occupational therapists, and psychotherapists.

Jason has a long history of inappropriate and offending behaviours, which first came to the attention of services when he was 12. At this age, teachers at his school for people with special educational needs expressed concerns about both inappropriate sexual behaviour and fire setting. Jason would regularly expose his genitals and attempt to touch the genitals of both male and female pupils. He would also set fire to waste bins and the school bags of other pupils, and the police arrested him for setting fire to a large haystack. At this stage he was referred to both the children's community learning disability team and the Child and Adolescent Mental Health Service (CAMHS). Both teams assessed Jason, and some services where offered. These included respite care and structured care plans that required family involvement. At this stage, learning disability nurses and other members of the multidisciplinary team gathered together important information that could explain some of the reasons why Jason displayed these behaviours of concern.

Jason lived in an overcrowded house, provided by social housing on a deprived estate. He has six siblings who have three different fathers. It became evident that Jason, and all of his siblings, had been sexually, physically, and psychologically abused by his father and by the fathers of his siblings. It was noted that Jason's mother colluded with the abuse and attempted to justify it by blaming her children for it. At this time, Jason's father was serving a prison sentence for abuse and there

(*continued*)

Case Study 7.1

was no contact with the fathers of his siblings. Because of this, it was recommended that Jason should remain in the family home as the risk of abuse had been considerably reduced.

Jason had regular contact with learning disability nurses from this stage. Jason's sexually inappropriate behaviour was assessed and treated by members of the community learning disability team and CAHMS. His behaviours did remain concerning, but were assessed as becoming less dangerous and more manageable. Jason's dangerous behaviour suddenly escalated when he was 18.

At this stage, Jason's father was due to be released from prison and Jason was just about to leave school. He was arrested by the police because he had set fire to two large waste bins outside a leisure centre, and he was seen by members of the public to try to 'grab' passing children while threatening to throw them into the burning bins. When he was interviewed by the police, a learning disability nurse who knew Jason was present as an appropriate adult. She was also the diversion from custody officer who was present in court where she advised that Jason would benefit from assessment and treatment in a specialist forensic unit.

Learning Activity 7.1

In the case study, Jason has been detained under the Mental Health Act in a medium-secure unit in which he has his own room. He has access to communal areas, involvement from the multidisciplinary team, and escorted trips into the community as part of his care plan. Consider what could be done to ensure that Jason is treated in as person-centred a way as is possible within this predominantly controlling environment. Make a list of your ideas and then go to Learning Activity 7.2.

Learning Activity 7.2

Learning Activity 7.1 requested that you consider and make a list of things that could be done so that Jason could be treated in person-centred ways. You should now think about the 'barriers' within forensic settings that could prevent you from implementing your ideas. Make a list of these barriers and then think of ways in which you can overcome them.

EPIDEMIOLOGY/PREVALENCE

Johnston (2005) and Harding et al. (2010) have commented that due to a combination of inter-linking factors, the prevalence and epidemiology of offending in learning disability is extremely difficult to accurately define. It is a fact that historically, and particularly in the first half of the twentieth century, there was a widespread belief that people with learning disabilities had a higher propensity to offend than did the general public. Johnston (2005) believes that this belief was to some extent the result of misconception, prejudice, and the stigmatisation of people with learning disabilities in general.

From approximately 1950, and particularly within the last 30 years, attempts have been made through research studies to more accurately ascertain the proportion of people with learning disabilities who offend within the population of people with learning disabilities, and compare this with that of the general public. Although this is the case, Johnston (2005) and Harding et al. (2010) have commented that a combination of variable factors can still lead to a degree of inaccuracy that can lead to people with learning disabilities receiving inappropriate support and admission to prison rather than specialist services (Talbot, 2011). These variables include applying the arbitrary IQ of 70 to include and exclude those studied, which can result in those with 'mild or borderline' learning disabilities with a forensic history being dealt with inappropriately. Other variables include the belief that people with learning disabilities who commit crimes are less likely to be able to conceal their offences than can people in the general public, and lack insight into their offending behaviour and its outcomes. They can be suggestible and therefore manipulated by others to commit offences, and an eagerness to please may make them more likely to confess to offences.

Harding et al. (2010) have attempted to summarise the evidence base in relation to the epidemiology of offending behaviour and people with learning disabilities. They suggest that there is some degree of correlation between learning disabilities and offending with people with mild learning disabilities being more likely than the general public to commit offences, and those with moderate or severe learning disabilities less likely to offend. It should be noted that Hodgins (1992) has reported that a birth cohort study indicated that women with learning disabilities are four times more likely to offend than women with an average IQ, and that the likelihood of committing a violent offence is 25 times greater. These figures are very different from those relating to the general public, as men are responsible for 90% of violent crimes.

Johnston (2005) has commented that there is a lack of clarity as to whether the personal characteristics of offenders who have learning disabilities are the same as those of the general public. It does seem to be the case that there are some comorbid factors associated with learning disabilities that predispose a propensity to offend, but also that many predisposing psychosocial factors are the same as those of the general public. Learning disability nurses working in forensic settings need to be aware of the factors that influence epidemiology so that they can effectively assess and plan care. A comprehensive knowledge of comorbid factors and broad psychosocial issues is therefore a requirement of forensic learning disability nursing.

SERVICE DEVELOPMENT AND CONFIGURATION

Beacock (2005) and Mason et al. (2010) have outlined the development of forensic learning disability services from historical and political perspectives. The overarching political and philosophical agenda of the closure of the large institutions to be replaced by care in the community has resulted in the contemporary provision of forensic learning disability services. This process can be tracked back in a timeline commencing with the publication in 1971 of *Better Services for the Mentally Handicapped*, followed by a plethora of subsequent key policy documents such as the Reed Report (1992), the NHS and Community Care Act (1990), *Valuing People* (2001), and *Valuing People Now* (2009). This chapter cannot focus in any depth on the specific detail of each of these reports and other similar documents. They have been mentioned to demonstrate that government policy and clinical practice agendas have resulted in the development of the current provision of forensic learning disability services and that this to a large extent dictates the way that learning disability nursing is practised in forensic settings. It should be noted that some of this policy guidance can be interpreted as being, at best, contradictory, and, at worst, difficult to implement within forensic settings. For example, a person with learning disabilities who has offended and is detained under a section of the Mental Health Act 1983 could be excluded from all four key principles from *Valuing People* (rights, independence, choice, and inclusion) as a result of their detention.

Mason and Phipps (2010) have suggested that the development of forensic learning disability service provision that resulted from the deinstitutionalisation of learning disability services that gathered pace in the 1980s lacked coordination and strategic planning. This has resulted in a range of forensic learning disability service provision that can vary in scope and remit depending on locality and the historical development of local services. The spectrum of forensic services that has developed includes high-, medium-, and low-secure units for inpatients and services that are part of the functions of the following

- Community learning disability teams
- Specialist community forensic mental health teams
- Generic mental health services
- Youth offending teams
- Child and adolescent mental health teams
- Specialist mental health teams for people with a learning disability
- Local multiagency networks involving police, probation, courts and diversion from custody schemes

Mason et al. (2010) have commented that these differing service models can create internal tensions between clinicians as a result of differing assumptions about the primary functions and purposes of forensic services. Forensic services can be seen to be influenced by the law, the medical model, politics, protection of the public, and therapeutic treatment. Irrespective of these sometimes contradictory factors, the primary purpose of forensic services and of learning disability nurses in forensic settings is to assess and treat people in therapeutic ways. Whereas this is the stated intention of forensic learning disability services, Mansell (2007) for the Department of Health has reported that in many instances inpatient units have become controlling mini-institutions that do not provide a therapeutic environment and often intensify mental distress. The most egregious example of this is provided by the recent gratuitous abuse of people at Winterbourne View (DH, 2012). It is evident that forensic learning disability nurses need to operate from an ethical value base and attempt to offer personalised care within systems that by their very nature can be extremely controlling.

So far, this chapter has begun to outline some of the complexities involved with nursing people with a learning disability in forensic settings. It would seem self-evident that there should be consensus in relation to the core competencies, requisite skills, and role expectations of learning disability nurses working in forensic settings; however, Kingdon (2010) has suggested that this is far from the case and that there is some confusion about the core competencies that learning disability nurses require in forensic settings and that an agreed definition of role has not been arrived at. Mason et al. (2010) have expressed concern about the preparation that learning disability nurses receive during their pre-registration nurse training and Kingdon (2010) has noted that there is a lack of standardisation of the core competencies required for forensic nursing within existing fields of practice programmes in pre-registration nurse education. Thus, it can be argued that the core competencies required for learning disability nursing in forensic settings have developed in practice settings to reflect the diverse and complex needs of the people being treated within them. A research study by Mason and Phipps (2010) have attempted to ascertain what practising learning disability and mental health nurses working in learning disability forensic settings considered to be the 10 most required core competencies for their role. In summary the skills and competencies identified were the following

1. Risk assessment and risk management
2. Multidisciplinary working
3. De-escalation
4. Identification of triggers
5. Management of aggression
6. Interventions to manage specific offences
7. Communication
8. Control and restraint
9. Early interventions
10. Clear boundaries

It is clear that some of these areas, such as multidisciplinary working and communication, can be linked directly to the generic domains of competence within the NMC standards (2010) and the An Bord Altranais domains of competence (2005). It is also evident that others, such as risk assessment and risk management, are linked to field-specific competencies. However, it should be noted that important issues such as interventions to manage specific offences are unlikely to be explicitly incorporated into NMC field-specific competencies. Because of this, learning disability nurses working within forensic settings should develop knowledge and skills relating to areas not covered by field-specific competencies through preceptorship and continuous professional development. The most common behaviours associated with people with learning disabilities in forensic settings, and which are unlikely to be incorporated in depth into field competencies, are destruction of property, self-injurious behaviour, arson, and sexually inappropriate behaviour. The chapter will now offer an exploration of sexual offending and arson, which are the two areas of offending behaviour associated with learning disabilities that result in the involvement of forensic services.

INAPPROPRIATE SEXUAL BEHAVIOUR

Riding (2005) has commented that, although on balance research findings can be equivocal, people with learning disabilities are more likely to enter the criminal justice system as a result of sexual offending than the general public. One significant factor to consider that relates to epidemiology is that whereas it is acknowledged that women with learning disabilities do commit sexual offences, men commit the vast majority of such offences. It is certainly the case that sexually inappropriate behaviour and offending behaviour constitute one of the major reasons for why people with learning disabilities are involved with forensic learning disability services.

The assessment and treatment of people with learning disabilities who exhibit sexually inappropriate behaviour presents some extremely difficult and complex challenges to nurses working within forensic environments. Riding (2005), Hepworth and Wolverson (2006), and Bennet and Henry (2010) have all stressed the necessity of person-centred and holistic care planning in relation to people with learning disabilities who display sexually inappropriate behaviours. Person-centred and holistic care planning using the nursing process (assessment, planning, implementation, and evaluation) is explicitly covered both within the generic domains and field-specific competencies detailed within the NMC standards (2010) and the An Bord Altranais domains of competence (2005). Learning disability nurses working within forensic settings will therefore be expected to be able to engage in holistic, person-centred care planning. Because there are some specific skills and areas of knowledge that relate to care planning and sexually inappropriate behaviour, nurses working in forensic settings will, at post-qualification, be required to expand their knowledge and skills base to effectively assess and treat people with learning disabilities who display sexually inappropriate behaviour.

Sexually inappropriate and offending behaviour encompasses a wide range of manifestations. Riding (2005) has explained that sexual offences can be divided into three areas as follows

- Behaviour that involves another person or people regardless of whether there has been physical contact
- Behaviour where there are issues of consent
- The illegality or unacceptable deviance of a behaviour, irrespective of whether this has resulted in a conviction

Within these categories specific examples of sexually offending behaviours include rape (vaginally, orally, and anally), touching of body parts, paedophilia, bestiality, voyeurism, exhibitionism, and the downloading of obscene images from the Internet. This list of offending behaviours serves to illustrate not only the diverse nature of offending behaviour but also the serious nature of these offences and how these often elicit moral revulsion from members of the public and nurses.

The generic domains within the NMC standards (2010) and the An Bord Altranais domains of competence (2005) reinforce the necessity of treating clients in non-judgemental and therapeutic ways, and these competencies often need to be reinforced when working with people who have committed sexual offences such as paedophilia.

The causation and development of sexually inappropriate and offending behaviours displayed by people with learning disabilities can be highly complex and multifactorial. Hepworth and Wolverson (2006) have emphasised the necessity of using global and robust assessment processes to ascertain the cause(s) of an individual's sexually inappropriate behaviour. Effective formulations and appropriate interventions can only be arrived at and implemented when based on thorough and accurate assessment. Bennet and Henry (2010) have pointed out that the reasons why people with learning disabilities commit sexual offences can be similar or the same as those that apply to the general public, but there are some specific factors relating to people with a learning disability that increase the propensity to commit sexual offences.

It has been suggested that people with learning disabilities who commit sexual offences can be categorised into two sub-types of offender. Type I offenders are those who commit sexual offences for the same reasons as members of the general public, and type II offenders are those who commit offences as a result of some aspects of their learning disability. Learning disability nurses in forensic settings should be aware of both the common and specific factors when assessing and planning care.

Type I offenders with learning disabilities may have deviant ideas about sexuality and have some understanding that these are socially unacceptable or illegal. Bennet and Henry (2010) explain how various models can be applied in an attempt to understand type I offending. Finklehor's model, which was originally proposed in relation to sexual offences against children, is used as the basis of the prison services Sex Offender Treatment Programme and has been adapted so that it can be used with people who have a learning disability. The model has four components as follows

1. The motivation to sexually abuse, or the 'thinking stage', which includes having a strong sexual attraction to children and fantasising about sexual activity with them.
2. Overcoming moral restraint: This involves 'rationalising' sexual offences by providing cognitive distortions or 'excuses', such as the victim 'enjoyed' the sexual contact or 'deserved' it due to their provocative behaviour.
3. Overcoming external barriers or creating the opportunity for sexual assault: This involves overcoming the victim's resistance and planning where the offence will take place.
4. Overcoming the victim's resistance: This can include grooming, threats, or force (Finklehor, 1986).

Wolf (1988) has proposed a similar model, which is often applied to people with learning disabilities who commit sexual offences. This model explains sexual offending as a 'vicious cycle' that leads to repetitive offending. The cycle begins with an individual experiencing a negative self-concept and low self-esteem, which leads to social isolation and the expectation of sexual rejection. To manage these negative emotions, and in the absence of appropriate coping strategies, the individual engages in deviant escapist fantasies, which will eventually lead to stages 2, 3, and 4 of the Finklehor model. Riding (2005) has suggested that having a physical disability alongside learning disabilities may compound associated factors that lead to low self-esteem and therefore entrench the 'vicious cycle' outlined within Wolf's model.

Some other causative factors of sexual offending apply equally to the general public and people with learning disabilities. It is widely recognised that a dysfunctional family upbringing can lead to sexual offending, particularly where sexually inappropriate behaviour is accepted (McBrien et al., 2010). It has been proposed that the experience of an individual being the victim of abuse may be a causative influence in the development of sexually inappropriate behaviour, although Riding (2005) cautions that this is unlikely to be a single causative factor. Other causative theories are the following

- Poor anger management
- Poor impulse control
- The self-perception that the individual does not conform to stereotypical views of masculinity

Type II offenders are perceived to be naïve offenders who commit offences as a result of not understanding that their behaviours are illegal or unacceptable. Sexual offending that occurs as a result of this has come to be known collectively as 'counterfeit deviance' (Griffiths et al., 2013), and some specific aspects of this are

- Lack of opportunity to develop appropriate sexual relationships.
- Poor sex education.

Box 7.1 *The potential organic causations of sexually inappropriate behaviours*

- Damage to the frontal lobe of the brain
- Side effects of medication
- Neurological abnormalities
- Klinefelter's syndrome
- Temporal lobe epilepsy
- Acquired brain injury

- Limited interpersonal and social skills.

- Sexual naivety.

- Lack of appropriate role models or lack of encouragement to adopt appropriate behaviour

- Relating to paedophilia: It has been suggested that the psychosexual developmental age of the offender is congruent with the age of those that they commit offences against.

- Sexually inappropriate behaviour lacks a sexual motive and serves a communicative function: This is particularly so for people with poor verbal skills, who may use inappropriate sexual behaviour to draw attention to abuse, 'escape' from uncomfortable situations, or to gain attention.

Most research findings relating to sexual offending in learning disabilities focuses on psychosocial causative factors. Although this is the case, it should be noted that there are some potential organic causations, which are listed in Box 7.1. In the case of Jason, a thorough assessment indicated that there was no apparent organic causation; it did reveal a combination of psychosocial causations relating to his learning disability and history of abuse. Jason did have some awareness that his offending behaviour was illegal; however, his learning disability also contributed to his offending as a result of some aspects on counterfeit deviance, particularly his limited interpersonal skills, lack of appropriate role models, and lack of opportunity to form appropriate sexual relationships.

Assessment

The discussion of the causative factors that can lead to an individual with a learning disability committing a sexual offence indicates the complex and diverse nature of this behaviour. To reflect this complexity and to plan targeted interventions it is therefore imperative that learning disability nurses working in forensic settings have the necessary competencies to be involved in the assessment of individuals who have committed sexual offences. Bennet and Henry (2010) and Hepworth and Wolverson (2006) have suggested that the assessment process should include the following

- Appropriate risk assessment to include the risk of reoffending (there are some specific risk assessment tools for this purpose such as SONAR [Hanson et al., 2005], SORAG [Quinsey et al., 2005], and STATIC-2002 [Hanson et al., 2010]).

- Psychometric testing using tools that have been adapted for use with people with learning disabilities. These include the Questionnaire on Attitudes Consistent with Sex Offences (QACSO), which is used to assess the extent to which individuals hold distorted beliefs that they use to rationalise their offending (Lindsay et al., 2006). This assessment is consistent with Stage 2 of Finklehor's model outlined earlier in this section.

- Assessment of the level of sexual knowledge. Specific assessments for this include the Socio-Sexual Knowledge and Attitudes Test (SSKAT) (Wish et al., 1980) and Sex and the 3R's (McCarthy and Thompson 1994).

- The gathering of personal history details from multiple sources, such as family, police, probation, and other supporting agencies. Areas of an individual's life that should be covered are personal, family, school, previous service involvement, and sexual behaviour including any previous offending. These should be examined in as much detail as possible so that a formulation can be arrived at that could explain the reasons for the offending behaviour.

Formulation

Formulation is the process of drawing together all of the information gathered from assessments and reports so that hypotheses can be made that explain why an individual engages in offending behaviour and which treatments might be the most effective to implement (Sturmey and McMurren, 2011). Formulas and flowcharts are often used to aid this process (Nezu et al., 1998; Murphy, 1997). Formulation can be interpreted as a form of applied functional analysis, and some methods of doing this use the S.T.A.R. approach, which involves organising assessment information into setting conditions, triggers, action, and results. Formulation can be used to form hypotheses relating to both long-term setting conditions and fixed functions, as well as more immediate situations (see Box 7.2 for an example).

In the case of Jason, the S.T.A.R approach enabled staff to develop a formulation in relation to the complex causation and functions of his sexually inappropriate behaviour (see Box 7.2).

Box 7.2 The S.T.A.R approach to formulation			
Setting – The environment/social context (both long term and immediate).	Triggers.	Action – Give a detailed description of the incident.	Responses – What happened after the incident, what impact did the responses have on the individual and others within the setting.
History of dysfunctional family dynamics and sexual abuse. Limited interpersonal skills and lack of appropriate role models. Difficulties with the transition after leaving school.	Father's imminent release from prison.	Setting fire to two large waste bins outside of a leisure centre. Attempting to grab passing children while threatening to throw them into the burning bins.	Arrested by the police and sectioned under the Mental Health Act. Detention in a medium-secure unit.

Source: Zarkowska, E., Clements, J., *Problem Behaviour and People with Severe Learning Disabilities; the S.T.A.R Approach (2nd ed.).* London: Chapman and Hall, 1994.

A range of hypotheses were drawn from the information collected in the S.T.A.R chart with a consensus emerging that Jason's dysfunctional family background and exposure to sexual abuse, alongside his learning disability, were clearly causative factors in the development of his sexually inappropriate behaviour. Formulation also led to an understanding that his sexually inappropriate behaviour served a variety of functions, including an expression of emotional distress, poor anger management, displaced aggression, and desperate attempts to 'escape' from his current situation.

Formulation is a recognised tool that structures clinical decision making of learning disability nurses working in forensic settings, and as such it has clear links to the NMC standards (2010), and the An Bord Altranais domains of competence (2005).

Treatment

Riding (2005) has suggested that until the early 1980s treatment options were limited to close supervision, use of libido-lowering medications, and elimination of deviant sexual arousal. From the early 1980s onwards, a spectrum of largely psychosocial treatments has been developed and tested in forensic learning disability services (Newton et al., 2011). This spectrum includes the following

- Developing appropriate interpersonal skills
- Challenging offence-related attitudes
- Self-monitoring and control techniques
- Developing victim empathy
- Strategies for relapse prevention
- Cognitive restructuring
- Increasing sexual knowledge and competence
- Decreasing inappropriate arousal and increasing appropriate arousal
- Cognitive behavioural therapy (Riding, 2005; Hepworth and Wolverson, 2006; Newton et al., 2011)

Many of the fundamental aspects of the causation and maintenance of sexually inappropriate behaviour, and the assessment and treatment of it also apply to other manifestations of offending behaviour such as arson, which will now be discussed.

ARSON

As is the case for offending in general and in relation to sexual offences, there has been an historical belief that there was a correlation between learning disabilities and fire setting. It was also thought that women, and particularly pubescent girls with learning disabilities and psychosocial difficulties, were more likely to deliberately set fires than men with learning disabilities and members of the general public (Chaplin, 2010). Raesaenen et al. (1994) and Rowe and Lopes (2003) have stated that people with learning disabilities are more likely to commit arson than other groups of people, although Hall et al. (2010) have suggested that accurate numbers and comparisons are difficult to ascertain. What is clear is that arson, alongside sexual offending, is one of the two most common offences that lead to admission to forensic learning disability services (Hall et al, 2010).

Arson is a complex phenomenon that may arise due to a combination of psychosocial causative factors, and it may serve a variety of functions for the perpetrator. As such, the assessment, treatment, and management of arson demand a skilled nursing approach from learning disability nurses working in forensic settings. Some of the NMC 2010 generic and field competencies and An Bord Altranais domains of competence (2005) will help prepare learning disability nurses to practise safely and offer effective and appropriate care planning skills in relation to arson. Generic and field-specific field standards for competence that support this are within Domain 2 competencies 3.1, 4, and 4.1, and within Domain 3 competencies 1, 3, and 3.1.

Causation

The causation of arson is multifactorial, and Chaplin (2010) has explained that there are two typologies of arsonist who have different motivations for committing the offence. They are the following

1. *Non-pathological arson*: This is often a single offence, with the motivation of deliberately using arson as method for achieving an outcome. Examples of this include concealment of another crime, to claim insurance, to make a political statement, or for revenge.
2. *Pathological arson*: This often involves a repeated pattern of fire setting, with high rates of recidivism. It can be associated with mental ill health, personality disorder and psychosocial issues associated with learning disabilities.

The likelihood is that learning disability nurses working in forensic settings will be involved in the assessment and treatment of people who are diagnosed as 'pathological arsonists'. It is worth noting that the terms non-pathological and pathological arson is the terminology of choice in the United States, and that 'pyromania' is a diagnosis in the DSM V (American Psychiatric Association, 2013) and the ICD-10 (World Health Organisation, 1992). In the DSM V, pyromania is categorised as a disruptive, impulse control, and conduct disorder. Although the term pyromania is rarely used in practice, it illustrates that there is a belief that arson can be strongly linked to mental disorder and mental illness, and this can add to the complexity of care planning.

Chaplin (2005), Hepworth and Wolverson (2006), and Hall et al. (2010) have all outlined a range of psychosocial factors that can lead to an individual with learning disabilities committing arson. Learning disability nurses working in forensic settings will be involved in the assessment of psychosocial factors that predispose an individual to commit arson and the subsequent functional analysis of this behaviour. Jackson et al. (1987) proposed that for the perpetrator the function of arson can be to cope with intolerable situations or emotions. These intolerable situations can be subdivided into external factors, such as being controlled by others, harassment, bullying, and internal factors, such as intrusive or distorted thoughts, low self-esteem, and poor regulation of emotions.

Some other suggested psychological motivations for arson include the following

- Seeking sensational impacts from fire setting and fantasising about being involved in fire fighting.
- Seeking sexual release and pleasure from fire setting.

- Exerting power.

- Displaced aggression: The individual can display aggression without direct contact with other people.

Other personal and social characteristics that can predispose an individual to commit arson are social isolation/deprivation and an inability to communicate effectively. It can also be the case that an individual with learning disabilities may not fully understand the potentially devastating consequences of arson and may not intend to cause harm as a result of fire setting. The case study provided by Jason demonstrates how a combination of personal and social characteristics, particularly low self-esteem, poor regulation of emotions, and displaced aggression can explain his propensity to commit arson.

Assessment

There are some specific assessment tools that can be used as part of a global assessment process. There is the Fire Assessment Schedule (Murphy and Clare, 1996), which is a structured interview divided into two sections that help to assess an individual's pre- and post-fire setting thought processes. A broader global multidisciplinary/agency range of assessments will also be necessary. In essence, these should incorporate the components already outlined earlier in this chapter in relation to sexual offending with some added assessment criteria to reflect some arson-specific issues. These criteria are that people with a learning disability are the following

- More likely than other people with a learning disability to commit other offences

- Extremely likely to re-offend if convicted for arson for a second time

- Often have a history of long-term behavioural problems that are most likely to be related to the destruction of property rather than direct aggression toward people

As with the discussion of sexual offending, findings from the assessment process should be amalgamated into a formulation to help explain the development of fire-setting behaviour so that appropriate treatment can take place. This can be based on a broad behavioural functional analysis incorporating a timeline of events as outlined in the S.T.A.R. approach (see Box 7.2). Box 7.3 outlines the components of behavioural analysis in relation to fire setting.

Box 7.3 The components of behavioural analysis

Antecedents: Assessment of the psychosocial setting and circumstances, such as family background, and history of behavioural difficulties and fire setting. The presence of a mental disorder. Peer pressures, coping strategies, and impulsivity. Immediate triggers.

Behaviour: How was the offence committed? What did the individual do during the fire? Were accelerants used, and did the individual commit the offence alone?

Consequences: What did the individual gain from the fire setting, and how did he or she feel?

Interventions

Some of the treatments and interventions, particularly those based on cognitive behavioural approaches and victim empathy, are very similar to those already outlined in the discussion of sexual offending and can be applied to people who have committed arson. Specifically, components for the treatment of arson include the following

- Helping individuals to understand the link between emotions and fire setting and to develop alternative and appropriate ways of coping with emotions, reducing impulsivity and problem solving
- Treating any underlying mental disorder

It is most important to note that people with a learning disability who commit arson are perceived to be dangerous and that they constitute a significant risk to the public. Although this is the case, they often present as being passive within forensic settings (Hall et al., 2005). Because of this, learning disability nurses working in forensic settings will need to be able to assess and manage risk. The next section of this chapter discusses risk management in forensic settings in a general way; however, it should be noted that the risk presented by people who commit arson is managed by some practical measures within forensic settings. These involve policies and procedures that apply to patients, staff, and all visitors for removing and searching for any inflammable materials.

RISK ASSESSMENT AND RISK MANAGEMENT

The discussion of sexual offending and arson has indicated that learning disability nurses working in forensic settings must be aware of and have the necessary ability to assess and manage risk specific to forensic settings. Some of the An Bord Altranais (2005) and NMC (2010) generic and field-specific standards for competence will help learning disability nurses to effectively assess and manage risk in forensic settings. The most relevant NMC standards are within Domain 3 standards 6 and 9, and within Domain 4 standard 6. These standards and competencies relate, to some extent, to the general management of risk and being accountable for this.

The most usual and simplest definition of risk is that risk is the combination of the chance that something may occur and the harm that this could cause (Fisher and Scott, 2013). Alaszewski and Alaszewski (2011) have argued that there is a range of more complex and culturally specific definitions of risk including that of balancing person-centred positive risk taking within risk-averse services, such as forensic settings. This is an important point, because learning disability nurses may be working in forensic settings that place more emphasis on the minimisation of the risks presented by patients than on person-centred therapeutic risk taking. The National Patient Safety Agency (2007) has explained that risk assessment is a sequential process based on the following five steps

1. Identify the risk, e.g., aggression.
2. Decide who might be harmed and how, e.g., the patient, other patients, physical or emotional harm.

3. Evaluate the risk and decide on precaution(s), e.g., how significant is it, how often does it occur.

4. Record findings and implement them, including monitoring of existing risk, change in patterns of behaviour, and emergent risks.

5. Regularly review the assessment and revise as required.

Risk assessment should involve the gathering together, from as many sources as possible, of as much information as possible that relates to the level of dangerousness an risk an individual poses. Some assessment tools such as the Sainsbury Centre Risk Management Tool are particularly comprehensive in collecting together important information enabling robust and effective risk assessment and planning. Hepworth and Wolverson (2006) listed the components of effective risk assessment and these can be seen in Box 7.4.

These general components should underpin risk assessment and risk management in forensic settings, and they can form part of a global risk strategy alongside specific assessments for specific behaviours, such as those already mentioned for sexual offending and arson. Another useful assessment tool, which Lindsay et al. (2004) have reported to be reliable, is the Dynamic Risk Assessment and Management System (DRAMS). DRAMS predicts risk in relation to psychotic symptoms, mood, self-regulation, and compliance with routines.

As well as individual risk assessments, learning disability nurses working in forensic settings will also need to be aware of, and be accountable for, some aspects of managing environmental risk. An example of this has already been provided in relation to the management of access to flammable materials in the case of arson. These procedures can apply both within forensic environments and when clients are on escorted leave. Other examples can be seen in Box 7.5.

Box 7.4 *The components of robust risk assessment*

- The collecting together of as much personal history as possible
- A multidisciplinary approach with named professionals being given responsibility for key tasks
- Clear identification and prioritisation of behaviour(s) most likely to constitute a risk to self and others
- Identification of immediate, short-term, and long-term risk
- Patient involvement whenever possible
- Identification of factors that could increase or decrease future risk
- Identification of factors that are likely to trigger dangerous behaviour
- Contingency options
- Arrangements for regular evaluation and revision of risk management plan

Source: Hepworth, K, Wolverson, M., In: Gates, B. (Ed.), *Care Planning and Delivery in Intellectual Disability Nursing*, Oxford: Blackwell Publishing, pp. 125–157, 2006.

> ### Box 7.5 Practical precautions for managing risk in forensic settings
>
> - Observing levels and ratio of staff to clients
> - Using safety alarms
> - Monitoring and preventing where required access to vulnerable groups such as children
> - Ensuring, if necessary, that the client is in sight at all times or that 'sight lines' within forensic units are kept clear
> - Minimising control or preventing access to materials that could cause harm to the client or others, such as CD cases, batteries, aerosols, and cutlery
> - Controlling or preventing access to materials that could be used for inappropriate arousal, e.g., magazines containing images of children or photographs of children

Learning disability nurses working in forensic settings are likely to take a lead role in assessing and managing risk, and they may have some responsibility for delegating tasks in relation to this. NMC Domain 4 (2010) underpins some of the skills involved with this area of practice, as do the field-specific competencies 4.1.1 and 4.6.1. These field-specific competencies and some of the generic standards can also support learning disability nurses and their involvement as named care coordinators or by contributing to other components of the Care Programme Approach (CPA).

CPA is a comprehensive, person-centred, systematic, and integrated approach to multi-agency care planning that also involves the management of risk. CPA was introduced originally in 1991 as a result of public concerns relating to the perceived lack of supervision of people who were known to mental health services and who had been previously sectioned under the Mental Health Act 1983. A main component of the original CPA was that the supervision of CPA care plans would be the responsibility of named care coordinators, and these were often in the past and today remain nurses.

The CPA was amended and strengthened somewhat in 2001, and its remit was broadened again in 2008 as a result of the policy document 'Reinforcing the Care Programme Approach' (DH, 2008). This broadened the scope of CPA to include a wider range of people who could benefit from it. To receive CPA an individual must be assessed against a list of criteria, and a list of the criteria that are most likely to indicate that an individual is involved with forensic services follows

- Severe mental disorder (including personality disorder) with a high degree of clinical complexity

- Current or potential risk (s) of suicide, self-harm, harm to others (including history of offending), relapse history requiring urgent response, disinhibition, physical/emotional abuse, cognitive impairment, child protection issues

- Current or significant history of severe distress/instability or disengagement

- Presence of learning disabilities

- Current/recent detention under the Mental Health Act

- Multiple service provision from different agencies including criminal justice

The chapter has discussed that the criteria outlined above are often characteristics associated with people with learning disabilities who are involved with forensic services. Because of this, learning disability nurses working in forensic settings will need to develop the requisite skills and use their competencies to act as CPA care coordinators. Further practice-based learning will usually be required to develop competence in this role.

THE MENTAL HEALTH ACT

The broad purpose of the Mental Health Act is to compel people with a mental disorder to be assessed and treated for that disorder. The Mental Health Act is the most important and influential piece of legislation relating to learning disability nursing within forensic settings. It dictates fundamental aspects of how people detained under the Act must be treated. It also instructs and guides the operational function of nurses treating people who are detained under the Act. When working in forensic settings nurses should develop their knowledge of the most relevant sections of the Act that relate to the people in their care and ensure that they operate within the legal parameters set out in the Act.

Before 2007 the scope of the learning disability nurse to act autonomously within the Act was limited to being able to detain people for six hours under Section 5.4 (see Box 7.6 for details of this) and to involvement with CPA as a provision of Section 117 (as outlined in the previous section). After much political debate the Mental Health Act 1983 was amended in 2007. The amendments to the Mental Health Act 1983 (amended 2007), most of which went into effect in November 2008, have provided some new opportunities and challenges for learning disability nurses working in forensic settings. The amendments to the Act were intended to limit the impact of mental disorder

---

Box 7.6 Section 5.4: Nurses' Holding Powers

This section of the Mental Health Act authorises registered mental nurses and registered learning disability nurses to prevent a person from leaving an inpatient setting if it is considered to be in the best interests of the individual or others. This holding power can last for six hours. Nurses who intend to use Section 5.4 should base the decision to do so on the following

- Likelihood of the patient harming themselves or others
- Patient's expressed intentions
- Evidence of disordered thinking
- Recent disturbances on the ward
- Likelihood of the individual being violent
- Whether the individual has received any disturbing news from relatives or friends
- Changes in usual patterns of behaviour
- Relevant involvement with other patients
- History of impulsivity or unpredictability
- Formal risk assessments that have been conducted and other relevant information from the multidisciplinary team

on the individual and society, including safeguards against the abuse of process and access to independent review. The amendments that impact most on learning disability nursing within forensic settings will be explained, in turn, beginning with the change of definitions used within the Act.

One fundamental amendment to the Act relates to the definitions used to apply to people who could be treated under the Act. Before the 2007 amendments, the Act attempted to define the types of mental disorder that might require an individual assessed as having that disorder to be treated under the Act (see Box 7.7 for these definitions). The two definitions most pertinent to learning disabilities were 'severe mental impairment' and 'mental impairment'. These definitions alone were not a reason for detention under the Act unless they were 'associated with abnormally aggressive or seriously irresponsible conduct of the person concerned'. However, it should be noted that no other specific client group was specifically identified within the 1983 Act, and this was perceived to be potentially stigmatising for people with mental impairments/learning disabilities. Mental impairment and severe mental impairment are no longer definitions within the amended Act, and there is now only one definition of mental disorder. Mental disorder is now defined as 'any mental disorder of the mind'. It should be noted that, whereas this definition includes autism spectrum conditions, learning disabilities alone is no longer categorised as a mental disorder. This amendment therefore excludes people with a learning disability from treatment or guardianship orders unless an individual's learning disability is 'associated with seriously irresponsible or abnormally aggressive conduct'.

A further amendment that directly applies to learning disability nurses is the changes to professional roles (National Institute for Mental Health in England, 2008). Before the amended Act, learning disability nurses could only autonomously detain a person under Section 5.4 of the Act and other than this had very limited involvement with the decision to detain an individual under the Act. Prior to the amendments to the Act, the Responsible Medical Officer (RMO) and Approved Social Worker (ASW) were responsible for making applications and recommendations for detention

---

Box 7.7 Definitions within the Mental Health Act 1983

Mental disorder: This included mental illness, arrested or incomplete development of mind, psychopathic disorder, or disability of mind.

The Act then offers three subcategories of mental disorder as follows:

1. *Severe mental impairment*: A state of arrested or incomplete development of mind, which includes severe impairment of intelligence and social functioning, and is associated with abnormally aggressive or seriously irresponsible conduct on the part of the person concerned.
2. *Mental impairment*: A state of arrested or incomplete development of mind (not amounting to severe impairment), which includes severe impairment of intelligence and social functioning, and is associated with abnormally aggressive or seriously irresponsible conduct on the part of the person concerned.
3. *Psychopathic disorder*: A persistent disorder or disability of mind (whether or not including significant impairment of intelligence), which results in abnormally aggressive or seriously irresponsible conduct on the part of the person concerned.

Box 7.8 The role and function of the Approved Mental Health Professional

A core responsibility of the Approved Mental Health Professional (AHMP) is to conduct an independent assessment about whether to make an application to have a person compulsorily admitted to hospital. Unlike doctors, it is not the responsibility of the AHMP to diagnose a mental disorder but to decide whether the use of compulsory powers are the only way a person can receive the treatment and care required. The AHMP should make an application for someone to be detained under the Act only if the AHMP is satisfied that detention in hospital is the most appropriate way of providing treatment. Other duties include the following

- Formal engagement with a person's nearest relative
- Taking or arranging for a person to be taken to hospital when an application has been made
- Returning a person who has been absent without leave
- Interviewing someone detained under Section 136 by the police
- Involvement in deciding whether to continue or end a Community Treatment Order

under the Act and for making reports to Mental Health Act Tribunals. The amended Act broadens the scope of professionals who can apply and train to become an Approved Mental Health Professional (AMHP).

The AMHP can now take on some of the functions previously limited to the RMO and ASW. The professional groups that can apply to become AMHPs are social workers, occupational therapists, chartered psychologists, mental health nurses, and learning disability nurses. The role and functions of AMHPs are similar to those undertaken by the ASW before the amendments to the Act (see Box 7.8 for an outline of the role and function of the AMHP) with some added responsibilities relating to Section 17, Supervised community treatment (see below).

Registered medical practitioners (doctors) and the professional groups that can apply to become AMHPs can also apply to become 'approved clinicians' (ACs). An AC has the authorisation to conduct specific duties under the Act that cannot be carried out by anyone else, such as writing court reports on some patients and being responsible for certain treatments. An AC who is given overall responsibility for an individual's case becomes a responsible clinician (RC), and the functions of this role replace those of the RMO in the amended Act. To become an approved clinician/responsible clinician, it is necessary to undertake post-registration training, and to demonstrate key competencies. The competencies for approved clinicians include the following

- Assessment skills, such as being able to identify and evaluate the severity of mental disorder and to determine whether this requires compulsory treatment
- Ability to assess risk
- Ability to include biological, psychosocial, and cultural factors within the assessment process
- Ability to consider different treatment options

- Demonstration of a high level of skills in determining capacity to consent
- Ability to effectively work within a multidisciplinary context
- Ability to make decisions without supervision in complex cases
- Report writing and presenting evidence to courts and tribunals

Clearly the functions of the role of the AMHP and approved clinician/responsible clinician are demanding and complex and require post-qualification training. However, it is important to note that many of the NMC generic and field-specific standards of competence can underpin the competencies required to become an AC/RC as outlined previously. These new roles require post-qualifying experiences and a lengthy training course before they can be applied for, and it is therefore unlikely that many learning disability nurses are fulfilling these roles as yet. However, it should be noted that learning disability nurses are the only professional group with a specific qualification that equips them to work with people with learning disabilities. Because of this, the competencies gained as part of their nurse training provide a good level of underpinning skills that make them ideally suited to develop into the new roles. This is acknowledged within the Mental Health Act Code of Practice (2008), which states

> **Wherever possible, an approved mental health professional (AMPH) who assesses a patient with a learning disability under the Act should have training and experience in working with people with learning disabilities. The patient's person centred plan and health action plan may also inform the assessment process.**

> *(Mental Health Act Code of Practice, 2008, p. 310)*

Section 17: Supervised community treatment— Compulsory Treatment Orders (CTOs)

Another major change to the Mental Health Act 1983 was the introduction of compulsory treatment orders (CTOs). CTOs allow for people with a mental disorder to be compulsorily treated outside of hospital. An intention of this was to prevent the multiple readmissions to and discharges from hospital of 'revolving door' patients. A CTO imposes 'conditions' on the individual who is to be compulsorily treated outside of hospital. Two conditions are obligatory and are that the individual must make themselves available for medical examination

- If consideration is needed to extend the CTO
- By second opinion doctor if required

People who are compulsorily treated under a CTO can be recalled to hospital if there is a risk to the health and safety of the individual or a risk to other people. The clinical decision-making skills of the AHMP and the AC/RC are vital to the CTO process. It is the RC who has the responsibility for making the order to discharge an individual onto a CTO, and the AHMP must agree that it is appropriate. The RC with agreement from the AHMP can also set additional conditions other than the two obligatory ones so that the individual receives treatment for his or her mental disorder or to prevent harm to him or her or other people. The RC can recall an individual to hospital by serving notice in writing. If the individual requires more than 72 hours to be in hospital for treatment the RC should consider revoking the CTO and the AHMP must agree to this.

Section 37: Hospital Order

If an individual is convicted of an offence punishable by a prison sentence, a court can authorise detention in hospital under section 37 of the MHA 1983, if it is satisfied that the offender has a mental disorder, and this includes learning disabilities (mental impairment). Before the 2007 amendments, this mental impairment must have been associated with seriously irresponsible or abnormally aggressive conduct, which was likely to alleviate or prevent deterioration in the individual's condition. This became known as the 'treatability test', and it has caused a degree of controversy, as it was seen to exclude some individuals from treatment.

The 2007 amendments replaced the 'treatability test' with an 'appropriate treatment test'. This requires that 'appropriate treatment' must be available in a hospital before an individual can be detained under section 37. The definition of 'appropriate treatment' is very wide and considers psychosocial factors relating to the individual such as gender, ethnicity, and culture. Learning disability nurses working in forensic settings have many of the requisite skills to respond to the demands of the diverse, person-centred, and holistic treatments that fall within the 'appropriate treatment' test. Some of the generic and field standards for competence such as NMC field-specific competence 3.1 and Domain 2.2 of the An Bord Altrainais will have prepared learning disability nurses for this complex and multidimensional role.

The Mental Capacity Act (MCA) 2005 Deprivation of Liberty Safeguards (DOLs)

The Mental Capacity Act Deprivation of Liberty Safeguards, which came into effect in April 2009, do not apply to people who are under a section of the Mental Health Act. The MCA DOLS provide legal protection from harm for individuals who lack capacity to give informed consent for their care or treatment, and who might be deprived of their liberty in hospitals or care homes. Further elements of the MCA DOLS are that people are cared for in the least restrictive ways, and that it must be in their best interests if they are deprived of their liberty. When a care home or hospital identifies a person as being at risk of being deprived of his or her liberty, then that entity must apply to a supervisory body for authorisation of the deprivation of liberty. For care homes, the supervisory body is the local authority and for hospitals, it is the health authority. For authorisation to be granted, the supervisory body must obtain six assessments, which are conducted by assessors. Nurses are one of the professional groups identified as being suitable assessors for this purpose. One key assessment is in relation to best interests, and learning disability nurses working in forensic settings will need to demonstrate well-developed decision-making skills based on often competing ideas about what constitutes an individual's best interests.

DE-ESCALATION AND CONTROL AND RESTRAINT

Learning disability nurses working in forensic settings are likely to be involved in the management of threatening, hostile, and, at times, aggressive behaviour. All clinical guidance at the national and local level demands that the management of aggressive behaviour be managed in the least restrictive ways possible and that physical restraint must be the last option. De-escalation involves responding to changes in an individual's emotional arousal level before he or she becomes physically aggressive, thus avoiding physical restraint. Kaplan and Wheeler (1983) linked de-escalation to what they termed the 'assault cycle'. The assault cycle involves changes in physiology, such as the increased production of adrenaline, which results in heightened levels of emotional arousal and can result in overt aggression. De-escalation is a proactive response that involves observing and identifying changes in an individual's usual or 'baseline' behaviour (Pickard et al., 2010). Some common changes to baseline behaviour include the following

- Changes in usual communication such as raised volume, muttering, making verbal threats
- Changes in physical presentation and activity such as dilated pupils, pallor, rapid breathing, pacing, and increasing agitation
- Changes in levels of interaction such as increased demands and invading personal body space

Learning disability nurses in forensic settings can use a range of communication skills to respond to these changes in arousal. Egan (2010) has developed the SOLER model of body language that can be used as a basis for how to approach an individual with increased levels of emotional arousal. The definition of SOLER follows

S—Face the individual squarely but at a slight angle
O—Adopt an open posture with arms unfolded
L—Lean slightly forward toward the individual
E—Maintain eye contact but do so intermittently as constant eye contact can be threatening
R—Model relaxed, calm, and non-threatening body language

Broader de-escalation techniques related to communication involve understanding that some individuals may have communication and comprehension difficulties, and responding to these differences in ways that ensure individuals feel listened to. One practical consideration is that if several members of staff are present, then one member of staff should take the lead in communicating with an aroused individual and use short, simple, and comprehensible words and language. Chapter 15 of the Mental Health Act Code of Practice offers guidance on best practice in relation to control and restraint and states the following

> **…Physical restraint, rapid tranquilisation, seclusion and observation should be used only where de-escalation alone proves insufficient.**
>
> **…any such intervention must be used in a way that minimises any risk to the patient's health and safety and that causes minimum interference to their privacy and dignity.**
>
> *(DH, 2008, p. 114)*

Learning disability nurses working in forensic settings will need the required competencies to implement physical restraint, seclusion, and rapid tranquilisation. Rapid tranquilisation involves the administration of PRN medication. The NMC generic and field standards and the An Bord Altranais domains will have, to some extent, prepared nurses for these tasks. Specific examples are NMC field standard 3.1 and An Bord Altranais Domain 2.2. NMC approved nursing courses within the United Kingdom and Ireland have a mandatory requirement that nursing students cover de-escalation and control and restraint. Competent medications management, including the use of PRN medication, is also a requirement for entry to nursing registers. Specific NICE guidelines for 2012 state that only suitably trained staff can implement these procedures. These required skills and competencies can be developed further as part of preceptorship and in-house training in forensic settings.

CONCLUSION

This chapter has attempted to explore the evolving role and contemporary practice of learning disability nursing for people with learning disabilities in their contact with forensic services. The implications of legislation and how this can lead to tensions between managing risk and maintaining a secure environment and person-centred approaches has been discussed. The clinical manifestations of sexual offending and arson have been used to highlight best practices and the complexities of assessment and care planning for people with learning disabilities who are involved with forensic services.

This chapter has made evident that learning disability nursing in forensic settings is an increasingly specialised role that requires the development of a specifically focused knowledge base and the mastery of nursing competencies. It has been discussed that people with learning disabilities in forensic settings are a stigmatised, marginalised, and often vulnerable client group. Further, it has been argued that learning disability nurses are the only specifically trained professionals with the requisite skills and knowledge that can advocate on behalf of this stigmatised client group and offer some degree of person centeredness within controlling environments.

REFERENCES

Alaszewski, A., Alaszewski, H. 2011. Positive risk taking. In: Atherton, H., Crickmore, D. (Eds.), *Learning Disabilities: Toward Inclusion* (6th ed.). London: Churchill Livingstone, pp. 179–195.

American Psychiatric Association. 2013. *Diagnostic and Statistical Manual of Mental Disorders DSM – V.* Washington, DC: American Psychiatric Association.

An Bord Altrainais. 2005. *Requirements and Standards for Nurse Registration Education Programmes* (3rd ed.). Dublin: Dublin Stationary Office.

Beacock, C. 2005. The policy context. In: Riding, T., Swann, C., Swann, B. (Eds.), *The Handbook of Forensic Learning Disabilities*. Padstow: Radcliffe Publishing, pp. 1–14.

Bennett, C., Henry, J. 2010. Working with sexual offenders with learning disabilities. In: Chaplin, E., Henry, J., and Hardy, S. (Eds.), *Working with People with Learning Disabilities and Offending Behaviour: A Handbook*. Brighton: Pavilion Publishing, pp. 97–108.

Chaplin, E. 2010. Working with fire setters with learning disabilities. In: Chaplin, E., Henry, J., and Hardy, S. (Eds.), *Working with People with Learning Disabilities and Offending Behaviour: A Handbook*. Brighton: Pavilion Publishing, pp. 109–120.

Department of Health and Social Security and Welsh Office. 1971. *Better Services for the Mentally Handicapped*. London: HMSO.

Department of Health. 1990. *The NHS and Community Care Act. London:* HMSO.

Department of Health. 1992. *Reed Report: Review of Mental Health and Social Services for Mentally Disordered Offenders and Others Requiring Similar Services: Vol. 1 Final Summary Report.* London: HMSO.

Department of Health. 2001. *Valuing People: A Strategy for Learning Disability for the 21st Century.* London: TSO.

Department of Health. 2007. *Services for People with Learning Disabilities and Challenging Behaviour or Mental Health Needs.* London: TSO.

Department of Health. 2007. *The Mental Health Act 1983 (amended 2007).* London: The Stationary Office.

Department of Health. 2008. *Refocusing the Care Programme Approach: Policy and Positive Practice Guidance.* London: Department of Health.

Department of Health. 2008. *Revised Mental Health Act Code of Practice.* London: Department of Health.

Department of Health. 2009. *Valuing People Now: A New Strategy for People with Learning Disabilities.* London: TSO.

Department of Health. 2012. *Transforming Care: A National Response to Winterbourne View Hospital: Department of Health Review: Final Report.* London: Department of Health.

Egan, G. 2013. *The Skilled Helper: A Problem Management and Opportunity Development Approach to Helping* (10th ed.). Stamford, CT: Cengage Learning.

Finklehor, D. 1986. *A Source on Child Sexual Abuse.* Beverley Hills, CA: Sage.

Griffiths, D., Hinsburger, D., Hoath, J., and Ioannou, S. 2013. 'Counterfeit deviance' revisited. *Journal Of Applied Research in Intellectual Disabilities*, 26:471–480.

Hall, I., Clayton, P., and Johnson, P. Arson and learning disability. 2005. In: Riding, T., Swann, C., Swann, B. (Eds.), *The Handbook of Forensic Learning Disabilities.* Padstow: Radcliffe Publishing, pp. 51–72.

Hanson, R.K., Harris, A.J.R., Scott, T.L., and Helmus, L. 2005. *Assessing the Risk of Sex Offenders on Community Supervision: The Dynamic Supervision Project.* Ottawa: Public Safety Canada.

Hanson, R.K., Helmus, L., and Thornton, D. 2010. Predicting recidivism among sexual offenders: A multi-site study of STATIC 2002. *Law and Human Behavior*, 34:198–211.

Harding, D., Deeley, Q., and Robertson, D. 2010. History, epidemiology and offending. In: Chaplin, E., Henry, J., and Hardy, S. (Eds.), *Working with People with Learning Disabilities and Offending Behaviour: A Handbook.* Brighton: Pavilion Publishing, pp. 13–20.

Hepworth, K., Wolverson M. 2006. Care planning and delivery in forensic settings for people with intellectual disabilities. In: Gates, B. (Ed.), *Care Planning and Delivery in Intellectual Disability Nursing.* Oxford: Blackwell Publishing, pp. 125–157.

Hodgins, S. 1992. Mental disorder, intellectual deficiency, and crime: Evidence from a birth cohort. *Archives of General Psychiatry*, 6:476–483.

Jackson, H.F., Glass, C., Hope, S. 1987. A functional analysis of recidivistic arson. *British Journal of Clinical Psychology*, 26:175–185.

Johnston, S. Epidemiology of offending in learning disability. 2005. In: Riding, T., Swann, C., Swann, B. (Eds.), *The Handbook of Forensic Learning Disabilities*. Padstow: Radcliffe Publishing, pp. 15–30.

Kaplan, S.G. and Wheeler, E.G. 1983. Survival skills for working with potentially violent clients. *Social Case Work: The Journal of Contemporary Social Work*, 64(6):339–346.

Kingdon, A. Forensic learning disability nursing practice. 2010. In: Jukes, M. (Ed.), *Learning Disability Nursing Practice: Origins, Perspectives and Practice*. Huntingdon: Quay Books MA Healthcare Ltd., pp. 361–372.

Lindsay, W.R., Murphy, L., Smith, G., Murphy, D., Edwards, Z., Chittock, C., Grieve, A., and Young, S.J. 2004. The dynamic risk assessment and management system: An assessment of immediate risk of violence for individuals with offending and challenging behaviour. *Journal of Applied Research in Learning Disabilities*, 17:267–274.

Lindsay, W.R., Michie, A.M., Whitefield, E., Victoria, M., Grieve, A., and Carson, D. 2006. Response patterns on the questionnaire attitudes consistent with sex offending in groups of sex offenders with intellectual disabilities. *Journal of Applied Research in Intellectual Disabilities*, 19(1): 47–53.

Mason, T., Phipps, D., Melling, K. 2010. Forensic learning disability nursing role analysis. *British Journal of Learning Disabilities*, 39:121–129.

Mason, T. and Phipps, D. 2010. Forensic learning disability nursing skills and competencies: A study of forensic and non-forensic nurses. *Issues in Mental Health Nursing*, 31:708–715.

McBrien, J., Newton, L., and Banks, J. 2010. The development of a sex offender assessment and treatment service within a community learning disability team (the SHEALD project): Mapping and assessing risk. *Tizard Learning Disability Review*, 15(1):31–43.

McCarthy, M. and Thompson, D. 1994. *Sex and the 3 Rs: Rights, Responsibilities and Risks - A Sex Education Package For People Working With People with Learning Disabilities*. Brighton: Pavilion Publishing.

Mental Capacity Act. 2005. *Deprivation of Liberty Safeguards. Code of Practice to Supplement the Main Mental Capacity Act 2005 Code of Practice*. London: TSO.

Mental Health Act. 2007. *New Roles: Guidance for Approving Authorities and Employers on Approved Mental Health Professionals and Approved Clinicians 2008*. National Institute for Mental Health in England. London: TSO.

Murphy, G.H., Clare, I.C.H. 1996. Analysis of motivation in people with mild learning disabilities (mental handicap) who set fires. *Psychology Crime and Law*, 2:153–164.

Murphy, G. 1997. Assessing risk. In: Churchill, H., Brown, H., Craft., Horrocks, C., (Eds.), *There Are No Easy Answers: The Provision of Continuing Care to Adults with Learning Disabilities Who Sexually Abuse Others*. Chesterfield/Nottingham: ARC and NAPSAC, pp. 103–108.

National Institute of Clinical Effectiveness. 2012. Using control and restraint and compulsory treatment. Available at www.nice.org.uk/guidance/qualitystandards/service-user-experience-in-adult-mental–health/usingControlAndResrtraintAndCompulsoryTreatment.jsp (accessed August 23, 2014).

National Patient Safety Agency. 2007. *Healthcare Risk Assessment Made Easy.* London: National Patient Safety Executive.

Newton, L., Bishop, S., Ettey, J., and McBrien, J. 2011. The development of a sex offender assessment and treatment service within a community learning disability team (the SHEALD Project): part 2. *Tizard Learning Disability Review*, 16(3):6–16.

Nezu, C.M., Nezu, A.M., and Dudek, J. 1998. A cognitive behavioural model of assessment and treatment for intellectually disabled sex offenders. *Cognitive Behavioural Practice,* 5:25–64.

Nursing and Midwifery Council. 2010. *Standards for pre-registration nursing education.* London: NMC.

Pickard, M., Henry, J., and Yates, D. 2010. Working with violent offenders with learning disabilities. In: Chaplin, E., Henry, J, and Hardy, S. (Eds.), *Working with People with Learning Disabilities and Offending Behaviour: A Handbook.* Brighton: Pavilion Publishing, pp. 121–132.

Quinsey, V.L., Harris, G.T., and Rice, M.E., and Cormier, C.A. 2005. *Violent Offenders: Appraising and Managing Risk* (2nd ed.). Washington DC: American Psychological Association.

Riding, T. 2005. Sexual offending in people with learning disabilities. In: Riding, T., Swann, C., and Swann, B. (Eds.), *The Handbook of Forensic Learning Disabilities*. Padstow: Radcliffe Publishing, pp. 31–50.

Raesaenen, P., Hirvenoja, R., Hakko, H., and Vaeisaenen, E. 1994. Cognitive functioning ability of arsonists. *Journal of Forensic Psychiatry*, 5:615–620.

Rowe, D., Lopes, O. 2003. People with learning disabilities who have offended in law. In: Gates, B. (Ed.), *Learning Disabilities: Toward Inclusion* (4th ed.). Edinburgh: Churchill Livingstone, pp. 237–252.

Sturmey, P., McMurren, M. (Eds.). 2011 *Forensic Case Formulation*. Chichester: Wiley & Sons, pp. 3–33.

Talbot, J. 2011. Working with offenders. In: Atherton, H. and Crickmore, D. (Eds.), *Learning Disabilities*: *Toward Inclusion* (6th ed.). London: Churchill Livingstone Elsevier, pp. 339–356.

Wish, J.R., McCombs, K.F., and Edmonson, B. 1980. *The Socio-Sexual Knowledge and Attitudes Test*. Stoelig: Wood Dale.

Wolf, S.C. 1998. A model of sexual aggression/addiction (Special issues: the sexually unusual guide to understanding and helping). *Journal of Social Work and Human Sexuality*, 7:131–148.

World Health Organisation. 1992. *ICD – 10 Classifications of Mental and Behavioural Disorder: Clinical Descriptions and Diagnostic Guidelines*. Geneva: World Health Organisation.

Zarkowska, E., Clements, J. 1994. *Problem Behaviour and People with Severe Learning Disabilities; The S.T.A.R Approach* (2nd ed.). London: Chapman and Hall.

FURTHER READING

Bennett, C., Henry, J. 2010. Working with sexual offenders with learning disabilities. In: Chaplin, E., Henry, J., and Hardy, S. (Eds.), *Working with People with Learning Disabilities and Offending Behaviour: A Handbook*. Brighton: Pavilion Publishing, pp. 97–108.

Chaplin, E., Henry, J., and Hardy, S. (Eds.). 2010. *Working with People with Learning Disabilities and Offending Behaviour: A Handbook*. Brighton: Pavilion Publishing.

Craig, L.A., Lindsay, W.R., and Browne, K.D. (Eds.). 2010. *Assessment and Treatment of Sexual Offenders with Intellectual Disabilities: A Handbook.* Chichester: Wiley-Blackwell.

Fisher, M. and Scott, M. 2013. *Patient Safety and Managing Risk in Nursing.* London: Sage.

Murphy, R. and Wales, P. 2013. *Mental Health Law in Nursing.* London: Sage.

Sturmey, P. and McMurren, M. (Eds.). 2011. *Forensic Case Formulation*. Chichester: Wiley & Sons.

Swann, C. and Swann, B. (Eds.). 2005. *The Handbook of Forensic Learning Disabilities*. Padstow: Radcliffe Publishing.

USEFUL RESOURCES/ADDRESSES

Risk assessment

Sainsbury Centre for Mental Health: Helpful information and a list of useful contacts.

Department of Health: Positive practice outcomes: A handbook for professionals in the criminal justice system working with offenders with learning disabilities (2010)

Website on the treatment and care of offenders with a learning disability: http://www.bild .org.uk

Publications and training

British Institute of Learning Disabilities: http://www.bild.org.uk

Tizard Centre: http://www.kent.ac.uk/tizard/.

Guide to the Mental Health Act: http://.dh.gov.uk/en/Publications-statistics/Publications/ PublicationsPolicyAndGuidance/DH_088162

Mental health and learning disability: http://www.connects.org.uk/index.cfm?js=@dom=1

Abuse of people with learning disabilities

The Ann Craft Trust
Centre for Social Work
University of Nottingham
University Park
Nottingham NG7 2RD

8 Community learning disability nursing

Kay Mafuba

INTRODUCTION

Community learning disability nurses now work with a wide cross-section of people with learning disabilities and agencies. This chapter will explore current and changing roles of learning disability nurses working in the community. This will be contextualised within the Nursing and Midwifery Council for the United Kingdom (2010) and An Board Altranis (2005) standards for competence.

Dependent upon the local configuration of services, community learning disability nurses often occupy a number of new and exciting roles. Many work as specialist practitioners, and will work on time-limited interventions that can include personal and sexual relationships in learning disabilities, challenging behaviours, teaching direct carers, managing groups, dealing with loss and bereavement issues, working in multidisciplinary teams, assessing individuals, supporting clients, working as epilepsy specialists, facilitating self-advocacy groups, and helping people access mainstream services. This chapter will serve as a template for good care planning within the context of community learning disability teams, or where nurses are attached to local authorities or NHS Trusts.

Current health and social policy, for example, clinical commissioning, will inevitably make further demands on the development of the everyday practice of learning disability nurses working in the community. Seemingly the public health agenda is becoming central to the role of this group of health care workers. Implications for all fields of nursing and midwifery will be outlined with reference to the NMC (2010) and An Bord Alranais (2005) standards for competence.

This chapter will focus on the following issues:

- Key concepts and policies
  - What is community nursing?
  - What is community learning disability nursing?
  - Community learning disability nursing roles in the United Kingdom
- A brief history of community learning disability nursing
  - Policy frameworks in the United Kingdom
- Community learning disability nursing practice
  - Models of community care

NMC Competences and Competencies

Domain 1: Professional values - Field standard for competence and competencies – 1.1; 2.1; 3.1; 4.1.

Domain 2: Communication and interpersonal skills - Field standard for competence and competencies – 1.1; 2.1; 4.1.

Domain 3: Nursing practice and decision-making - Field standard for competence and competencies – 1.1; 3.1; 5.1; 8.1.

Domain 4: Leadership, management and team working - Field standard for competence and competencies – 1.1; 1.2; 2.1; 6.1; 6.2.

An Bord Altranais Competences and Indicators

Domain 1: Professional/ethical practice – 1.1.1; 1.1.2; 1.1.3; 1.1.5; 1.1.6; 1.1.8; 1.2.6.

Domain 2: Holistic approaches to care and integration of knowledge – 2.1.1; 2.1.2; 2.1.3; 2.1.4; 2.2.1; 2.31; 2.3.2; 2.2.4.

Domain 3: Interpersonal relationships – 3.1.2; 3.1.3; 3.2.1; 3.2.2.

Domain 4: Organisation and management of care – 4.1.2; 4.2.3; 4.3.1.

Domain 5: Personal and professional development – 5.1.3.

KEY CONCEPTS AND POLICIES

What is community nursing?

There is no universal definition of 'community nursing'. This is because the word community means different things to different people. To understand what 'community nursing' might mean, there is a need to understand the many definitions of what 'community' means. According to Laverack (2009), there are four main characteristics of a 'community', and these are the following

1. Geographical location of a place
2. Shared identities or interests of groups of people
3. Social interactions that bond people together
4. Common needs

The dialogical and operational definition of community nursing has tended to incorporate some or all of the four key characteristics (Chilton, 2012). What is important to note is the social construction of community nursing, which suggests that their roles may be defined and influenced by others (Kelly and Symonds, 2003).

What adds to the challenges of having a unified definition of community nursing is the range of specialities of community nursing practice. District nursing, health visiting, school nursing, community learning disability nursing, community mental health nursing, occupational health nursing, and practice nursing are all variations of community nursing (Butterworth, 1988). Within and between each of these nurses, there may be varied perceptions of their 'community nursing' roles.

What is community learning disability nursing?

Community learning disability nursing in the United Kingdom can be traced back to the 1970s. However, there is no legal or professional definition of community learning disability nursing. Furthermore, the four countries of the United Kingdom do not provide a working definition of community learning disability nursing.

The Royal College of Nursing has attempted to define community learning disability nursing (RCN, 1992). This definition has traditionally been accepted in practice, but it is constraining and no longer adequate. This is because the role of community learning disability nurses has evolved and continues to evolve in the practice setting (Boarder, 2002; Mobbs et al., 2002; and Barr, 2006). In addition, although no specific studies have investigated the drivers of these changes, recent reviews of policies for people with learning disabilities has led to the re-organisation of services across the United Kingdom (DH, 2001; Department of Health, Social Services and Public Safety, 2004; Scottish Executive, 2000). Furthermore, the *NHS Knowledge and Skills Framework* has outlined role expectations for community learning disability nurses in the United Kingdom (DH, 2004). The meaning of 'community learning disability nursing' is more likely to be influenced by the roles the nurse undertakes. These roles have evolved significantly in the recent past and will continue to evolve and increasingly focus on meeting the complex physical and health care needs of people with learning disabilities and their families (Barr, 2009). In this book, 'community learning disability nurse' refers to a Nursing and Midwifery Council 'learning disability nurse' RN5 or RNLD registrant whose role involves provision of nursing care to people with learning disabilities in a wide range of community settings. In current practice, the 'community learning disability nurse' works in a multidisciplinary team, holds a caseload, and admits and discharges people with learning disabilities who have health needs.

Community learning disability nursing roles in the United Kingdom

The creation of community learning disability nursing roles was partly influenced by deinstitutionalisation. Community learning disability nursing roles were first described in studies undertaken in the 1980s and 1990s (Mackay, 1989; Parahoo and Barr, 1994; Parahoo and Barr, 1996). Although these studies did not clearly describe community learning disability nursing roles at the time, they detailed the complex needs of people with learning disabilities who were supported in the community by the nurses. Broadly, these roles were focused on meeting the health and social care needs of people with learning disabilities living in the community.

Boarder (2002) in a study detailed the roles of community learning disability nurses as health maintenance; care planning; health promotion group work; team working; needs assessment; staff and carer training and support; advocacy; supporting community living, maintaining a place in the community; direct work with people with challenging behaviour, autism, mental illness, sensory, and communication difficulties; service development; working with play groups and schools; living skills development; personal relationship education and counseling; bereavement counseling; and research. In England, Mobbs et al. (2002) cites as the key roles of community learning disability nurses needs assessment and health screening, provision of advice and support, health monitoring, provision of direct nursing care, counseling, ongoing health promotion, direct clinical procedures, crisis intervention, care reviews, health education and teaching, respite care provision, child protection work, supporting access to leisure and recreation, and other direct work with people with

Paul is a young man with a moderate learning disability living in a staffed residential home. Paul has diabetes for which he is on insulin. He also has epilepsy for which he takes 200 mg QDS sodium valproate and 200mg QDS carbamazepine.

He has been prescribed antibiotics for a urinary tract infection, but he has refused to take his medication and refused to discuss any issues with care staff. Whilst on duty one day, you hear one of the care staff trying to explain the importance of the antibiotics to Paul. You then hear this staff member say, '*You are not having your coffee until you take your medication*'. Paul then takes the medication.

Some time later Paul is admitted to an acute medical ward in a general hospital to receive intravenous antibiotics and other treatments for his infection. He does not present any problems, but the busy nurses find it time-consuming to persuade him to take his medication. Paul tells the nurses that he would like to take his medication but needs constant reassurance. Subsequently, nurses crush his tablets and put them in his food without his knowledge.

a. Identify the roles of the community learning disability nurse in meeting Paul's health and health care needs.

b. Compare the roles you have identified with those that apply to your country in Table 8.1.

c. Identify relevant NMC/An Bord Altranais competencies that are applicable in this scenario.

learning disabilities. In a study undertaken in Northern Ireland, Barr (2006) identified as some of the key roles of community learning disability nurses health monitoring, provision of advice and support, direct clinical procedures, care reviews, needs assessment and health screening, education and training, care management/care coordination, health promotion, delivery of direct nursing case, counseling, respite care provision, child protection, and support with leisure and recreation. Mafuba and Gates (2013) have detailed the public health role of community learning disability nurses (see Chapter 4 and Table 8.1).

What is clear from these studies (Boarder, 2002; Mobbs et al., 2002; Barr, 2006; and Mafuba and Gates, 2013) is the increasing focus of the roles of community learning disability nurses in meeting the complex health care needs of people with learning disabilities. Brown et al. (2011), in a study of learning disability health liaison nurses, highlighted this increasing focus on meeting the continuing health and health care needs of people with learning disabilities.

These studies demonstrate significant developments in clarifying the roles and contributions to meeting the complex health and health care needs of people with learning disabilities by community learning disability nurses. However, a number of challenging issues need to be noted here. A study by Hames and Carlson (2006) have highlighted that local primary health care staff did not know about community learning disability teams. In addition, primary care staff lacked knowledge of the roles of local community learning disability teams, and there was confusion regarding the professionals within specialist community learning disability teams. Lack of clarity of the health promotion and health facilitation roles of community learning disability nurses was also highlighted.

Table 8.1 Community nursing roles

England	Northern Ireland	Wales
Child protection	Care management/care coordination	Advocacy
Clinical procedures	Counseling	Bereavement counseling
Counseling	Delivery of direct nursing care	Care planning
Crisis intervention	Direct clinical procedures; care reviews	Direct work (autism, mental illness, sensory and communication difficulties, challenging behaviour)
Education and teaching	Education and training	Health maintenance
Health monitoring	Health monitoring	Health promotion
Needs assessment and health screening	Health promotion	Living skills development
Nursing care	Needs assessment and health screening	Maintaining a place in the community
Ongoing health promotion	Provision of advice and support	Needs assessment
Other work with people with learning disabilities	Respite care provision; child protection	Personal relationships
Provision of advice and support	Support with leisure and recreation	Research
Provision of respite care	Other	Service development
Reviews		Sex education and counseling
Support with leisure and recreation		Staff and carer training, and support
		Supporting community living
		Team working
		Work with play groups and schools

Source: Mobbs, C. et al., *British Journal of Learning Disabilities*, 30(1):13–18, 2002; Barr, O., *Journal of Clinical Nursing*, 15:72–82, 2006; Boarder, J.H., *Journal of Learning Disabilities*, 6(3):281–296, 2002.

Agenda for Change (DH, 1999), *The NHS Knowledge and Skills Framework (NHS KSF)*, and *The Development Review Process* (DH, 2004) attempted to clarify the roles of community learning disability nurses in the United Kingdom. Mafuba (2013) noted a lack of consistency in role expectations for community learning disability nurses in the United Kingdom, suggesting that the evaluation of community learning disability nurses' roles through *Agenda for Change* had failed to adequately highlight the importance of these roles. In addition, Welbourne and Trevor (2000) suggested that there has been a failure to articulate the health contributions of community learning disability nurses; this is likely to have implications on community learning disability nursing roles.

Another important point is the constantly changing structures of services in which community learning disability nurses work. In the recent past there have been multiple organisational change agendas in the U.K. health system. These involved the creation of new structures, organisations, ideology, and roles (Ashburner et al,. 1996). The multi-agency nature of community learning disability nursing practice, with associated organisational cultural differences between health and social care may affect how community learning disability nurses undertake their roles. According to Davies (2002), differing professional and organisational cultural practices underlie day-to-day role enactment by health professionals. Scott et al., (2002) have argued that complex and multi-level organisational culture is inherent in the U.K. health system, and is likely to affect how community learning disability nurses undertake their roles.

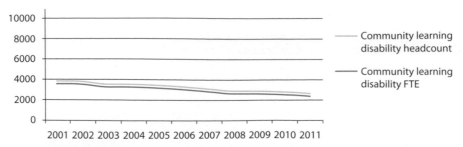

Figure 8.1 Community learning disability nurses in England. (From RCN. 2012. *The Community Nursing Workforce in England*. London: Royal College of Nursing, p. 6, 2012.)

While overall community nursing statistics and those for certain specific areas of community nursing practice in the last decade show gradual increase in relation to the re-orientation of health care toward preventative care, community learning disability nursing numbers have been characterised by a gradual and consistent long-term decline (RCN, 2012) (see Figure 8.1).

Although there are no clearly defined statutory roles, and limited studies regarding the roles of community learning disability nurses, important lessons emerge from literature. First, the complexity and increasingly specialised roles of the community learning disability nurses (Mobbs et al., 2002) need to be understood by the nurses themselves, employers, and other health and social care professionals. Second, community learning disability nurses make an important contribution to meeting the health and health care needs of people with learning disabilities in the community and primary care (Bollard, 2002; Marshall and Moore, 2003; and Barr et al., 1999). Third, other primary care professionals have positive regard for community learning disability nurses' roles in meeting the health and health care needs of people with learning disabilities (Stewart and Todd, 2001). However, the lack of in-depth research to evaluate and validate the roles of community learning disability nurses needs to be addressed to make clear their positive contributions to meeting the health and health care needs of people with learning disabilities in the community. What also needs to be addressed is the lack of clarity of community nursing roles among community learning disability nurses themselves, among other health care professionals, and among wider health and social care organisations (Boarder, 2002; Hames and Carlson, 2006; Mobbs et al., 2002; and Stewart and Todd, 2001). Making clear the roles of community learning disability nurses is important because a lack of role clarity may lead to confused and ambiguous expectations between health care professionals, resulting in reduced quality of care for people with learning disabilities in the community (Taylor, 1996).

A BRIEF HISTORY OF COMMUNITY LEARNING DISABILITY NURSING

Learning disability nurses' role in meeting the health needs of people with learning disabilities can be traced back to the 1960s (Jukes, 1994). In the 1980s, several attempts were made to identify and clarify the contribution of community learning disability nurses to health promotion (RCN, 1985). The Griffiths Report (Griffiths, 1988) and the NHS and Community Care Act (DH, 1990) emphasised the contribution of community learning disability nursing in meeting the health and health care needs of people with learning disabilities. However, there is a lack of clarity as to what this role entails and how the role is supposed to be carried out in practice.

As a result, this role has evolved differently across the United Kingdom (Mobbs et al., 2002; Boarder, 2002; Barr, 2006). In addition, health care and social care services have a differing understanding of the role and contribution of community learning disability nurses to meeting the health and health care needs of people with learning disability in the community (McGarry and Arthur, 2001).

Recent studies have highlighted the professional roles of community learning disability nurses, such as advocacy (Gates, 1994; Jukes, 1994; Mansell and Harris, 1998; Stewart and Todd, 2001; Alaszewski, 1977; Mobbs et al. 2002; Llewellyn and Northway, 2007) and generic community nursing roles (Holloway, 2004; Melville et al., 2005; Thornton, 1996; Thornton, 1997; Boarder, 2002; Powell et al., 2004).

Policy frameworks in the United Kingdom

The policy agenda for the provision of health care for people with learning disabilities in the United Kingdom and the Republic of Ireland can be traced back to the beginning of the twentieth century (see Table 8.2). In England, the Mental Deficiency Act 1913 provided a distinct legal identity for people with learning disabilities.

Negative reports regarding segregated health care provision for people with learning disabilities (Department of Health and Social Security, 1969; Morris 1969) led to a new policy direction through

Table 8.2 Community care policy development timeline in the United Kingdom and the Republic of Ireland

Year	United Kingdom	Year	Republic of Ireland
1913	Mental Deficiency Act	1945	The Mental Treatment Act 1945
1957	Royal Commission on the Law Relating to Mental Illness and Mental Deficiency 1954–57	1947–2004	Government of Ireland - Health Acts 1947 to 2004
1963	Health and Welfare: The Development of Community Care (Ministry of Health)	1990	Needs and Abilities: A Policy for the Intellectually Disabled (Department of Health [DOH])
1969	Report of the Committee of Inquiry into Allegations of Ill-Treatment and Other Irregularities (Howe Report)		
1971	Better Services for the Mentally Handicapped (DHSS White Paper) Social Services Departments established (England and Wales) Social Work Departments established (Scotland)		
1979	Report of the Committee of Enquiry into Mental Handicap Nursing and Care (Jay Report)	2001	Quality and Fairness: A Health System for You (Department of Health and Children)
1981	Care in the Community (DHSS White Paper)		
1984	Registered Homes Act	2004	The Education of Persons with Special Educational Needs Act (Government of Ireland)
1989	Government Objectives for Community Care (DHSS White Paper)	2008	Government of Ireland - Mental Health Act 2008
1990	NHS and Community Care Act	2005	Disability Act (Government of Ireland)
		2007	Government of Ireland - Health Act 2007

(*continued*)

Table 8.2 Community care policy development timeline in the United Kingdom and the Republic of Ireland (*continued*)

Year	United Kingdom	Year	Republic of Ireland
2000	The Same as You (Scottish Executive)	2006	A Vision for Change (Ireland's national mental health policy framework) (Department of Health and Children)
2001	Valuing People (DH White Paper)	2009	Vision Statement for Intellectual Disability in Ireland for the 21st Century (National Federation of Volunatry Bodies)
2002	Review of Mental Health and Learning Disabilities (Northern Ireland) (Department of Health and Social Services)	2011	Time to Move on from Congregated Settings: A Strategy for Community Inclusion (Health Services Executive)
2003	Fulfilling the Promises (Welsh Assembly)	2012	Your Voice, Your Choice (National Disability Authority)
		2012	Value for Money and Policy Review of Disability Services in Ireland (Department of Health)
		2013	National Standards for Residential Services for Children and Adults with Disabilities
2012	Health and Social Care Act (England)	2006–2015	Towards 2016: Ten-Year Framework Social Partnership Agreement 2006-2015 (Department of the Taoiseach)

Better Services for the Mentally Handicapped (Department of Health and Social Security, 1971). This policy shift had two significant effects in relation to the roles of community learning disability nurses. The first effect was the shift of service provision from institutions to the community. The second effect was that learning disability nurses had to realign their roles with the new models of service provision based in the community. As de-institutionalisation gathered pace in the 1980s and 1990s, community learning disability nursing roles focusing on meeting the health needs of people with learning disabilities in the community began to emerge.

Health Services for People with Learning Disabilities (Mental Handicap) (NHS Executive, 1992) highlighted the need for people with learning disabilities to access generic health care services. It could be argued that this position contributed to the development of some community learning disability nursing roles. *Signposts for Success* (NHS Executive, 1998) outlined care pathways for people with learning disabilities in mainstream services. This was an acknowledgement that people with learning disabilities were experiencing poor access to services in the NHS. The emphasis was on ensuring that people with health care needs for learning disabilities were met through mainstream services. However, the policy document recognised the need for continued specialist health and health care provision in areas such as mental health, epilepsy, and complex needs.

Another important policy development was *Once a Day* (NHS Executive, 1999). This policy highlighted the challenges people with learning disabilities faced in accessing health services. The policy also provided guidance for primary health care teams on how support could be provided to people with learning disabilities in order for them to access health promotion and health screening services through primary care services.

Chapter 6 of *Valuing People: A New Strategy for Learning Disability for the 21st Century* (DH, 2001) highlighted the need to improve the health of people with learning disabilities in

England and Wales (*The Same as You* in Scotland) (Scottish Executive, 2000). The complexity of the health care needs of people with learning disabilities are acknowledged, and the inadequacies of existing models of health care provision for people with learning disabilities in generic community health care settings highlighted. In Scotland, the *Health Needs Assessment Report: People with Learning Disabilities in Scotland* (NHS Health Scotland, 2004) highlighted the needs of people with learning disabilities and provided guidance to health care professionals on how these could be met.

A number of initiatives relevant to policy implementation and community nursing roles of learning disability nurses were proposed in *Valuing People* (DH, 2001). To improve the implementation of health policy initiatives and access to services for people with learning disabilities, health action planning was introduced (DH 2002; DH 2009). Health facilitation and health liaison were also introduced (DH, 2001). These policy initiatives affected the community nursing roles of community learning disability nurses.

COMMUNITY LEARNING DISABILITY NURSING PRACTICE

Models of community care

Community nursing is at the heart of this model of care and in response community nursing services have developed into complex, multi-disciplinary teams. The work of nurses in the community encompasses the promotion of health, healing, growth and development, as well as the prevention and treatment of disease, illness, injury and disability.

(RCN, 2012, p. 1)

The future of community learning disability nursing

The current structures of community health and health care services in the United Kingdom and Ireland are complex and present significant challenges on how community learning disability nurses meet the health and health care needs of people with learning disabilities. The current fragmentation of health services for people with learning disabilities between primary care and specialist learning disability services leads to unnecessary philosophical and inter-agency tensions. As the shift toward '*upstreaming*' (RCN, 2012) and more preventive health in the United Kingdom gathers pace, the public health roles of community learning disability nurses need to be made more explicit in the organisations in which such nurses work. Clarity about, and development of new models of how community learning disability nurses will enact their community nursing roles in the future needs to have a strategic impetus (see Figure 8.2).

Understanding the distribution of the population and morbidity rates of people with learning disabilities is becoming more important for community learning disability nurses to deliver targeted and appropriate community services for people with learning disabilities. The importance of the accuracy of demographic information on the roles of community learning disability nurses in the future cannot be over-emphasised for a number of reasons. First, demographic intelligence is important in the investigation and diagnosis of the epidemiological problems that affect people with learning disabilities. In addition, this would be useful in facilitating prioritisation of health programmes for people with learning disabilities. Furthermore, this would enable better targeting of community health initiatives. Demographic intelligence would also be useful in monitoring and evaluating the impact of health programmes and strategies targeted at the population of people

John is a 34-year-old male with moderate learning disabilities. He was observed experiencing full body convulsive movements whilst at his work placement. An ambulance was called, because the day care workers had not previously witnessed him having a tonic–clonic seizure. No medication was administered, as the seizure had ended by the time paramedics arrived. John has a diagnosis of epilepsy and is known to experience tonic–clonic seizures. On average, he has one seizure every three months with a duration of approximately 30 seconds to 1 minute, usually late in the day just prior to going to bed at 10:30 p.m. His epilepsy was diagnosed when he was a child and he has been successfully managed on sodium valproate 500 mg twice daily and carbamazepine 200 mg thrice daily for the past five years. This has been assessed as providing him with the best seizure control. Since his father died three months ago from a myocardial infarction, John now lives with his mother. He is able to communicate verbally and generally demonstrates an ability to understand information given to him. Information needs to be explained appropriately, and he needs to be given time to consider it. He also needs to be given an opportunity to ask any questions. He is unable to read or write. Since his referral to the Community Learning Disability Team (CTLD) his mother reports that he has been very confused and agitated and keeps saying he 'does not know what is happening' and this is 'just like what happened to Dad'. He is reported to have been displaying a lack of motivation, disengagement with usual company, general restlessness, and a disturbed sleep pattern over the last four to six weeks. John is prescribed no other medication other than anticonvulsants.

- Explore the role of the community learning disability nurse in meeting John's health and health care needs.
- Explore and justify any assessment you might need to carry out, using a recognised assessment tool(s). You will need to consider and highlight the role(s) of other professionals in the assessment process.
- Using the information obtained during the assessment process, draw up a health action plan. You will need to clearly provide a rationale for your approach to health action planning (see Chapter 4). You will need to clearly identify John's needs, proposed interventions, and expected outcomes. You will need to clearly identify the role of the multi-disciplinary team.
- Identify relevant NMC/An Bord Altranais competencies that are applicable in this case.

with learning disabilities. Finally, demographic intelligence is likely to be key to ensuring that health programmes and strategies for people with learning disabilities are evidence-based.

The *'health liaison'* role of community learning disability nurses in the delivery of health services for people with learning disabilities is becoming increasingly important (Powell et al., 2004). There is evidence indicating that this role is increasingly being based in acute services (Brown et al., 2011). There is need for this role to be more prominent in the delivery of health services for people with learning disabilities by community learning disability nurses.

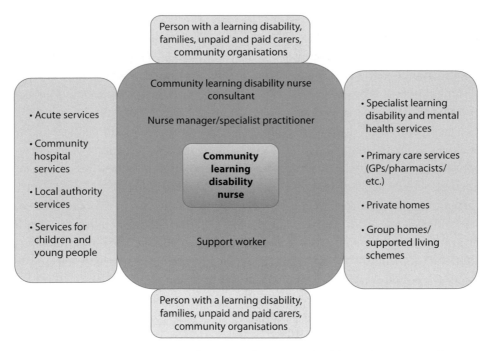

Figure 8.2 Model of community care. (From Elliott, L. et al., 2012. *Study of the Implementation of a New Community Health Nurse Role in Scotland.* Edinburgh: Scottish Government Social Research, p. 12, 2012.)

Community learning disability nurses' roles in meeting the health and health care needs of people with learning disabilities are more complex and include health care delivery, health protection, health prevention, health surveillance, research, and leadership, in addition to the public health roles identified in previous studies (Mafuba, 2013). However, the lack of strategic clarity of community learning disability nurses' roles in meeting the health and health care needs of people with learning disabilities needs to be addressed. A lack of role clarity for community learning disability nurses may lead to role confusion and ineffective implementation of health services for people with learning disabilities (Fyson, 2002; Ross, 2001). Ensuring strategic role clarity of community learning disability nurses could result in improved flexibility and responsiveness to the health and health care needs of people with learning disabilities in both primary and acute services.

There is an increasing acceptance of the importance of the health facilitation role of community learning disability nurses among other professionals within primary and acute healthcare settings. This development has evidently enhanced the roles of community learning disability nurses. The increasing genericisation of the delivery of health care for people with learning disabilities and the shift from treatment to preventive health indicates a need for community learning disability nurses to focus on enhancing their health facilitation knowledge and skills. This change in roles has been noted before (Barr, 2006), and is inevitable and unavoidable. It is clear that supporting people with learning disabilities to access acute and other mainstream services is becoming an important role for community learning disability nurses.

Community learning disability nurses are expected to work with other primary health and social care agencies to reduce health inequalities by facilitating access to health services, including public health services. This will require community learning disability nurses to establish partnerships working with local primary care services and work in collaboration with various primary care agencies to mitigate the impact of health inequalities on people with learning disabilities. However, to be effective in working in partnership and in collaboration with other agencies, community learning disability nurses need to be aware that the health needs of people with learning disabilities may not necessarily be a priority for other agencies. In addition, this will require that community learning disability nurses provide leadership in enhancing and improving access to generic health services, promoting inclusion in generic public health services, preventing ill health, promoting equality of access, improving the quality of life of people with learning disabilities, and working to reduce the adverse impacts of the circumstances of individuals with learning disabilities.

For '*effective collaboration*', community learning disability nurses need to engage with health action planning, health facilitation, and health liaison. Castledine (2002) has noted that community learning disability nurses could play a significant role in the development of coordinated approaches to delivering health services for people with learning disabilities. In addition, Jukes (2002) has argued that community learning disability nurses could be key in developing appropriate pathways and protocols for access to health and health care for people with learning disabilities. These roles need to focus on the development of health action plans, effective systems of liaison, and the development of learning environments for other professionals, agencies, and people with learning disabilities and their carers.

CONCLUSION

The variation of the public health roles discussed here demonstrate the intricacies of how public health services are organised, and the challenges that people with learning disabilities face when accessing these services. The health facilitation and professional advocacy roles of community learning disability nurses highlight their responsibility to challenge public health services to improve accessibility for people with learning disabilities. In addition, community learning disability nurses need to collaborate and work in partnership with others to fulfil these roles (Broughton and Thompson, 2000). To work effectively as agents of change, community learning disability nurses need to have '*leadership*' skills at all levels. Community learning disability nurses will need to assume '*leadership roles*' in implementing preventive health programs, developing appropriate services, planning, and develop shared care with primary and secondary health services. These leadership skills are important to influence others and facilitate the collaboration that is essential to developing appropriate public health pathways and implementation of public health policies for people with learning disabilities. The importance of the leadership roles of community learning disability nurses in the development of appropriate services for people with learning disabilities have been highlighted previously (Powell et al., 2004).

REFERENCES

Alaszewski, A.M. 1977. Suggestions for re-organisation of nurse training and improvement of patient care in a hospital for the mentally handicapped. *Journal of Advanced Nursing*, 2(5):461–477.

An Bord Altranais. 2005. *Requirements and Standards for Nurse Registration Education Programmes* (3rd ed.). Dublin: An Bord Altranais.

Ashburner, L., Ferlie, E., and FitzGerald, L. 1996. Organisational transformation and top-down change: The case of the NHS. *British Journal of Management*, 7(1):1–16.

Barr, O. 2009. Community learning disability nursing. In: Sines, D., Saunders, M., and Forbes-Burford, J. (Eds.), *Community Health Care Nursing* (4th ed.). Chichester: Wiley-Blackwell.

Barr, O. 2006. The evolving role of community nurses for people with learning disabilities: Changes over an 11-year period. *Journal of Clinical Nursing*, 15:72–82.

Barr, O., Gilgunn, J., Kane, T., and Moore, G. 1999. Health screening for people with learning disabilities by a community learning disabilities nursing service in Northern Ireland. *Journal of Advanced Nursing*, 29(6):1482–1491.

Boarder, J.H. 2002. The perceptions of experienced community learning disability nurses of their roles and ways of working. *Journal of Learning Disabilities*, 6(3):281–296.

Bollard, M. 2002. Health promotion and learning disabilities. *Health Education*, 16(27):47–55.

Brown, M., MacArthur, J., McKechanie, A., Mack, S., Hayes, M., and Fletcher, J. 2011. Learning disability liaison nursing services in south-east Scotland: A mixed-methods impact and outcome study. *Journal of Intellectual Disability Research*. doi: 10.1111/j.1365-2788.2011.01511.x.

Butterworth, T. 1988. Breaking the boundaries. *Nursing Times*, 84:47.

Castledine, G. 2002. The important aspects of nurse specialist roles. *British Journal of Nursing*, 11(5):350.

Chilton, S. 2012. Nursing in a community environment, In: Chilton, S., Bain, H., Clarridge, A., and Melling, K, *A Textbook of Community Nursing*. London: Hodder & Stoughton.

Davies, H.T.O. 2002. Understanding organisational culture in reforming the NHS. *Journal of the Royal Society of Medicine*, 95(3):140–142.

Department of Health and Social Security. 1969. *Report of the Committee of Inquiry into Allegations of Ill-Treatment of Patients and Other Irregularities at the Ely Hospital, Cardiff* (Cmnd 3975). London: HMSO.

Department of Health and Social Security. 1971. *Better Services for the Mentally Handicapped* (Cmnd 4683). London: HMSO.

Department of Health, Social Services and Public Safety. 2004. *Equal Lives*: Draft Report of *Learning Disability Committee*. Belfast: Department of Health, Social Services and Public Safety.

DH. 1990. *NHS and Community Care Act*. London: HMSO.

DH. 1992. *The Health of the Nation: A Strategy for Health in England*. London: HMSO.

DH. 1995. *The Health of the Nation: A Strategy for People with Learning Disabilities*. London: HMSO.

DH. 1999. *Agenda for Change: Modernising the NHS Pay System*. London: Department of Health.

DH. 2001. *Valuing People. A New Strategy for the 21st Century*. London: TSO.

DH. 2002. *Action for Health: Health Action Plans and Health Facilitation*. London: Department of Health.

DH. 2004. *The NHS Knowledge and Skills Framework (NHS KSF) and the Development Review Process*. London: Department of Health

DH. 2007. *Good Practice Guide in Learning Disabilities Nursing*. London: Department of Health.

DH. 2009. *Health Action Planning and Health Facilitation for People with Learning Disabilities: Good Practice Guidance*. London: Department of Health.

DHSS. 1971. *Better Services for the Mentally Handicapped* (Cmnd 4683). London: HMSO.

DHSSPSNI. 2002. *Investing for Health*. Belfast: DHSSPSNI.

Elliott, L., Kennedy, C., Rome, A., Cameron, S., Currie, M., Pow, J., and Mackenzie-Baker, M. 2012. *Study of the Implementation of a New Community Health Nurse Role in Scotland*. Edinburgh: Scottish Government Social Research.

Fyson, R.E. 2002. 'Defining the Boundaries: The Implementation of Health and Social Care Policies for Adults with Learning Disabilities'. Unpublished PhD thesis, University of Nottingham.

Gates, B. 1994. *Advocacy: A Nurses' Guide*. London: Scutari Press.

Griffiths, R. 1988. *Community Care: Agenda for Action. Report for the Secretary of State for Social Services*. London: HMSO.

Hames, A. and Carlson, T. 2006. Are primary care staff aware of the role of community teams in relation to health promotion and health facilitation? *British Journal of Learning Disabilities*, 34(1):6–10.

Holloway, D. 2004. Ethical dilemmas in community learning disabilities nursing: What helps nurses resolve ethical dilemmas that result from choices made by people with learning disabilities? *Journal of Learning Disabilities*, 8(3):283–298.

Jukes, M. 1994. Development of the community nurse in learning disability. *British Journal of Nursing*, 3(15):779–783.

Kelly, A. and Symonds, A. 2003. *The Social Construction of Community Nursing*. Basingstoke: Palgrave MacMillan.

Laverack, G. 2009. *Public Health: Power, Empowerment and Professional Practice* (2nd ed.). Basingstoke: Palgrave MacMillan.

Llewellyn, P. and Northway, R. 2007. The views and experiences of learning disability nurses concerning their advocacy education. *Nurse Education Today*, 27(8):955–963.

Mackay, T. 1989. A community nursing service analysis. *Journal of Intellectual Disability Research*, 40(4):336–347.

Mafuba, K. 2013. Public health: Community learning disability nurses' perception and experience of their role. Unpublished PhD thesis, University of West London.

Mafuba, K. and Gates, B. 2013. An investigation into the public health roles of community learning disability nurses. *British Journal Learning Disability*. doi: 10.1111-bld.12071.

Mansell, I. and Harris, P. 1998. Role of the registered nurse learning disability within community support teams for people with learning disabilities. *Journal of Learning Disabilities for Nursing, Health and Social Care*, 2(4):190–194.

Marshall, D. and Moore, G. 2003. Obesity in people with intellectual disabilities: The impact of nurse-led health screenings and health promotion activities. *Journal of Advanced Nursing*, 41(2):147–153.

McGarry J. and Arthur A. 2001. Informal caring in late life: A qualitative study of the experiences of older carers. *Journal of Advanced Nursing*, 33(2):182–189.

Melville, C.A., Finlayson, J., Cooper, S. A., Allan, L., Robinson, N., Burns, E., Martin, G., and Morrison J. 2005. Enhancing primary healthcare services for adults with intellectual disabilities. *Journal of Intellectual Disability Research*, 49(3):190–198.

Mental Deficiency Act 1913. London: HMSO

Mobbs, C., Hadley, S., Wittering, R., and Bailey, N.M. 2002. An exploration of the role of the community nurse, learning disability, in England. *British Journal of Learning Disabilities*, 30(1):13–18.

Morris, P. 1969. *Put Away*. London: Routledge and Kegan Paul.

NHS Executive. 1992. *Health Services for People with Learning Disabilities (Mental Handicap)*. London: Department of Health.

NHS Executive. 1998. *Signposts for Success in Commissioning and Providing Health Services for People with Learning Disabilities.* London: DH.

NHS Executive. 1999. *Once a Day*. London: HMSO.

NHS Health Scotland. 2004. *Health Needs Assessment Report: People with Learning Disability in Scotland*. Glasgow: NHS Health Scotland.

NMC. 2010 *Standards for Pre-Registration Nurse Education*. London: Nursing and Midwifery Council.

Parahoo, K. and Barr, O. 1996. Community mental handicap nursing services in Northern Ireland: A profile of clients and selected working practices. *Journal of Clinical Nursing*, 5(4):221–228

Parahoo, K. and Barr, O. 1994. Job satisfaction of community nurses working with people with a mental handicap. *Journal of Advanced Nursing*, 20(6):1046–1055.

Powell, H., Murray, G., and McKenzie, K. 2004. Staff perceptions of community learning disability nurses' role. *Nursing Times*, 100(19):40-42.

RCN. 1985. *The Role and Function of the Domiciliary Nurse in Mental Handicap*. London: Royal College of Nursing.

RCN. 1992. *The Role and Function of the Domiciliary Community Nursing for People with a Learning Disability*. London: Royal College of Nursing.

RCN. 2012. *The Community Nursing Workforce in England*. London: Royal College of Nursing.

Ross, J. 2001. 'Role Identification: An Impediment to Effective Core Primary Healthcare Teamwork'. Wellington: Victoria University of Wellington (Unpublished MA thesis).

(Online). Available at http://researcharchive.vuw.ac.nz/handle/10063/85 (accessed December 30, 2008).

Scott, T. Mannion, R., Davies, H.T.O., and Marshall, M.N. 2002. Implementing culture change in healthcare—theory and practice. *International Journal of Quality in Healthcare*, 15(2):111–118.

Scottish Executive. 2000. *The Same as You*. Edinburgh: Scottish Executive.

Stewart, D. and Todd, M. 2001. Role and contribution of nurses for learning disabilities: A local study in a county of Oxford-Anglia region. *British Journal of Learning Disabilities*, 29(4):145–150.

Taylor, J.C. 1996. Systems thinking boundaries and role clarity. *Clinical Performance and Quality Healthcare*, 4(4):198–199.

Thornton, C. 1996. A focus group inquiry into the perceptions of primary healthcare teams and the provision of healthcare for adults with learning disability living in the community. *Journal of Advanced Nursing*, 23(6)1168–1176.

Thornton, C. 1997. Practice. Meeting the healthcare needs of people with learning disabilities. *Nursing Times*, 93(20):52–54.

Welbourne, T.M. and Trevor, C.O. 2000. The roles of departmental and position power in job evaluation. *Academy of Management Journal*, 43(4):761–771.

FURTHER READING

Chilton, S., Bain, H., Clarridge, A., and Melling, K. 2012. *A Textbook of Community Nursing*. London: Hodder & Stoughton.

Evans, D., Coutsaftiki, D., and Fathers, C.P. 2011. *Health Promotion and Public Health for Nursing Students*. Exeter: Learning Matters Ltd.

Hubley, J. and Copeman, J. with Woodall, J. 2013. *Practical Health Promotion* (2nd ed.). Cambridge: Polity Press.

Jukes, M. (Ed.) 2009. *Learning Disability Nursing Practice—Origins, Perspectives and Practice*. London: Quay Books.

Kelly, A. and Symonds, A. 2003. *The Social Construction of Community Nursing*. Basingstoke: Palgrave MacMillan.

Sines, D., Saunders, M., and Forbes-Burford, J. (Eds.). 2013. *Community Health Care Nursing*. (4th ed.). Chichester: Wiley-Blackwell.

Welbourne, T.M. and Trevor, C.O. 2000. The roles of departmental and position power in job evaluation. *Academy of Management Journal*, 43(4)761–771.

USEFUL RESOURCES

An Bord Altranais: http://www.nursingboard.ie/en/reqs_stds_reg.aspx

BILD: http://www.bild.org.uk/

Contact a Family: http://www.cafamily.org.uk/medical-information/conditions/

Enable Scotland: http://www.enable.org.uk/Pages/Enable_Home.aspx

Foundation for People with Learning Disabilities: http://www.learningdisabilities.org.uk/

General Medical Council: http://www.gmc-uk.org/learningdisabilities/

Inclusion Ireland: http://www.inclusionireland.ie/

Intellectual Disability Info Web Pages: http://www.intellectualdisability.info/

Learning Disabilities Observatory: https://www.improvinghealthandlives.org.uk/publications

Mencap: http://www.mencap.org.uk/

Mencap Northern Ireland: http://www.mencap.org.uk/northern-ireland

Mencap Wales: http://www.mencap.org.uk/wale

Nursing and Midwifery Council: http://standards.nmc-uk.org/Pages/Welcome.aspx

9 Challenging and distressed behaviour in people with learning disabilities: The role of learning disability nursing

Bob Gates and Kay Mafuba

INTRODUCTION

The support of people with learning disabilities who present with challenging or distressed behaviour by learning disability nurses has never been so important. This chapter will promote the unique contribution that learning disability nursing can provide in promoting holistic support, whilst drawing from a strong value and professional base. Understanding of challenging or distressed behaviour in people with learning disabilities is problematic, and managing such behaviours has been the subject of much past and recent controversy. Recent controversy has included inappropriate use of medication; there remains a persistent problem of over-prescribing psychoactive

This chapter will focus on the following issues:

- A note on terminology
- Prevalence of behavioural difficulties
- Understanding behaviour from differing theoretical perspectives
  - Psychodynamic, behaviourist, and humanistic theory
  - What divides the theorists?
  - The philosophical view
  - Internal and external forces
  - The concept of self
  - Awareness and consciousness
  - Thoughts, feelings, and behaviour
  - The past, present, and future

- The psychodynamic model
  - Object relations theory
  - Product and author
  - External and internal worlds
  - All behaviour is logical
  - Emotional development
  - Application and limitation
- Behaviourism
  - Operant conditioning
  - The application of behaviourism
- The humanistic model
- Methods of measurement
- Therapeutic approaches to behavioural difficulties
  - Psychotherapeutic approaches
  - Behavioural approaches
  - Humanistic approaches
  - Positive behaviour support
  - Other therapeutic approaches

medication for this population (Reiss and Aman, 1998), along with wholly inappropriate and, at times, illegal, means of managing people who have supposedly presented with challenging behaviours (Flynn, 2012). In relation to medication it is imperative that before anything else is done, an assessment is undertaken to identify the reasons for a person's challenging behaviour and to exclude physical or mental ill health. Even when medication is used, it should only be given with the person's consent (or if the person is a child, the parents' consent). In the case of an adult lacking capacity to make a decision about taking medication, it may be administered as long as the decision is made within the framework of a 'best interests' decision (see Chapter 5).

The term 'challenging behaviour' was most likely introduced into the United Kingdom from North America during the 1980s. It was a term originally used to describe behaviours in people with learning disabilities that were, up until this point, referred to as behavioural problems. And therein lies a central problem, because over the years all behaviours exhibited by people with learning disabilities that present as remotely 'testing' have come to be called 'challenging behaviour'; this now, wrongly, seems to incorporate distressed behaviours. Distressed behaviours are not challenging behaviours in the sense that they require some kind of special intervention; they are 'normal' behavioural responses to stressful situations. Examples include being in a hospital setting, and not wanting a doctor to examine someone, or administer an injection, or being unco-operative when a dentist is trying to undertake an oral examination. Behavioural responses to such situations might include shouting, head banging, biting, scratching, and spitting. Similarly, in other settings, they might include a similar behavioural response to abuse, bullying, boredom, physical pain (e.g., toothache, migraine, appendicitis), or discomfort. The point being made here is that some behavioural responses should be considered normal and should not be described as challenging behaviour in the special sense that it is used for that group of people who present with behavioural management issues. Learning disability nurses have a clear role in educating health and social care professionals about the hazards of using inappropriate terminology. Challenging behaviour is reported to negatively affect a variety of quality-of-life outcomes for individuals with learning disabilities (Lloyd and Kennedy, 2014). In a recent paper a useful and contemporary review about the current status of research relating to the assessment and treatment of challenging behaviour for people with learning disabilities has been presented (Lloyd and Kennedy, 2014). They outline the functions of challenging behaviour, functional behaviour assessment, and reinforcement-based interventions. These issues will be outlined in more detail in the final section of this chapter. The management and support of individuals with learning disabilities who present with challenging behaviours is of critical importance to learning disability nurses, and this is because the collective professional integrity of this specialist field of nursing can easily be contaminated by the few who choose not to practice within an ethical and legal framework of nursing practice. That is why this chapter focuses on the knowledge and practical skills that such nurses will require to meet the needs of people with learning disabilities who present with challenging or distressed behaviours; this will be contextualised within the Nursing and Midwifery Council for the United Kingdom (2010) and An Bord Altranais (2005) standards for competence.

Competences

NMC Competences and Competencies

Domain 1: Professional values - Field standard competence and competencies – 1.1; 2.1; 3.1; 4.1.

Domain 2: Communication and interpersonal skills - Field standard competence and competencies – 3.1; 4.1.

Domain 3: Nursing practice and decision making - Field standard competence and competencies – 1.1; 3.1; 5.1; 8.1.

Domain 4: Leadership, management and team working - Field standard competence and competencies – 1.2; 2.1; 6.1; 6.2.

An Bord Altranais Competences and Indicators

Domain 1: Professional/ethical practice – 1.1.2; 1.1.3; 1; 1.1.5; 1.1.6; 1.1.7; 1.1.8; 1.2.4; 1.2.5; 1.2.6.

Domain 2: holistic approaches to care and the integration of knowledge – 2.1.1; 2.1.2; 2.1.3; 2.1.4; 2.2.1; 2.2.3; 2.2.4; 2.3.1; 2.3.3; 2.3.4; 2.4.1; 2.4.2.

Domain 3: Interpersonal relationships – 3.1.1; 3.1.2; 3.1.3; 3.2.1; 3.2.2.

Domain 4: Organisation and management of care – 4.1.3; 4.1.4.

Domain 5: Personal and professional development – 5.1.1; 5.1.2; 5.1.3.

A NOTE ON TERMINOLOGY

An immediate problem that learning disability nurse practitioners face in studying or managing challenging behaviour (behavioural difficulties is our preferred term) is being able to adequately operationalise its meaning. The term '*challenging behaviour*' has now long replaced the previously used term 'behavioural problems' or 'behavioural difficulties'. The problem with this is that the term 'challenging behaviour' has become conflated with a wide variety of other behavioural manifestations, making the isolation of people with specific behavioural difficulties complex. Current-day usage of the term 'challenging behaviour' is extremely sensitive to overtones of '*political correctness*'. It is suggested that reasons for concern for appropriate terminology lay in the potential for some terms to evoke powerful and negative imagery (Hastings and Remington, 1993). This, however, has a potential corollary, which is that a range of other behaviours are also becoming known as challenging behaviour. Of these and most problematic is 'distressed behaviour', which is often demonstrated in strange or unfamiliar settings or toward people not well known—and behaviour that is not challenging in the sense that some kind of intervention is required. These manifestations are 'normal' behavioural responses to stressful situations. Examples have already been given and primarily represent a communication of distress when someone lacks the necessary range of verbal communication skills to express his or her distress. This can be particularly so for people with profound learning disabilities and complex needs, and those who lay on the spectrum of autistic conditions.

A number of definitions are now explored that identify the scale of difference about what is meant when nurses or researchers refer to challenging behaviour, as far back as the mid-1980s Blunden and Allen (1987) maintained the following

> **We have decided to adopt the term challenging behaviour rather than problem behaviour or severe problem behaviour since it emphasises that such behaviours represent challenges to services rather than problems which individuals with learning difficulties in some way carry round with them.**
>
> *(Blunden and Allen, 1987, p. 14)*

Later the Department of Health described challenging behaviours as the following

> **People with learning disabilities who have challenging behaviours form an extremely diverse group, including individuals with all levels of learning disability, many different sensory or physical impairments and presenting quite different kinds of challenges. The group includes, for example, people with mild or borderline disability who have been diagnosed as mentally ill and who enter the criminal justice system for crimes such as arson or sexual offences; as well as people with profound learning disability, often with sensory handicaps and other physical health problems, who injure themselves, for example by repeated head banging or eye poking.**
>
> *(DOH, 1992)*

Finally, Emerson (1995) helped to focus the nature of challenging behaviour and described it as the following

> **. . . culturally abnormal behaviour of such an intensity, frequency or duration that the physical safety of the person or others is likely to be placed in serious jeopardy, or behaviour which is likely to seriously limit use of, or result in the person being denied access to, ordinary community facilities**
>
> *(Emerson, 1995)*

All of these definitions, even the latter, are very broad, and that is why in this chapter we focus upon what we refer to as behavioural difficulties, and we will consistently make a distinction between behavioural difficulties and distressed behaviours. And whereas these definitions are by no means exhaustive of the plethora that are currently found in the literature, they do serve to illustrate the differing ways in which the term 'challenging behaviour' is used. Definitions concerning challenging behaviour can be grouped into two distinct categories. The first uses the term to identify a collection of behaviours and a state of being that challenge service providers. This group could be said to be comprised of people with learning disabilities with additional disabilities, or handicaps, who may or may not display behavioural difficulties. The second usage of the term appears to be reserved for those people with learning disabilities who predominantly demonstrate behavioural difficulties. An example here is a study by Scorer et al. (1993) that sought to evaluate a pilot project support team and used the term 'challenging behaviour', even though it is clear from the case studies presented that each of the individuals had a history of behavioural difficulties. Another study by Chamberlain et al. (1993) that looked at the relationship of communication problems to challenging behaviour uses the term 'challenging behaviour' but uses it exclusively to refer to people with behavioural difficulties. Clearly the implications of this are important both to providers, both statutory and private, as well as commissioners of health care, where the management of behavioural difficulties predominantly rests. Clifton and Brown (1993) made this point as far back as the mid-1990s and identified that the term 'challenging behaviour' had become so general that in practice a wide variety of definitions were being used. They identified that this would be particularly unhelpful when commissioners sought to provide training to meet a person's specific needs. In addition to this, there is an issue here concerning confusion between provider and clinical commissioning groups about services for people with challenging behaviour. It might be the case that a provider would offer a service for people with challenging behaviour that included provision for people with profound learning disability with additional sensory or motor handicaps, whereas commissioners thought that they were commissioning services for people with behavioural difficulties. This is one reason why it is suggested that the term 'behavioural difficulties' should be adopted when referring to people with a learning disability who predominantly manifest with care challenges that amount to challenges of behavioural management. This section has attempted to illustrate that the term 'challenging behaviour' is so inclusive of a wide variety of states that it makes the identification of particular groups within such a term difficult and that this has implications for calculating the prevalence of behavioural difficulties as a distinct group; its use therefore should be judiciously applied.

PREVALENCE OF BEHAVIOURAL DIFFICULTIES

Prevalence of a particular disorder or disease is calculated on the basis of measurement, and herein lays a paradox. This is because, as previously stated, with inadequate operationalisation of the nature of challenging behaviour it is difficult to be reassured concerning the prevalence of behavioural difficulties. The prevalence of behavioural difficulties would appear to be subsumed in the overall calculation of this, or more specifically, challenging behaviour. Data on people with learning disabilities who exhibit behavioural difficulties is crucial for research and care planning and management purposes, and it is not always clear whether special needs registers hold such information and that even if they do whether such information is reliable (Dagnan and Kroese, 1993). This has resulted in considerable scepticism concerning the reliability or validity of claims made about the prevalence of challenging behaviour or behavioural difficulties in the population of people with learning disabilities. In 1980, the DHSS calculated incapacity associated with learning disability, and it was suggested that within a general population of 1,00,000 aged between 0 and 15+, 34.28% of these individuals had behavioural difficulties that required constant supervision. This epidemiological data provided analysis of both 'within hospital or other residential care and home settings'. No supportive evidence is provided as to method or instrument(s) used in measurement, therefore the degree of confidence that one may place on such a calculation is problematic.

Kiernan and Moss (1990) found that 40% of people with a learning disability at a large hospital exhibited moderate or severe behavioural difficulties. On the basis of this study, it was calculated that behavioural problems were present in community settings to a slightly lesser extent. No empirical or epidemiological evidence for this assumption was offered. The appropriateness of using measurement from a hospital setting and applying it to another setting is of doubtful value, because there is an issue of ecological validity, which concerns the generalisablity of research conclusions from one setting to another.

Qureshi and Alborz (1992) estimated that 30% of people with learning disabilities in a hospital setting presented with some form of challenging behaviour. Harris (1993) identified that 17.6% of people with a learning disability within one health district had aggressive behaviour. The DH (1992) has suggested that (i) between 25% and 50% of adults have additional mental health needs; (ii) 12% to 15% have significant impairment of sight; (iii) 8% to 20% have significant impairment of hearing; and (iv) at least 50% will have significant impairments of communication or social ability. This report calculated that 20 adults with a learning disability per 1,00,000 total population present a significant challenge. Given the earlier definition from the DH (1992), it is difficult to know the prevalence of behavioural difficulties within this overall group of people.

This discussion brings into sharp relief two emergent issues. Firstly, there are considerable variations between researchers who have identified prevalence of challenging behaviour and/or behavioural difficulties. Reasons for this lie in the ways in which the term 'challenging behaviour' has been operationalised to encompass a heterogeneous group of people. Second, fundamental and unprecedented change to the context in which support or care is now provided to people with learning disabilities means that data gathered in the past in large learning disability hospitals cannot be assumed to be valid indicators of the prevalence of behavioural difficulties within new community settings (Lloyd and Kennedy, 2014).

UNDERSTANDING BEHAVIOUR FROM DIFFERING THEORETICAL PERSPECTIVES

People observe others, and from these observations they develop theories about why these others behave as they do, and how they are different. For professional carers it is necessary to have some means of predicting how people are going to behave in general, even if each is treated as an individual. Effective, safe, and compassionate nursing care needs to be built on a coherent theory, but it must be remembered that this in itself is built on a number of basic assumptions. Nursing actions need to be grounded in some kind of theory if they are not to be random and incoherent. For learning disability nursing practice to be more effective, it needs to make explicit underlying assumptions and theoretical position/s that otherwise remain implicit and hidden in the ways in which we work with others.

Psychodynamic, behaviourist, and humanistic theory

This next section explores three theoretical approaches to understanding behaviour that are commonly used in a learning disability nursing context—the psychodynamic, behaviourist, and humanistic theories. Each of these has arisen in a particular context for a particular purpose, and each makes a significant contribution to our understanding of the complexity of human nature and behaviour. In this chapter we concentrate on the different basic concepts, principles, assumptions, and applicability of each theory. This should help you as a student of nursing to articulate and compare your own personal theory-making with that of other specialists in the field and potentially gain new insights into understanding how we view behaviour demonstrated by others, particularly when it is described as challenging, difficult, or distressed.

What divides the theorists?

There are six basic issues that divide theorists (Pervin, 2001), and which reflect the personal life experiences of the theorists, as well as the social and scientific zeitgeist current at the time of their work. The way that these issues are addressed affects the way a person is viewed and, more importantly, which aspects of human functioning are chosen for emphasis and investigation. This has particular relevance when we work with people with learning disabilities who are said to have challenging behaviours (behavioural difficulties).

The philosophical view

People rarely need to articulate to each other the values and beliefs that underlie their view of the world, and yet we all have them. Any coherent theory of the person is built upon a philosophical view about human nature. One theory will emphasise instinctive forces, whereas another emphasises social factors. One will pose as problematic whether we believe people are driven, or are they free, whether they are rational or compulsive in nature, whether they are self-seeking or capable of altruism, and whether they are they spiritual or biological beings. These issues and others have been debated throughout history and are at the root of any major shift in the perception of patients in receipt of treatment regimes.

When seeking to understand a philosophical model, it is useful to consider its philosophical base. The model that best suits an individual will be influenced by personal factors, life experiences, and culture, as well the social validity of approach, in a sense just as the original proponents of each model were so influenced. For example, psychodynamic model has its origins in Sigmund Freud's (Freud, 1986) ideas that are grounded in seeing the person as a product of early experiences; Burrhus Frederic Skinner's (1938) behaviourist view purports that behaviour is a response to a person's environment and the feedback received from it. And, finally, Carl Rogers' (1970) humanistic or person-centred view is that each individual is a self-actualising organism who has a positive drive toward health and happiness.

Internal and external forces

A second and related issue is whether the causes of behaviour are inside of a person or outside in the environment. The extreme views are easy to recognise. Freud, for example, believed that unknown internal forces within the unconscious control human beings, whereas Skinner suggested that a person does not act upon the world, the world acts upon him or her, that is, environmental forces control him or her. To a certain extent, all views are interactive, but it is worth asking whether the focus of any one view is on internal, personal factors or on external, environmental factors.

The concept of self

To be a distinct person is to have some coherent, consistent pattern and organisation of thought, feeling, and behaviour. To account for this aspect of human functioning the concept of 'self' is used. Awareness of self is an important part of experience. The way an individual feels about himself or herself affects that individual's outlook on the world, as well as his or her behaviour toward others. Here theorists differ considerably in their use of the self. Rogers makes it the central integrating concept as the person seeks to make the self and experience congruent with each other. Skinner in principle avoids the very notion of self as a vague, romantic and fanciful idea.

Awareness and consciousness

It is generally recognised by psychologists that potential exists for different states of consciousness in human experience. Nevertheless, there is strong disagreement as to whether the concept of the unconscious, as used in psychology, is useful or necessary to explain the diverse phenomena of this experience. How are dreams accounted for? Can people give an accurate account of themselves, or are large parts of their thoughts, feelings, and behaviour outside their awareness? The answers to these and other questions determine how we communicate, and how we interpret the behaviour of others. So, if a learning disability nurse asks someone with learning disabilities about his or her sense of wellness, should such a nurse take that person's answer at face value, or should other factors to be taken into account?

Thoughts, feelings, and behaviour

Theorists differ in the relative weight they give to each of these areas of functioning. From the psychodynamic view, all behaviour is a product of thought and feeling. Behaviourists focus on overt behaviour and reject any investigation of internal processes. Other theorists argue that thoughts are primary and cause both feelings and behaviour. Still others argue that emotions are primary and can direct thought and behaviour. Although there is a growing acceptance that all three aspects influence each other, the relative emphasis of one over the others distinguishes one model of the person from another.

The past, present, and future

Is behaviour determined by the past or by expectations of the future or solely by factors in the present? This is another issue that divides theorists. The distinguishing feature in each of the different theories is how the links between all three – past, present, and future – are conceptualised. If people are viewed as being determined by their past with little hope for change, they are unlikely to be treated differently, with a more optimistic view of the future. A learning disability nurse's whole basis for intervention with someone with learning disabilities is built on their view of the relation between their past and present state of affairs, and prospective future is.

Having examined the basic issues that divide theorists, these three theoretical models can now be examined in more detail and these issues are shown diagramatically in Figure 9.1.

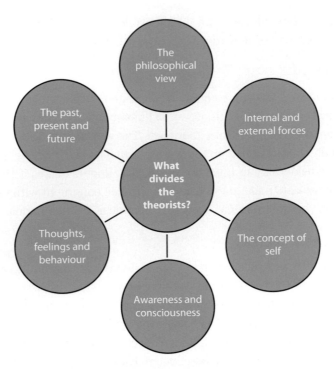

Figure 9.1 Concepts that divide theorists in understanding behaviour.

THE PSYCHODYNAMIC MODEL

Psychodynamic understanding of the person is derived from the origins of work by Sigmund Freud (Freud, 1986). Freud's theories and psychoanalytic techniques have provided a rich source of ideas that many others have since developed and modified. This has given rise to a vast and complex literature involving many different schools of thought, which can be confusing and overwhelming to a new reader.

The term 'psychodynamic' is useful because it refers not to one theory but to a collection of theories that owe their origins to the pioneering work of Freud. The two parts to the word offer some insight into the focus of the model. 'Psyche' is generally used to refer to mind, but it might be better to think about it as referring to the whole of a person's inner world of feelings, thoughts, and experiences. Older words, such as soul and spirit, need to be added to give the full sense of meaning to the word 'psyche'. 'Dynamic' refers to a view that the psyche is seen as active and not static, not relating only to other people but also active within itself, relating to itself. Reflection on experience, and the way we describe experience, for example, *'I just did it. I don't know why, and now I feel so cross with myself'*, often reveals a person's internal relationships, which are full of feeling, and not necessarily linked to other people at all. Thus, the dynamic is both internal and external, and the word 'psychodynamic' applies to the internal world of experience, which in turn affects the external world. The ways that we relate to ourselves with compassion, hatred, fear, or envy are expressed outside in the way we relate to others.

Object relations theory

Freud's original theory emphasised the instinctive drives of the individual alone. Object relations theory, a development from Freud, puts at centre stage the need for human beings to relate to each other and explains how early relationships become internalised and repeated in the ways that a person relates to himself or herself and others. The term 'object' can be somewhat confusing initially because it usually refers to persons and relationships rather than objects as 'things'.

Product and author

Individuals are generally viewed as products of their environment as well as their time and place in history. People develop conceptions about themselves, about whether they are, for example, lovable, clever, and good-looking, or unlovable, stupid, or ugly. These perceptions enable the person to make sense of the world and make it predictable. An expectation of being rejected will affect the interaction with the next unfamiliar person we meet. This tendency will result in the achievement of the 'self-fulfilling prophecy'.

Harder to accept is the fact that these adult feelings and behaviours have roots in the much earlier experiences of childhood and infancy. Patterns of relating to our earliest figures, usually parents, are internalised, resulting in an internal world dominated by feelings of anxiety and fear or confidence and worth. These early experiences are beyond normal memory, leaving unconscious constructions and expectations about later life. Conscious and deliberate interpretations are made about what is happening in the present, and it is these factors that actively contribute to shaping our behaviour. So individuals are both product and author of their own history.

Those in the caring professions often have to live with a tension of ambivalent feelings toward their patients. Knowing that, to some extent, patients are victims of circumstances arouses a desire to help and serve that patient's best interests by understanding and compassion. However, it is common to see quite clearly how much a patient is contributing to his present condition, sometimes consciously but often quite unconsciously. It is difficult for a patient to hold both 'product and author' in mind, and to take some appropriate responsibility for his or her present condition. It is also difficult for carers when the patient will not take responsibility and will not cooperate.

External and internal worlds

The second assumption makes the reality of the unconscious mind a centrepiece. It can safely be said that the unravelling of the workings of the unconscious was one of Freud's major contributions to understanding the human person. All sorts of things can be unconscious, such as drives and wishes, conflicts, fears, values, aims, defences, images of people, and the self, as well as our relationships.

Psychodynamic theorists such as Klein (1963) have suggested that unconscious phantasy underlies all thinking and feeling, not just the feelings of conscious awareness. Such phantasy begins very early in childhood and is concerned primarily with bodily processes and relating to others. It becomes more and more symbolic and elaborate during growth and development, but it never loses its primitive roots in infancy. Phantasies about being abandoned, lost, or heroically saved, for example, seem to exist independently of whether any of these things actually happened. They appear to be products of the mind rather than of direct experience, even though such events might actually happen.

This internal world constantly interacts with the external one, and people live simultaneously in both. When both worlds are in harmony, there are no problems in living. It is when conscious and unconscious wishes and aims differ that conflict and confusion are experienced. If the boundary between the two worlds becomes blurred, it is possible to misconstrue people and events in potentially disastrous ways. Because of its origins in infancy, the unconscious internal world is energetic. And when it surfaces, it does so with the force of infantile feeling that can be highly disturbing.

How might the psychodynamic view of a practitioner affect the way he or she interprets behavioural difficulties in people with learning disabilities?

All behaviour is logical

Yet a third assumption asserts that all behaviour has meaning if examined. What appears to be bizarre behaviour in the present is usually derived from the demands of the unconscious breaking through the defence structure, from patterns of long ago in childhood, or as a result of living in a permanently defensive way. At some time in the past, coping strategies may have been necessary and comforting but are now anachronistic. The present behaviour derived from them now seems senseless or maladaptive, but if the whole historic picture were to be known it would make sense. The term defence is used to refer to the ways in which the human psyche has evolved to protect itself from the feelings of anxiety that inevitably arise from unconscious forces; these are sometimes referred to as ego defence mechanisms.

Such defence mechanisms have a positive aspect in that they help the individual control and understand emotional experiences. When defences are down, the person may be unable to function and feel overwhelmingly vulnerable. Defence mechanisms, however, also have a negative aspect when they are so strong that they make it difficult to act spontaneously or with trust. Thus, potentially rewarding experiences may be inaccessible to the over-defensive person.

Emotional development

A fourth assumption points to the fact that growth that is linked to the passage of time, such as physical development and ageing, has a given and irreversible quality about it. Emotional development, on the other hand, is not linear nor is it steady, and it has many detours and reversals. The term 'fixation' is applied if emotional development stops altogether and 'regression' is applied if there is a reversion to an earlier state or way of functioning. Patients frequently show regressive behaviour, that is, they act and feel as if they were much younger, especially when they are stressed, as is the case when they are ill. Being helpless and dependent may make the strongest of patients feel so anxious that they may well regress to a more infantile state, and it is then likely to feel the other anxieties of that stage, such as unrealistic fears of danger or abandonment.

The psychodynamic model of the person uses many concepts that have found their way into everyday language but which are here used here in a technical and restricted way, for example, phantasy, defence, and regression. Another important concept is transference. This is the process by which one person unconsciously relates to another in present circumstances in ways that are derived from the past. So, someone with learning disabilities, for example, might react to a learning disability nurse practitioner as if the practitioner were that person's mother. He or she may know that the nurse is not at all like their mother but nevertheless find that they have familiar feelings whenever a nurse or carer talks to or looks at them.

Application and limitation

The psychodynamic concepts and assumptions outlined here interrelate to give a coherent picture of a person. Such a view is helpful when trying to understand complex behaviours and their manifestations.

In such understanding, behaviour with or toward others may have a component of indirectness, of something alluded to but not made explicit. When things are straightforward, there is no need to resort to the concepts of the unconscious to help explain behaviour. It is worth remembering that ill or (dis)stressed people are likely to behave in ways that might be atypical of their normal behaviour, and it is useful to have some ideas available that can potentially make sense of what is happening.

Although it can help to be aware of psychic mechanisms in communication with others, a deeper exploration with a patient into his or her feelings and the meaning of his or her behaviour is likely to need a great deal of time and skill. This type of help is more the remit of counselling and psychotherapy. Nevertheless, given that treatment of illness and communication with patients is now seen to involve a relationship between patient and carer, it is not surprising that certain writers in the field, for example, Balint (1964), have suggested that an understanding of psychodynamic processes is required to effectively treat a person's entire illness rather than the disease or symptoms alone.

BEHAVIOURISM

At the turn of the century, a group of psychologists became dissatisfied with the psychodynamic approach to explain and understand the person, and developed a new school of psychology known as behaviourism. Pivotal to this perspective was the theory that all behaviour rested on learned responses to given stimuli, often referred to as associative, connectionist, or behavioural theory. This relationship between stimulus and response by an organism is accounted for by an understanding of both classical and operant conditioning.

The behavioural model

The behavioural perspective of understanding the person is grounded in early psychological research into the nature of learning. This approach to understanding learning was first postulated by a neurophysiologist called Pavlov, who in 1902 described a relationship between unconditioned responses and unconditioned stimuli. The response was called unconditioned because it was almost reflexive in nature, meaning that it was an integral component of the organism's repertoire of behaviour. The most famous example of this is the response of a dog's salivation when in the presence of food. In a series of experiments on dogs, Pavlov found that if an unconditioned stimulus were paired with a conditioned stimulus, then it would be possible to elicit a conditioned response. This is demonstrated in Figure 9.2 as occurring in three stages. In Stage 1, the unconditioned stimulus of food causes the dog to respond by salivating. If this unconditioned response (Stage 2) is paired for a sufficient time with a conditioned stimulus (the bell), then eventually the response of salivation can be obtained by using the conditioned stimulus alone. That is, the response becomes conditioned to the sound of the bell.

The work of Pavlov was extremely important at the turn of the century in shaping the thinking of the emerging group of American psychologists now referred to as behaviourists. Of these the psychologist John Watson became credited as the founder of behaviourism. He believed that for psychology to become a science, its data had to be objective and measurable. He was not concerned with introspective, hypothetical causes of behaviour but with public, observable, and measurable causes. Watson argued that behaviour was the direct result of conditioning. He believed that this conditioning emanated from the environment in which the organism was located and that this environment would shape an organism's behaviour by reinforcing specific behaviours.

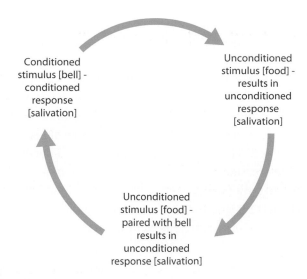

Figure 9.2 Classical conditioning.

He further believed that simple chains of stimulus/response connections formed into longer, more complex, strings of behaviour. These strings of behaviour, he argued, explained how a person thought and what motivated him or her. In addition, these strings of behaviour accounted for personality, emotion, learning, and remembering. Such beliefs were clearly articulated by Watson (1924) when he said

> **Give me a dozen healthy infants, well-formed, and my own specified world to bring them up in and I'll guarantee to take any one at random and train him to become any kind of specialist I might select—lawyer, artist, merchant, chief and yes even a beggar man and thief, regardless of his talents, penchants, abilities, vocations, and race of his ancestors**

(Watson, 1924)

Such a belief can be seen to be in complete contrast to the psychodynamic approach. From this early work on behaviourism emerged, amongst others, the work of Skinner (1938). His work, known as operant conditioning, later became known as behaviour modification. Skinner's contribution in this area is important because he was the first psychologist to point to the clinical and social relevance of operant conditioning (Bellack et al., 1982). The next section provides examples of the application of behaviourism, which has been used as a therapeutic strategy to deal with psychological disorder and to improve or develop communication.

Operant conditioning

Operant conditioning suggests that when an organism makes a connection between a stimulus, the elicited response and the subsequent rewards or punishment, then its behaviour is reinforced negatively or positively.

Behaviourists believe that if behaviour is reinforced positively, then the incidence of that behaviour will increase. Conversely, if a behaviour is negatively reinforced the incidence of that behaviour will decrease. The essential difference between operant and classical conditioning is that in the latter the behaviour is a part of the organism's repertoire of behaviour. For example, salivation is a naturally occurring response of some organisms to food that can become conditioned

---

Box 9.1 Behavioural explanation for language acquisition

1. *Echoic response:* Early on in development, an infant mimics a noise made by others, who in turn reinforce the infant's behaviour.
2. *Mand response:* Later, the infant engages in initiating sound—but without meaning. The meaning is attached by others; once again reinforcement of the behaviour is provided by others.
3. *Tact response:* At this stage, a child moves on to making an attempt to use a word to name something that is present in the environment. When a child does this successfully, the behaviour is reinforced.

---

by the repeated pairing of a conditioned stimulus (a bell, for example) with an unconditioned stimulus (food, for example), as described previously. In operant conditioning, however, the behaviour is not a part of the animal's repertoire of behaviour. The deliberate or otherwise use of reinforcement will result in a new behaviour.

In 1957, Skinner postulated a behavioural explanation for the acquisition of language in children. He argued that if an infant's vocalising was positively reinforced, then that infant would increase the frequency of that behaviour. Skinner (1957) outlined three ways in which the process of language acquisition might be achieved, as shown in Box 9.1.

Although greatly simplified, the process outlined here seeks to demonstrate how the behavioural model would explain the acquisition of language.

The application of behaviourism

Operant conditioning, as an approach to understanding learning and behaviour, has had an enormous impact upon nursing and the ways in which some client groups are cared for. For example, one behavioural treatment used in the field of mental health, for phobic conditions, is systematic desensitisation. This technique consists of pairing a response that inhibits anxiety, for example, muscle relaxation, with something that provokes anxiety. Consider the case of an individual suffering from arachnophobia (a fear of spiders). In desensitisation, a therapist would pair the anxiety-provoking event in a graduated manner with relaxation techniques. So, for example, the therapist would commence desensitisation by showing the patient a photograph of a spider coupled with relaxation exercises. Eventually the therapist would show the patient a living spider and perhaps get him to touch the spider, which again would coupled with relaxation exercises. In between these two extremes are a series of graduated stimuli that could cause a corresponding graduated fear response. This fear response is shown in Figure 9.3.

Repeated pairing of the stimuli with relaxation would eventually bring about a different response to fear at the sight of spiders. Instead a patient would feel more comfortable and relaxed, because he or she would associate the relaxation with the spider instead of the anxiety and fear.

For a description of this type of therapeutic intervention, the reader is advised to see Paul and Bernstein (1976) or McLeod (2000). Bellack (1982) has described the use of behaviourism as a mediator in a number of studies of social skills training for schizophrenic patients. He suggested that

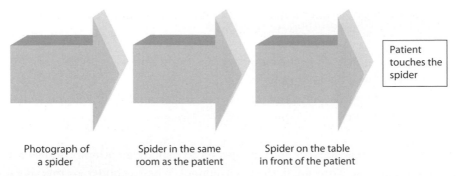

| Photograph of a spider | Spider in the same room as the patient | Spider on the table in front of the patient | Patient touches the spider |

Figure 9.3 Systematic desensitisation.

social skills were deficient in schizophrenic patients, resulting in social isolation. One study comprised targeting and improving the assertiveness of two chronic schizophrenic patients. Eye contact, speech duration, smiles, requests, and compliances were reinforced positively. Results demonstrated that the targeted behaviours significantly improved and that these improvements remained for some weeks after the skills training.

Another example of the use of behavioural interventions to improve communication is recorded by Lovass (1977). Here, a series of steps was taken to train children with autistic conditions in vocal imitation. In Step 1, the therapist increased the child's vocalisations by reinforcing him (usually with food) contingent on such behaviour. In Step 2, the child was trained in temporal discrimination: His vocalisations were reinforced only if they were in response to the therapist's speech, that is, if they occurred within five seconds of the therapist's vocalisation. In Step 3, finer discriminations were reinforced. For example, the child was reinforced for making successively closer approximations to the therapist's speech until the child could match the particular sound given by the therapist; Lovass (1977) has presented a detailed account of how new behaviour was reinforced, leading to increased vocalisation in the children.

The examples provided serve to demonstrate how a behaviourist view of the person may influence the ways in which nurses communicate with their patients. McCue (2000) has demonstrated very clearly how the behavioural approach can be used to help people with both learning disabilities, and challenging behaviours. Having briefly outlined the behavioural approach to understanding the person, let us now consider the third of the three approaches, that of the humanistic model.

THE HUMANISTIC MODEL

Finally, Nolen-Hoeksema et al. (2009) have suggested that during the first half of the last century the psychodynamic and behavioural approaches to understanding the person were dominant. However, during the late 1950s and early 1960s a group of psychologists developed a new and radical approach based on phenomenology in which the humanistic approach to understanding the person is central. Phenomenology rejects the behavioural approach to understanding the person where behaviour is seen as the result of associations or connections between stimuli and responses. It also rejects the suggestion that behaviour is controlled by unconscious impulses, located in our past, as suggested by the psychodynamic approach. Instead, humanism asserts the unique, subjective, and lived experience of each individual.

From the humanistic approach came the work of Maslow (1954) who described a system of hierarchy of needs in the person. These needs range from basic physiological needs such as food, water, and air to complex psychological needs such as security, belonging, and self-esteem. The pinnacle of this hierarchy is self-actualisation—the individual's need to find fulfilment and develop to his own potential.

Another important contributor to the humanistic approach is Carl Rogers (see Rogers, 1970). His ideas emerged from his therapeutic work with people in need of psychotherapy. Rogers believed that people have an innate tendency to develop and grow in maturity, which will lead an individual to actualise all the capacities he has. If a person's development is stunted, it is likely that it is due to relationships in which their experiencing was denied, defined, or discounted. What is healing is a relationship in which the person feels fully accepted and valued, the famous core conditions for therapeutic change vis á vis unconditional positive regard (acceptance), empathy, and genuineness. Central to this approach is a fundamental philosophical belief in the individual to develop to his full potential.

It can be seen from the examples given in this section that the philosophical position underlying the theory of the person is inclined to determine the nature of the intervention chose, and this can occur at the level of the individual practitioner or professional grouping. Having outlined issues of measurement, the following section addresses some of the thornier aspects of measurement.

METHODS OF MEASUREMENT

Before considering therapeutic approaches, this chapter now briefly turns to issues of measurement that have implications for reliability and validity that the nurse practitioner should be aware of. Within the literature, three methods of measurement are advocated (see, for example, Yule and Carr, 1987; Iwata et al., 1990; McCue, 2000).

- *Indirect.* This style is probably the simplest approach used to obtain data. Carers are interviewed by a nurse or researcher about the frequency or absence of behaviours from a predetermined list. Such an approach is clearly dependent upon the carer being able to answer the questions posed and also having sufficient knowledge of the subject so that the relevant questions can be answered fully and reliably.

- *Descriptive.* This is a more objective approach that is undertaken through systematic analysis of behaviour following naturalistic observation. This is achieved through developing interval-based observation procedures, gathering objective data, and calculating for inter-observer reliability. Although time-consuming, Iwata et al. (1990) have stated that the descriptive approach is superior because it is more objective than verbal report and that, because it is quantitative, it allows for correlation calculation between variables. It is also thought to be superior because observation is conducted in a natural environment where a wide range of events can be observed and studied.

- *Functional analysis*. This approach requires the nurse or researcher to control for a number of variables whilst observation is conducted simultaneously. In a sense, this approach is experimental where at least one variable that is of interest to the nurse of researcher is manipulated in a highly controlled environment to bring about a reduction in an undesired behaviour. The purpose of assessment is therefore to demonstrate a cause-and-effect relationship between an environmental factor and behaviour.

In respect of these differing methods of measurement, Iwata et al. (1990) have stated the following

Although designed to serve the same purpose, these methods vary considerably in terms of both precision and complexity, and each method contains inherent strengths and weaknesses

(Iwata et al., 1990, p. 305)

It should be noted that the scales that are often used in indirect measurement have been criticised because often they have only been studied for inter-rater reliability, and other factors of reliability and validity have largely been ignored. In addition to the threats that the method of measurement might make to reliability and validity there are also difficulties associated with the type of measurement chosen. For example, commonly found in direct observational analysis are the following types of measurement

- *Frequency*. This form of measurement requires the nurse or researcher to identify the number of times that a target behaviour is observed within a predetermined period of time. The total of observed targeted behaviour can be divided by the period of observation time, to arrive at a mean calculation of frequency of that behaviour.

- *Duration*. If a target behaviour occurs infrequently, but for long periods of time, then observation may be required for extended periods of time. An example here may be bouts of screaming that occur relatively infrequently but with such intensity, and over such a long period of time, that it makes the behaviour extremely distressing for the individual and carers. It then becomes more appropriate to measure the total amount of time spent on such behaviour; this is known as a duration measurement.

- *Interval recording*. In this form of measurement, the nurse or researcher divides a period of observation into predetermined time intervals. This is useful when behaviours are of variable duration, for example, head banging, which may occur for a few seconds or last for several minutes. Each occurrence of the targeted behaviour that falls within the time interval is recorded. Such measurement provides relatively accurate information on the frequency of behaviour but only limited insight as to duration or intensity of behaviour.

- *Time sampling*. This involves identifying specific periods of time when target behaviour is to be measured. If the behaviour occurs at the time when sampling occurs, then it is recorded. A major strength of this approach is that it is less time-consuming than other approaches. Clearly, however, the measure may not be reliable in that target behaviour may occur outside of the sample frame and thus would not be recorded.

These methods of measurement are not exhaustive of the wide range of approaches used in learning disability nursing, but they do illustrate that there are a number of issues that the learning disability nurse should consider when making a choice. First, the reliability of the process of measurement is entirely dependent upon the observer rating the behaviour. Yule and Carr have discussed this issue

> **Observers are human, and human beings process their observations before recording them (therefore) simple observational measures of behaviour can become unreliable**
>
> *(Yule and Carr, 1987, p. 21)*

In addition to this, a number of studies have indicated anomalies in the reliability of raters. First, Taplan and Reid (1973) have found that raters behave differently when they are observed in reliability studies, than when they are on their own. Second, the choice of measures taken can also affect the reliability of any findings. For example, the use of time sampling by a nurse, whilst convenient and less demanding of resources, may provide unreliable data about the frequency or severity of behavioural difficulties. Given that behavioural difficulties and their management in the field of learning disabilities present significant care problems for parents and professional carers alike, therapeutic interactions that attempt to bring about remediation of effect must be based upon best outcomes. With carefully conducted measurement the learning disability nurse practitioner can achieve the following

- Evaluation of intervention/s against therapeutic goals
- Comparison of results achieved with others using the same treatment methods
- Exploration of self-reporting of improvements in measurement

Within the context of ever-limited, and limiting, resources for health care, and the consequent need for effectively targeting that resource, practice has to ensure that the most appropriate therapeutic strategies are adopted in managing people with a learning disability who exhibit behavioural difficulties. The importance of outcome studies in this area is very clearly articulated in Emerson et al. (1994), Wright et al. (1994), and Lloyd and Kennedy (2014).

THERAPEUTIC APPROACHES TO BEHAVIOURAL DIFFICULTIES

In broad terms, therapeutic approaches to the management of behavioural difficulties are to assess, intervene, and measure outcomes post-intervention. Given all that has been said in the previous section about challenges to the validity and reliability of assessments, a variety of tools should be used and these might include functional analysis, observations, and interdisciplinary assessment of competence skills, as well as standardised measures that might include questionnaires completed by the individual, informant-based measures, and those focused on staff perceptions and stress. Once physical or mental ill health has been excluded as the basis for presenting behavioural difficulties, clinicians must decide upon which therapeutic approach they will base their intervention; and it has to be said that to date the behavioural approach would appear to be the most efficacious (Lloyd and Kennedy, 2014).

Psychotherapeutic approaches

Psychotherapy and counselling applied to people with learning disabilities encompass a vast range of theories and potential approaches. Because of this, the reader is strongly advised to pursue the recommended further reading. Although there are many counselling and psychotherapeutic approaches available, they all, in essence, share a common theoretical basis, and they all share the same potential benefits.

This section briefly outlines some key approaches and their shared origins, and then outlines the key common benefits. Psychotherapeutic approaches are based on the belief that individuals can experience errors in thinking that are emotionally damaging and can result in distressed states of behaviour. Treatment approaches may vary between the different methods of psychotherapy/counseling, but they are likely to include the need for a thorough assessment that will involve the following

- A thorough exploration of the individual's history
- Functional analysis to include known triggers of distress
- Arousal levels, patterns of behaviour, and current coping strategies
- Psychological questionnaires and interviews
- Identification of errors in cognition
- The level of the individual's motivation to change, and his or her ability to follow a treatment plan

Therapeutic techniques include a range of approaches that might include some of the following

- Giving information and developing an understanding of specific disorders, paranoia, for example
- Social skills training involving role play and re-enactment of past triggers
- Relaxation techniques
- Problem solving
- Challenging errors in thinking
- Modelling
- Cognitive distraction, visualisation, for example
- Testing out coping strategies within a controlled environment
- Self-report methods
- Desensitisation to stressful situations
- Guided fantasies
- Dream work
- Brainstorming solutions

There are a number of common benefits of psychotherapy and counselling; however, a criticism of psychotherapy and counselling, in relation to their application to people with learning disabilities, is that many within this client group are not of a sufficient cognitive level of ability to benefit from such forms of therapy due to issues of communication, understanding, and engagement with the process. However, many people with learning disabilities will benefit from some of the common benefits of psychotherapy and counselling, which include the following

- The building of a relationship that is based upon trust, genuineness, and mutuality and one where an individual feels listened to and understood
- The development of a working alliance in which the individual and therapist feel they are working in partnership to achieve shared goals

- Support and reassurance
- The development of insight
- The development of a range of healthy and adaptive responses through the implicit reinforcement of appropriate behaviour/responses

Learning disability nurses may not be engaged in these approaches, as they are undertaken by trained psychotherapists and counsellors; however, many nurses do undertake post-qualifying training courses so that they can engage in this important area of care (James, 2014).

Behavioural approaches

A behavioural approach to the management of behavioural difficulties in people with learning disabilities is rooted in behaviour modification, and is based on the use of systematic analysis and application of reinforcers to modify behaviours. Reinforcement is a process where new responses are acquired and strengthened. It refers to a procedure of providing consequences for a given behaviour that increases or maintains frequency of a desired behaviour as opposed to an unwanted or undesirable behaviour. Reinforcers are defined by their power to bring about desired changes to behaviour. It is possible to develop very structured and detailed programmes of reinforcement that alter their schedule, ratio, and nature. Also restructuring an environment to remove significant contingent events may also be viewed as necessary; for example, social relationships associated with patterns of particular behavioural responses may be avoided until an individual appears more settled or confident about the environment that he or she is in, and this prevents reverting to former patterns of behaviour.

Assessment of challenging behaviours through the use of functional analysis can greatly assist in identifying alternative behaviours that will produce desirable consequences instead of challenging behaviour. The skills inherent in producing such alternative responses may need to be learned or shaped, as they may not be present in the individual's repertoire of behaviour (McCue, 2000)

Humanistic approaches

Gentle teaching (GT) is an excellent example of how the humanistic approach affects the ways in which nurses and other therapists work with people within the field of learning disability. GT is an approach that emphasises the importance of therapeutic bonding and functional communication and was mainly evident in the U.K. research and practice literature in the 1980s and 1990s. It is still practiced in the United States and other parts of Europe (for example, the Netherlands). However, in the United Kingdom, GT is now rarely referred to and has been predominantly replaced by a more general move toward more positive, non-aversive therapeutic approaches to working with people with learning disabilities. GT promoted the underlying philosophical approach of this intervention that all human beings need to participate in reciprocal loving relationships, and to participate with others in activities that comprise daily life. Thus, the success of GT was determined by the extent to which parties involved in a relationship moved toward a more functional form of interaction. In GT, the approach first focused on gathering information, which was undertaken to identify how best to begin the process of engagement, and explored the following:

- How the person participated
- How the person communicated
- How the person related to others

GT advocates introducing participation through the use of activities, which it saw as opportunities for engaging people; these activities should have the following aspects

- Be simple and easily broken down into steps
- Have repetitive sequences
- Call for the use of materials
- Be done in a variety of places
- Require active participation and two-way interaction
- Have built-in mini-breaks
- Be structured to find the 'entry point'

It was advocated that within each sequence of repeated steps in an activity, the GT practitioner observed the person's non-verbal cues closely to identify an 'entry point'. This was the point that the person found interesting or attractive, for example, he or she may increase eye contact or change his or her facial expression when that point occurred; it was felt that a person was more likely to engage in an activity at this stage more than at any other. Also advocated was an approach to dealing with behavioural difficulties through *'defusion'*. This term is used to describe a strategy used by GT practitioners to manage behavioural difficulties within the context of shared participation in activities and relationships. It is used to provide emotional and physical safety for both someone with learning disabilities as well as the practitioner. It involved the following

- Demands being placed on the person are reduced or removed.
- Mini-breaks are introduced to allow the person some time to relax.
- The practitioner gradually recommences the activity seeking an entry point.
- The focus is shifted from the person's behaviour to the calm, predictable safety of the shared activity.

Criticisms were levelled against GT, and these included, amongst others, that it was ineffective at reducing behavioural difficulties and that this was proved by research. It should be remembered that the focus and purpose of the GT approach was quite different from behavioural ones; GT concentrated on the whole person and relationships rather than on specific behaviours (Jones and Connell, 1993). Research to date has demonstrated some success for GT particularly in the areas of the following

- Communication
- Relationships
- Skill building

Problematic for some is that it is potentially 'aversive' and might be potentially distressing to people who experience difficulties engaging in relationships (those with autistic spectrum conditions, for example), or that those behavioural difficulties are motivated by a desire to escape interaction.

Problematic with GT was that the central tenets of this approach were never satisfactorily defined. (Jones and Connell, 1993) The 'Caregiver Interactional Observation System' (CIOS) and the 'Person Interactional Observation System' (PIOS) were developed as a measurement tool by practitioners to code the dyadic variables of interactional change. However, attempts to replicate these variables under research conditions have failed to find any significant differences in therapeutic effect between GT and other interventions. GT evolved out of behavioural approaches and adopted some of the techniques used in behavioural interventions, for example, positive praise, ignoring behaviour, shaping, extinction, reinforcement, fading, errorless learning, physically redirecting self-injury, restructuring the environment, maintaining normal conversation, and using physical and visual cues (O'Rourke and Wray, 2000). Lately, positive behaviour support (PBS) seems to have become the preferred approach to the management of challenging behaviour in people with learning disabilities. This approach seems to incorporate elements of all the theoretical perspectives to behaviour that have been outlined in this chapter.

Positive behaviour support

Positive behaviour support, or PBS, is a relatively new behaviour management system that attempts to understand what maintains an individual's so-called challenging behaviour. Challenging behaviours are often difficult to change because they serve a function in the sense that they often enable someone with limited communication skills or competence to make their wishes, anxieties, distress, and pain known. And problematic is that these behaviours can be supported and reinforced by the environment in which someone is located. For example, in the case of someone with profound learning disabilities and complex needs, the environment, in its widest sense, may reinforce undesired behaviour/s because the person will receive objects or attention because of their behaviour. In other words, the person's behaviour is reinforced. This is why a functional behaviour assessment (FBA) needs to be undertaken that can describe the behaviour/s, and identify the context (this will include the events, times, and situation) that predicts when behaviour/s may or may not occur and identifies the consequences that maintain the behaviour. The FBA also summarises and creates a hypothesis about the behaviour, directly observes the behaviour, and takes data to get a baseline. Readers should note that a caveat needs to be exercised here in relation to what has already been said in the preceding section concerning the reliability and validity of assessments undertaken. Notwithstanding, PBS incorporates the elements of goal identification, information gathering, hypothesis development, support plan design, implementation, and monitoring.

For techniques to work in decreasing undesired behaviour, they should include feasibility, desirability, and effectiveness. Carers and/or parents need successful strategies that they are able, and as importantly, likely to use that have an impact on an individual's ability to participate in activities. PBS is increasingly being recognised as a strategy that meets these criteria. Therefore, by changing stimuli and reinforcement in the environment, and by teaching the person to develop his or her competences, a person's behaviour can be changed. The three primary areas of competence deficit that are generally targeted include communication skills, social skills, and self-management skills. PBS focuses on what is referred to as re-directive therapy, which is particularly important in building

---

Learning Activity 9.3

Spend some time searching the World Wide Web to see what evidence you can find of the benefits of using the PBS approach in adults with learning disabilities with behavioural difficulties.

positive relationships between carers and people with presenting behavioural difficulties. There is a growing consensus of opinion that PBS within structured specialist teams has the potential to address challenging behaviour in people with learning disabilities (Allen, 2006).

Other therapeutic approaches

Music therapy: There have been published single-case studies that have demonstrated that music therapy can help in reducing challenging behaviours in people with learning disabilities (Liebman, 2000).

Multi-sensory therapy (Snoezelen): Although this is mainly a leisure and recreational facility, it has been advocated as having therapeutic value (Hulsegge and Verheul, 1987). It has also been suggested that multi-sensory therapy has been successful in helping with challenging behaviours (Slevin and McClelland, 1998).

Treatment and Education of Autistic and Related Communication Handicapped Children (TEACCH): Structured teaching using principles of TEACCH is widely used with people with communication difficulties, and especially with those on the autistic spectrum of conditions. This method is used not only when teaching such people new tasks and helping them to understand what is required of them, but also to help them become more independent and effective in their environments (home, school, community). The intervention is a lifelong approach that takes into consideration the person's strengths and difficulties. The developed programme considers the person and their functions as it is and then supports the person to develop his or her skills as much as possible (Schopler et al., 1982) and helpful with challenging behaviour (CB) (Sines et al., 1996; Barr et al., 2000).

Complementary therapies: These may also have value (Sayre-Adams, 1994). Aromatherapy, for example, may be useful for other client groups (Brooker et al., 1997; Cannard, 1996), but it is acknowledged that there is limited research in learning disabilities. Massage, for example, can assist in relaxation (Hegarty and Gale, 1996), and Corbett (1993) discussed how acupuncture and pressure massage can stimulate neural pathways to the brain. If these approaches could be used, for example, to actively induce relaxation in people who are hyperactive, aggressive, or self-injure, then people with learning disabilities could benefit from such approaches; however, it should be remembered that there is limited evidence to support these approaches.

CONCLUSION

In this chapter the support of people with learning disabilities who present with challenging or distressed behaviour by learning disability nurses has been placed centre stage. This chapter has advocated the unique contribution that learning disability nursing can provide in promoting holistic support, whilst drawing from a strong value and professional base. Our understanding of challenging or distressed behaviour in people with learning disabilities has been presented as problematic. It has also been advocated that distressed behaviours should not be seen as challenging behaviours in the sense that they require some kind of special intervention. Rather they should be seen as 'normal' behavioural responses to stressful situations. Learning disability nurses have a clear role in educating health and social care professionals about the hazards of using inappropriate terminology.

REFERENCES

Allen, D., Lowe, J., Jones, E., James, W., Doyle, T., Andrew, J., Davies, D., Moore, K., and Brophy, S. 2006. Changing the face of challenging behaviour services: The special projects team. *British Journal of Learning Disabilities*, 34(4):237–242.

An Bord Altranais. 2005. *Requirements and Standards for Nurse Registration Education Programmes* (3rd ed.). Dublin: An Bord Altranis.

Balint, M. 1964. *The Doctor, His Patient and the Illness* (2nd ed.). London: Tavistock/Routledge.

Barr, O., Sines, D., Moore, K., Boyd, G. 2000. Structured teaching. In: Gates, B., Gear, J., and Wray, J. 2000. *Behavioural Distress: Concepts and Strategies.* London: Baillière Tindall, pp. 185–214.

Bellack, A., Hersen, M., and Kazdin, A. 1982. *International Handbook of Behaviour Modification and Therapy.* New York: Plenum Press.

Blunden, R. and Allen, D. 1987. *Facing the Challenge: An Ordinary Life for People with Learning Difficulties and Challenging Behaviour*. Kings Fund Paper No. 74. London: Kings Fund Centre.

Brooker, D.J. and Snape, M. 1997. Single case evaluation of the effects of aromatherapy and massage on disturbed behaviour in severe dementia. *British Journal of Clinical Psychology*, 36(2):287–296.

Cannard, G. 1996. The effect of aromatherapy in promoting relaxation and stress reduction in a hospital. *Complementary Therapies in Nursing and Midwifery*, 2(2):38–40.

Chamberlain, L., Chung, M.C., and Jenner, L. 1993. Preliminary findings on communication and challenging behaviour in learning difficulty. *British Journal of Developmental Disabilities*, 39(77):118-125.

Clifton, M. and Brown, J. 1993. *Learning Disabilities, Challenging Behaviour and Mental Illness*. Research Highlights. London: English National Board for Nursing, Midwifery and Health Visiting.

Corbett, J. 1993. Healing the mind through the body. *Mental Handicap*, 21(3):82–86.

Dagnan, D. and Kroese, B.S. 1993. The uses of a special needs register for people with learning difficulties. *Mental Handicap*, 21:10–13.

DOH. 1992. *Services for People with Learning Disabilities, Challenging Behaviour or Mental Health Needs*. London: HMSO.

Emerson E., McGill P., and Mansell J. (Eds.). 1994. *Severe Learning Disabilities and Challenging Behaviours: Designing High Quality Services*. London: Chapman and Hall.

Emerson, E. 1995. *Challenging Behaviour. Analysis and Intervention in People with Learning Difficulties*. Cambridge: Cambridge University Press, p. 4.

Flynn, M. 2012. *Winterbourne View Hospital: A Serious Case Review*. Gloucester: Gloucestershire Safeguarding Adults Board.

Freud A. 1986. *The Ego and the Mechanisms of Defence.* London: Hogarth Press.

Harris P. 1993. The nature and extent of aggressive behaviour amongst people with learning difficulties (mental handicap) in a single health district. *Journal of Intellectual Disability Research*, 37:221–242.

Hastings, R. and Remmington, B. 1993. Connotations of labels for mental handicap and challenging behaviour: A review research evaluation. *Mental Handicap,* 6(3):237–249.

Hegarty, J.R. and Gale, E. 1996. Touch as a therapeutic medium for people with challenging behaviours. *British Journal of Learning Disabilities*, 24(1):26–32.

Hulsegge, J. and Verheul, A. 1987. *Snoezelen: Another World*. Chesterfield: ROMPA UK Publications.

Iwata B.A., Vollmer R., and Zarcone J.R. 1990. The experimental (functional) analysis of behaviour disorders: Methodology, applications, and limitations. In: Repp, A. and Singh, N. (Eds.), *Perspectives on the Use of Non-Aversive and Aversive Interventions for Persons with Developmental Disabilities*. Sycamore, IL: Sycamore Publishing, pp. 301–330.

James, C.W. and Stacey, J.M. 2014. The effectiveness of psychodynamic interventions for people with learning disabilities: A systematic review. *Tizard Learning Disability Review*, 19(1):17–24.

Jones, R. and Connell, E. 1993. Ten years of gentle teaching: Much ado about nothing? *The Psychologist*, 6:544–548.

Kiernan, C. and Moss, S. 1990 Behaviour disorders and other characteristics of the population of a mental handicap hospital. *Mental Handicap Research*, 3(1):3–20.

Klein, M. 1963. *Our Adult World and Its Roots in Infancy*. London: Pitman.

Liebman, M. 2000. The arts therapies. In: Gates, B., Gear, J., and Wray, J. 2000. *Behavioural Distress: Concepts and Strategies*. London: Baillière Tindall, pp. 107–130.

Lloyd, P. and Kennedy, H. 2014. Assessment and treatment of challenging behaviour for individuals with intellectual disability: A research review. *Journal of Applied Research in Intellectual Disabilities*, 27(3):187–199.

Lovaas, O.I. 1977. *The Autistic Child: Language Development through Behavior Modification.* New York: Irvington.

Maslow, A. 1954. *Motivation and Personality*. New York: Harper and Row.

McCue, M. 2000. Behavioural interventions. In: Gates, B., Gear, J., and Wray, J. 2000. *Behavioural Distress: Concepts and Strategies*. London: Baillière Tindall, pp. 215–256.

McLeod, J. 2000 *An Introduction to Counselling* (2nd ed.). Buckingham: Open University Press.

Nolen-Hoeksema, S., Fredrickson, B., Loftus, G., and Wagenaar, W. 2009. *Atkinson and Hilgard's Introduction to Psychology* (15th ed.). USA: Wadsworth Pub Co.

Noonan, E. 1983. *Counselling Young People*. London: Methuen.

Nursing and Midwifery Council. 2010. *Standards for Pre-Registration Nursing Education*. London: NMC.

O'Rourke, S. and Wray, J. 2000. Gentle teaching. In: Gates, B., Gear, J. Wray, J. *Behavioural Distress: Concepts and Strategies.* London: Baillere Tindall.

Paul, G. and Bernstein, D. 1976. Anxiety and clinical problems: Systematic desensitisation and related techniques. In: Spence, J., Carson, R., and Thibaut, J.W. *Behavioural Approaches to Therapy*. Morristown, NJ: General Learning Press.

Pavlov, I. 1902. *The Work of the Digestive Glands*. Trans. W.H. Thompson. London: Charles Griffin.

Pervin, L.A. 2001. *Personality: Theory and Research* (6th ed.). New York: John Wiley.

Qureshi, H. and Alborz, A. 1992. Epidemiology of challenging behaviour. *Mental Handicap Research*, 2:130–145.

Reiss, S. and Aman, M. 1998. *Psychotropic Medications and Developmental Disabilities: The International Consensus Handbook*. Columbus, OH: The Ohio State University Nisonger Centre.

Rogers, C.R. 1970. *On Becoming a Person: A Therapist's View of Psychotherapy*. Boston: Houghton Mifflin.

Sayre-Adams, J. 1994. Clinical complementary therapies therapeutic touch: A nursing function. *Nursing Standard*, 8(17):25–27.

Schopler, E., Mesibov, G. 1982. Evaluation of treatment for autistic children and their parents. *Journal of American Academy of Child Psychiatry*, 21(3):262–267.

Scorer, S., Cate, T., Wilkinson, L., Pollock, P., and Hargan, J. 1993. Challenging behaviour project team: A six month project evaluation. *Mental Handicap*, 21:49–53.

Sines, D. and Moore, K. 1996. *A Study to Evaluate the TEACCH Project (Treatment and Education of Autistic and Related Communication Handicapped Children) in the South Eastern Library Board Area of Northern Ireland*. Belfast: DHSS and University of Ulster.

Skinner, B.F. 1938. *The Behaviour of Organisms*. New York: Appleton-Century Crofts.

Skinner, B.F. 1957. *Verbal behavior.* Englewood Cliffs, NJ: Prentice-Hall.

Slevin, E. and McClelland, A. 1999. An evaluation of the relaxation effects of multi-sensory therapy in a person with learning disabilities: A single subject quasi-experiment. *Journal of Clinical Nursing*, 8(1)48–56.

Taplin, P.S. and Reid, J.B. 1973. Effects of instructional set and experimenter influence on observer reliability. *Child Development,* 44:547–554.

Watson, J.B. 1924. Behaviourism (revised edition, 1930). In: Stevanson, L. 1974. *Seven Theories of Human Nature*. Oxford: Oxford University Press.

Wright, K., Haycox, A., and Leedham, I. 1994. *Evaluating Community Care: Services for People with Learning Difficulties*. Buckingham: Open University Press.

Yule, W. and Carr, J. 1987. *Behaviour Modification for People with Mental Handicaps* (2nd ed.). London: Chapman and Hall.

FURTHER READING

Emerson, E. and Einfeld, S.L. 2011. *Challenging Behaviour* (3rd ed.). Cambridge: Cambridge University Press.

Gates, B., Gear, J., and Wray, J. 2000. *Behavioural Distress: Concepts and Strategies*. London: Baillièrre Tindall.

Hardy, S. and Joyce, T. 2011. *Challenging Behaviour: A Handbook: Practical Resource Addressing Ways of Providing Positive Behavioural Support to People with Learning Disabilities Whose Behaviour is Described as Challenging*. Brighton: Pavilion Publishing Ltd.

USEFUL RESOURCES

LSE Research Articles Online: http://eprints.lse.ac.uk/336/1/dp1930.pdf

The Knowledge Network - Scotland: http://www.knowledge.scot.nhs.uk/home/portals-and-topics/support-workers/topics/dealing-with-challenging-behaviour.aspx

The Challenging Behaviour Foundation: http://www.thecbf.org.uk/

Review of Mental Health and Learning Disability (Northern Ireland) Consultation: http://www.dhsspsni.gov.uk/learning-disability-consultation

SCOPE: http://www.scope.org.uk/support/families/diagnosis/behaviour

SENSE - Scotland: http://www.sensescotland.org.uk/media/857815/understanding_challenging_behaviour.pdf

10 The future of learning disability nursing

Kay Mafuba and Bob Gates

INTRODUCTION

Within the arena of an ever-changing context of health and social care that is dictated by political imperatives at policy level, both nationally and internationally, and with the ever-growing move toward citizenship, and the importance of human rights, learning disability nursing needs to place itself carefully—within the family of nursing and within a complex landscape of human service organisations, as well as the wider community of learning disabilities.

This chapter briefly reflects on the past but most importantly looks to the future of the modern learning disability nurse practitioner. It discusses issues affecting learning disability nursing, such as changing professional requirements, policy directions such as: Strengthening the Commitment (2012), and ever-growing opportunities for learning disability nurses to assert themselves in a widening practice arena.

Therefore, this chapter, focuses on the knowledge and practical skills that learning disability nurses will need to meet the needs of people with learning disability in the future, and this will be contextualised within the Nursing and Midwifery Council for the United Kingdom (2010) and An Bord Altranais (2005) standards for competence. The future of learning disability nursing is discussed in the context of policy directions, emerging roles, and learning disability nurses' clinical and other expertise, and their ability as individuals and as a profession to adapt, and work effectively in multidisciplinary and interagency settings.

This chapter will focus on the following issues:

- Challenges for professional identity
- The need for learning disability nursing
  - Need for health advocacy
  - Current health care policies and professional requirements
  - Enhancing health and health care outcomes for people with learning disabilities
  - Developing expertise and specialist knowledge
  - Enhancing interprofessional working
  - Providing leadership
  - Research
  - Managing change
  - Policy process
  - Workforce planning

- Future spheres of practice
- Emerging roles
  - Policy development
  - Policy implementation
  - Policy evaluation
  - Healthcare quality
  - Commissioning
  - Health surveillance
  - Health action planning
  - Health facilitation
  - Health liaison
  - Non-medical prescribing
  - Learning disability nurse consultant
  - School nursing
  - Criminal justice system

Competences

NMC Competences and Competencies

Domain 1: Professional values - Field standard for competence and competencies – 1.1; 3.1.

Domain 2: Communication and interpersonal skills - Field standard for competence and competencies – 3.1; 5.1.

Domain 4: Leadership, management and team working - Field standard for competence and competencies – 1.1; 1.2; 6.1; 6.2.

An Bord Altranais Competences and Indicators

Domain 1: Professional/ethical practice – 1.1.1; 1.2.2; 1.2.3; 1.2.6.

Domain 4: Organisation and management of care – 4.1.1; 4.1.2; 4.1.5; 4.3.1.

Domain 5: Personal and professional development – 5.1.1; 5.1.2.

CHALLENGES FOR PROFESSIONAL IDENTITY

The United Kingdom and Ireland are now the only countries to provide a specialist pre-qualification programme for nurses caring for people with learning disabilities. In both countries, learning disability nursing developed as a consequence of the medicalisation of the colony system for 'mental defectives' into mental deficiency hospitals, which required trained nurses. Since its inception in the early part of the twentieth century, like people with learning disabilities, learning disability nursing has been largely invisible, and its relevance and position within the nursing profession has been repeatedly questioned. Learning disability nursing's origins in large psychiatric institutions in the United Kingdom, and religious orders and mental asylums in Ireland, have resulted in the profession being associated with widely reported malpractice, and poor practice in these institutions. Events of the past few years, such as the abuses at Winterbourne View, demonstrate that standards of professional practice and integrity need to be high in relation to learning disability nurses, who support some of the most vulnerable people in society. Learning disability nurses have a collective professional responsibility to ensure that those who fail to safeguard, abuse, or commit criminal offences against vulnerable individuals with learning disability have no place in the profession.

Collectively, learning disability nurses may not have considered the full implications of such events, which have negatively affected the positive contributions they make to the lives of people with learning disabilities. This inability to focus on the positive contribution that learning disability nursing has made to the lives of people with learning disabilities has perhaps resulted in misunderstanding and confusion of its role among the wider health and social care communities. Perhaps even more significant is the resulting confusion among learning disability nurses themselves about what their role involves (Stewart and Todd, 2001). As a professional group, learning disability nurses need to take responsibility and a lead in defining their role and be instrumental in shaping the future of their sphere of practice. It could be argued that *Better Services for the Mentally Handicapped* (1971), *The Same as You* (2000), *Valuing People* (2001), *Requirements and Standards for Nurse Registration Education Programmes* (2005), *Healthcare for All* (2008), *Standards for Pre-registration Nurse Education* (2010), *Continuing the Commitment* (2012, *Confidential Inquiry into Premature Deaths of People with Learning Disabilities* (2013), *The Health Equalities Framework* (2013), and other recent policy documents, reports, and service re-organisations have, over the years, provided numerous opportunities for learning disability nurses to clarify their positive contributions to the lives of people with learning disabilities.

The challenge for learning disability nursing is to be proactive in defining its contribution to the lives of people with learning disabilities, to develop their skills, and to develop an evidence base that validates their contribution to the health and well-being of people with learning disabilities. If learning disability nurses are to continue to make a positive difference to the lives of people with learning disabilities, such nurses will need to collaborate and be proactive in articulating and validating their contributions to people with learning disabilities and the nursing profession.

THE NEED FOR LEARNING DISABILITY NURSING

Extent of the health and health care needs of people with learning disabilities

First, it is now widely accepted that people with learning disabilities have much greater and more complex health needs than the general population (Backer et al., 2009). For example, people with learning disabilities experience higher rates of mental disorders (Linna et al., 1999), visual impairments (Barr et al., 1999), epilepsy (Ryan and Sunada, 1997), hypertension and hypothyroidism (Barr et al., 1999), and obesity (van Schrojenstein Lantman-de Valk, et al. 2000), and they are more likely to die from preventable causes (Pawar and Akuffo, 2008). Second, the extent of the avoidable disparity (van Schrojenstein Lantman-de Valk et al., 2000) between the health and the health care needs of people with learning disabilities as compared to that of the general population (Kerr, 2004; DH, 2001) as a result of poor accessibility of health services for people with learning disabilities means that learning disability nurses will continue to play an important role in meeting those needs. As discussed in Chapter 4, studies have consistently shown that people with learning disabilities experience health inequalities (Scheepers et al., 2005; Melville et al., 2006), poor access to health care (Nocon et al., 2008; Brown et al., 2010), unequal access to health services (Kerr, 2004; DRC, 2006; Iacono and Davis, 2003; Janicki et al., 2002; Scheepers et al., 2005; Mencap, 2004), and inadequate diagnosis of treatable conditions (Hollins et al., 1998; Mencap, 2007; DH, 2007a; DH, 2007b; Durvasula et al., 2002), and are considered a low priority by health care professionals (Aspray et al., 1999). In addition, it has been highlighted earlier that international studies have demonstrated widespread concerns about the inequalities in health experienced by people with learning disabilities (Janicki, 2012; Scheepers et al., 2005) resulting from people with learning disabilities themselves, and how health services and systems are organised. Furthermore, it has been discussed in Chapter 4 that people with learning disabilities have complex health needs, and lifestyle-related comorbidity is common (Messent et al., 1999). International studies have demonstrated poor uptake of health services by people with learning disabilities (Beange et al., 1995; Wood and Douglas, 2007).

We also noted previously in this book that cognitive impairments can limit people with learning disabilities' ability to access services (Jones and Kerr, 1997); communication difficulties and limited understanding of the diagnostic and treatment issues for people with learning disabilities (Straetmans et al., 2007), and health care professionals' limited augmentative communication skills (Lennox and Diggins, 1999) limit effective diagnosis and treatment of people with learning disabilities. The complexity of the health and health care needs of people with learning disabilities, and the ever changing nursing practice environment means that learning disability nurses need to continue to adapt.

Need for health advocacy

It is clear that learning disability nurses will need to continue to develop effective health advocacy that will improve the health and health care outcomes for people with learning disabilities (Lennox et al., 2000; Llewellyn, 2005; Llewellyn and Northway, 2007). Internationally in the past few decades, efforts to depathologise learning disabilities have gathered pace. In the United Kingdom this has resulted in people with learning disabilities having to access mainstream health services. What has become increasingly clear and has been acknowledged by the increasing number of learning disability health liaison nurses in acute mainstream hospitals is the important contribution learning disability nurses make in improving access to health and health care for people with learning disabilities. The recent shift from treatment to preventive health care in the United Kingdom is a welcome development for people with learning disabilities. Delivering effective preventive health care through mainstream services for people with learning disabilities is challenging (Thomas and Kerr, 2011), and learning disability nurses will need to be proactive in assimilating new roles that arise from this re-orientation of services. Assimilating new roles in this area is important to ensure that provision of health services for people with learning disabilities is not opportunistic (McIlfatrick et al., 2011). This is a logical development in the absence of people with learning disabilities' ability to self-refer for health care (Felce et al., 2008). Recent international studies have shown that preventive interventions are effective in identifying the health and health care needs of people with learning disabilities (Beange et al., 1995; Webb and Rogers, 1999; Emerson and Glover, 2010; Emerson et al., 2011). Learning disability nurses need to work collectively to assimilate, clarify, and validate new roles that focus on preventive interventions for meeting the health needs of people with learning disabilities.

Lack of role clarity of the professionals, including learning disability nurses, working with people with learning disabilities has been consistently identified as one of the most common barriers to improving the health and health care outcomes for people with learning disabilities (Thornton, 1996; Powrie, 2003; NHS Health Scotland, 2004; Phillips et al., 2004; Melville et al., 2005). Phillips et al. (2004) have highlighted the importance of primary health care services in meeting the health and health care needs of people with learning disabilities. Learning disability nurses occupy a unique position to develop an evidence base that demonstrates the need for and their ability to address the barriers that people with learning disability experience when accessing generic primary and acute health services. It is therefore important for learning disability nurses to play an active role in implementing health initiatives for people with learning disabilities across all existing health care pathways. The extent of the health and health care needs of people with learning disabilities, and the current regulatory support for the profession, mean that learning disability nurses themselves need to address the lack of clarity of their positive contribution in meeting the health and health care needs of people with learning disabilities.

To continue to be relevant in modern-day practice, learning disability nurses need to be aware of the implications about how they enact their roles as a result of the major restructuring of health care organisations in the United Kingdom, Ireland, and globally, resulting from the political and economic challenges to contain the cost of health care. In the United Kingdom, these changes mean that learning disability nurses not only have to embrace an ever-increasing repertoire of new roles, but that they are also increasingly working in a wider range of complex and challenging environments. For learning disability nurses to continue to make meaningful contributions in meeting the health and health care needs of people with learning disabilities, it is imperative that such nurses are actively engaged with this change, engage in developing new knowledge and ways of working within and beyond the profession, and assimilate new roles in their traditional working environments and beyond existing working environments. Learning disability nurses at all levels need to create formal and informal opportunities to engage with colleagues in other health services to improve access to mainstream services for people with learning disabilities. Learning disability nurses need to exploit their unique professional position and take lead roles in influencing the continued development and delivery of mainstream and specialist health and health care services for people with learning disabilities.

Current health care policies and professional requirements

Current health care policies and health care professional education in the United Kingdom and Ireland recognise the contributions of and need for specialist learning disability health services and learning disability nurses. Such services, even in light of the significant shift toward the mainstreaming of health care for people with learning disabilities, particularly in the United Kingdom, mean that learning disability nurses now and in the future will continue to be important and have significant roles in assessing, treating, supporting, educating, and coordinating the delivery of care for people with learning disabilities. It is clear that the need for preventive interventions, primary care, and specialist learning disability services will remain an essential part of health care and professional education systems in both the United Kingdom and Ireland for the foreseeable future.

Although the shift from treatment to preventive interventions has resulted in questions and anxieties about the future roles of learning disability nurses, *Requirements and Standards for Nurse Registration Education Programmes* (2005), *Healthcare for All* (2008), *Standards for*

Pre-registration Nurse Education (2010), *Learning Disability Nursing: Task and Finish Group Report for the Professional and Advisory Board for Nursing and Midwifery - Department of Health, England* (2011), *Continuing the Commitment* (2012), *Confidential Inquiry into Premature Deaths of People with Learning Disabilities* (2013), and *The Health Equalities Framework* (2013) clearly demonstrate the continued professional need for, and political commitment to, learning disability nursing. What is perhaps important for learning disability nurses is for them to individually and collectively focus on the opportunities for enhancing the contributions they make in meeting the health and health care needs of people with learning disabilities.

Enhancing health and health care outcomes for people with learning disabilities

Among other things, Mafuba (2013) has noted the need for learning disability nurses to focus on developing their expertise and specialist knowledge of the health and health care needs of people with learning disabilities, developing the research evidence base for their practice, developing professional leadership, ensuring that pre-registration and post-registration learning disability nurse education reflects the changing needs of people with learning disabilities, and actively engaging with the health policy process to ensure that their unique knowledge and expertise shapes their future practice to improve the health and health care outcomes for people with learning disabilities (see Figure 10.1).

To enhance the health and health care outcomes for people with learning disabilities, learning disability nurses individually and collectively need to achieve a delicate balance of the activities illustrated in Figure 10.1 to influence the direction and relevance of the profession. Learning disability nurses are the only professional group in the United Kingdom and Ireland that is exclusively trained to work with people with learning disabilities across the lifespan.

Developing expertise and specialist knowledge

Learning disability nurses possess an unmatched breadth, depth of knowledge, and set of skills crucial to enhancing the health and health care outcomes of people with learning disabilities. Recent studies have highlighted the positive contributions of learning disability nurses (Bollard, 2002; Marshall and Moore, 2003; Barr et al., 1999), and the positive regard for learning disability nurses

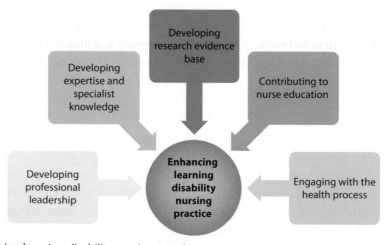

Figure 10.1 Enhancing learning disability nursing practice.

by other health care professionals (Stewart and Todd, 2001). Other health care professionals, people with learning disabilities, and their families have positive regard for learning disability nurses resulting from their extensive knowledge of learning disabilities (Gates, 2011). Learning disability nurses therefore need to continue to develop and translate their theoretical knowledge into daily practice and support other professionals to develop their own knowledge essential to improving the outcomes the health and health care needs of people with learning disabilities.

Enhancing interprofessional working

Increasing life expectancy for people with learning disabilities and developments in health and health care provision mean that learning disability nurses need to be actively involved in developing innovative pre-registration and post-registration curricula that not only influence how they will practice in the future, but also focus on enhancing interprofessional working and practice. To achieve this, learning disability nurses need to adopt fully the culture of lifelong learning to realise the opportunities occasioned by the rapidly changing knowledge and nature of health service provision for people with learning disabilities. Learning disability nursing curricula need to focus on the development of knowledge relevant for day-to-day practice.

Providing leadership

The current organisation of health care in the United Kingdom and Ireland highlighted previously suggest that the future direction of learning disability nursing is going to be influenced significantly by how learning disability nurses occupy positions of influence and leadership in a wide range of positions and organisations (Faugier, 2004). Learning disability nurses need to urgently address the absence of a clear leadership structure at local and national levels that may result in a professional leadership vacuum regarding the health and health care needs of people with learning disabilities. In the United Kingdom the learning disability nursing profession may benefit from developing a clear leadership structure, which incorporates the learning disability nurse consultant role and other emerging roles (Mafuba, 2013). The destiny of learning disability nurses is in their own hands. Learning disability nurses need to embrace the current opportunities provided by ongoing health care reorganisations by taking on lead roles at all levels when opportunities for such roles arise. The learning disability nursing profession needs leaders with highly developed personal qualities such as self-belief, intellectual competence and flexibility, political shrewdness and judiciousness, and proficiency and virtuosity in marshalling essential change (UK Learning Disability Consultant Nurse Network, 2006). This will require learning disability nurses to develop an extended repertoire of leadership skills and competencies. Learning disability nurses in positions of leadership and influence need to contribute meaningfully to the development of positive opportunities that will develop influential leaders of the profession, both now and for the future. For learning disability nursing to be sustainable in the long term, learning disability nurses themselves need to make succession planning an integral part of their professional structures.

Research

The Royal College of Nursing (2004) has noted that research and development of new ways of working underlie effective nursing practice. Learning disability nurses need to maximise the opportunities afforded by current collaborative arrangements between higher education and clinical practice to ensure that they develop a sound evidence base that informs their practice.

To engage effectively in research and development, learning disability nurses individually and collectively need to appreciate that research evidence underlies effective nursing practice. Without sound evidence that supports clinical practice, questions of clinical competence and credibility of learning disability nursing and questions about their professional relevance will continue unabated. Learning disability nurse researchers need to seek to enhance and develop the current evidence base of the contribution of learning disability nurses to meeting the health and health care needs of people with learning disabilities. Such research needs to explain and evaluate the skill base required for learning disability nurses to effectively enact their roles (Mafuba, 2013). In addition, learning disability nurses need to develop evidence that validates their interventions. Current and potential learning disability nursing research leaders need to seek to establish collaborative research centres that would be able to build the appropriate intellectual capacity necessary to undertake research of local, national, and international standing (Mafuba, 2013). Parahoo et al. (2000), in a study of research utilisation and attitudes toward research among learning disability nurses In Northern Ireland, concluded that learning disability nurses were less likely to be aware of the evidence for their practice than nurses in other fields of practice. Limited capacity and capability to undertake leading research has contributed to a limited evidence base in learning disability nursing practice. Therefore, learning disability nurses need to make strategic alliances with other nursing disciplines and other professions, nationally and internationally, to enhance their research capacity and outputs (Mafuba, 2013). Current efforts to establish the *Learning/Intellectual Disability Academics Network*, involving learning disability nursing academics and practitioners in the United Kingdom and Ireland, need to be pursued with strategic focus and tenacity. The *UK Modernising Learning Disabilities Nursing Review* (2012) has provided opportunities for collaborative working to enhance research activities among learning disability nurses, which they need to embrace. Learning disability nurses need to see their involvement in research activities as an integral part of their daily practice. This is relevant for all learning disability nurses individually and collectively irrespective of their area of practice. It is therefore important for learning disability nurses, particularly those in influential positions, service managers, commissioners, and education providers, to ensure that research and personal development activities are embedded in nursing roles at every level (Brimblecombe, 2004). To engage effectively with the research process, learning disability nurses need to develop their research competency.

Managing change

Ongoing broader changes in health service provision and organisation create challenges and opportunities for learning disability nurses. This can result in some learning disability nurses experiencing professional, managerial, organisational, and geographical isolation, both individually and collectively (Mafuba, 2013). Learning disability nurses need to actively engage with managing change that affects their practice. It is no longer sufficient for learning disability nurses to simply respond to change imposed by others, who in most cases lack a clear understanding of learning disability nursing roles, and the health and the health care needs of people with learning disabilities. Learning disability nurses who have gained greater autonomy and flexibility afforded by these changes need to ensure that they use such opportunities to influence not only their own practice but that of the learning disability nursing profession as a whole.

Learning disability nurses need political astuteness and awareness to be effective agents of change for their own future practice. This will require them to develop effective local, national, and international networks that will enhance their effectiveness as agents of change. In addition, learning disability nurses need to develop their capacity to think and act strategically to influence the direction and pace of change of their own practice. To be effective agents of change, learning disability nurses will need to influence health policies that affect the health and health care of people with learning disabilities.

Policy process

There is a need for learning disability nurses to be politically sensitised to the health policy processes in both the United Kingdom and Ireland. Learning disability nurses need to develop professional mechanisms to coordinate their contributions to health policy development and evaluation. The nature of U.K. health policy and policy implementation is that it is very much driven from central government (Ham, 2004). Historically, this has resulted in learning disability nurses and other nurses disengaging from the process. However, recent shifts toward the involvement of health professionals in health care design and commissioning in England have created opportunities for learning disability nurses to influence health policy development and implementation. Learning disability nurses will need to influence and contribute to health policy development, policy implementation, policy evaluation, and health policy research (Mafuba, 2013). They need to be aware of the immense influence of health policy on their practice. It is therefore important that learning disability nurses contribute meaningfully to policy consultations as individual practitioners and collectively. In the United Kingdom, formal consultation of both professionals and users of health services is part of the policy formulation process. Learning disability nurses need to collaborate with other professionals and groups of people with learning disabilities to ensure that health policies that affect the health and health care needs of people with learning disabilities are relevant. In addition, learning disability nurses need to develop mechanisms that will enable them collectively to gain access to policymakers of incumbent governments to articulate their contributions to meeting the health and health care needs of people with learning disabilities.

Workforce planning

The *Learning Disabilities Nursing Task and Finish Group* (Gates, 2011) and *Strengthening the Commitment* (2013) have demonstrated the need for strategic planning to ensure that learning disability nursing will continue to have the right numbers and appropriately skilled professionals. This is essential to ensure that the health and health care needs of people with learning disabilities are adequately met. The learning disability nursing profession needs to take the lead in ensuring that there are sufficient numbers of learning disability nurses who are competent, experienced, and skilled to meet the health and health care needs of people with learning disabilities in a wide range of settings. Learning disability nurses need to collaborate with commissioners and employers to develop the workforce. This is essential, because having skilled, competent, and experienced learning disability nurses will lead to improved health, and health care outcomes for people with learning disabilities. Learning disability nurses need to take responsibility for clarifying career pathways, so that new entrants into the profession can follow across the NHS, and other service-provider organisations, commissioning organisations, academia, and other organisations.

> **Learning Activity 10.1**
>
> Having read the section on the need for learning disability nursing in the United Kingdom and Ireland, identify and reflect on examples about how learning disability nurses in your own country and elsewhere have done the following
>
> - Contributed to developing expertise and specialist knowledge in learning disability nursing practice
> - Enhanced interprofessional learning and working
> - Provided professional leadership that made a significant difference to learning disability nursing practice
> - Undertaken research that has affected the learning disability nursing profession
> - Managed change that resulted in the enhancement of the roles of learning disability nurses at national or international levels
> - Contributed to health policy development that affected learning disability nursing practice or health and health care outcomes for people with learning disabilities
> - Contributed to workforce planning that enhanced learning disability nursing roles
> - Acted as a professional health advocate for people with learning disabilities, which resulted in improved recognition of learning disability nursing at national or international levels
> - Contributed to improved professional recognition and identity for learning disability nursing

FUTURE SPHERES OF PRACTICE

Requirements and Standards for Nurse Registration Education Programmes (2005), *Standards for Pre-registration Nurse Education* (2010), and *Continuing the Commitment* (2012), demonstrate professional and political recognition that learning disability nurses have much to contribute to current and future health care provision and development for people with learning disabilities. Learning disability nurses will need to take essential roles in initiatives targeted at developing health and health care services for people with learning disabilities. This is essential to facilitate partnerships with other professionals, organisations, people with learning disabilities, their families, carers, and other stakeholders. The complexities of the health and health care needs of people with learning disabilities, current models of health service provision, and challenges people with learning disabilities experience when they access health and health care services means that partnership working will be key to improving the health and health care outcomes for people with learning disabilities.

The population of people with learning disabilities is growing. This is characterised by children with learning disabilities and complex health and health care needs surviving into adulthood. In addition, the population of older adults with learning disabilities is increasing in line with overall life expectancy trends. This will have a significant effect on learning disability nursing as new health and health care challenges emerge and increase with the growing population. Learning disability nurses should focus on developing knowledge and skills that will equip them to work more effectively with people with learning disabilities across their lifespans. This will require learning disability nurses to take on new roles in non-traditional areas of their practice to effectively address the many complex and comorbid health needs of people with learning disabilities.

People with learning disabilities have a complex health profile that is different from that of the general population. As more people with severe learning disabilities and complex health and health care needs increases, there is likely to be an increase in complex comorbid health needs. Emerson and Baines (2010) have concluded that mental illness, autism spectrum disorder, behavioural challenges, and dementia are all more common in people with learning disabilities. As the population of people with learning disabilities increase, so too will the prevalence of these conditions. (Torr and Davis, 2007). Learning disability nurses need to be cognisant of these population trends so that they can develop new roles in new health care settings where services for people with learning disabilities with increasingly complex health needs will be delivered in the future.

People with learning disabilities experience significant barriers when accessing health services, resulting in poorer health outcomes as compared to people without learning disabilities (Cooper et al., 2011). This increasingly complex repertoire of needs will require increased and more frequent use of health care services. With mainstream professional health care education often lacking emphasis on the needs of people with learning disabilities (DoH, 2008), learning disability nurses need to develop new roles in mainstream health and health care services.

EMERGING ROLES

The emerging roles discussed here only represent a select few learning disability nursing roles that have emerged or significantly evolved since the beginning of the twenty-first century (see Figure 10.2).

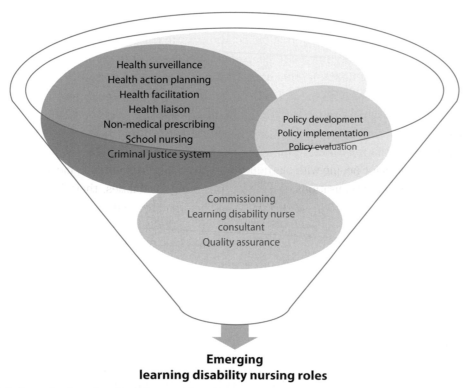

Health surveillance
Health action planning
Health facilitation
Health liaison
Non-medical prescribing
School nursing
Criminal justice system

Policy development
Policy implementation
Policy evaluation

Commissioning
Learning disability nurse consultant
Quality assurance

**Emerging
learning disability nursing roles**

Figure 10.2 Emerging learning disability nursing roles.

Policy development

The limited involvement of learning disability nurses in health policy development is likely to be reflective of the complexity of the health policy process. As the practice and policy landscape of health care provision becomes more complex, learning disability nurses need to be actively seeking to embrace new roles, which involve responsibility for policy formulation at local and national levels. The lack of strategic involvement by learning disability nurses in the development of health policy needs to be addressed to ensure the appropriateness of such policies to meeting the health and health care needs of people with learning disabilities. For health policies to be effective in meeting the health and health care needs of people with learning disabilities, learning disability nurses need to be meaningfully involved at every level in the policy process.

Policy implementation

Under the general practitioner (GP) contract in the United Kingdom, additional payments have been made available since 2008 to facilitate increased access to health screening services for people with learning disabilities. This was in recognition of the increased morbidity rates in the population of people with learning disabilities and the need for reasonable adjustments to improve the accessibility of primary and preventive health services by people with learning disabilities (Melville et al., 2006; NHS Health Scotland, 2004). If learning disability nursing is going to remain relevant in meeting the preventive and primary health care needs of people with learning disabilities, such nurses must actively collaborate with, and develop new roles in, primary care, and other areas to positively influence the implementation of such important policies.

Learning disability nurses are increasingly expected to be involved in implementing preventive health initiatives for people with learning disabilities in primary care settings (Mafuba, 2013), and learning disability nurses need to assimilate these new roles. This means that such nurses need to be prepared for significant changes in role expectations from traditional methods of working. It is important for learning disability nurses to keep abreast of the context in which their roles evolve. This context is undergoing fundamental change, particularly in England, with the transfer of the 'public health' function of the NHS to local authorities. In addition, the reorganisation of the English NHS means learning disability nursing roles are being transferred to acute NHS trusts, specialist mental health and learning disability NHS organisations, local authorities, and social enterprises. All of these changes will affect how learning disability nurses participate in the implementation of health policies for people with learning disabilities.

Policy evaluation

The evaluation of health policy implementation has been neglected (O'Toole, 2004), and particularly so for people with learning disabilities. The contribution of learning disability nurses in evaluating health policy effectiveness for people with learning disabilities is important in identifying areas of health care that need improvement. It is also likely to positively affect how people with learning disabilities experience and access health and health care services (Mafuba, 2013). Learning disability nurses' involvement with health policy evaluation will become increasingly important and significant in the future.

Health care quality

Following the BBC Panorama programme report in May 2011, which exposed the abuses that had taken place at Winterbourne View hospital in Bristol, the Care Quality Commission announced a programme of unannounced inspections of health and social care services providing care for people with learning disabilities and challenging behaviours (CQC, 2012). The Care Quality Commission is the independent regulator of health and adult social care services provided by hospitals, dentists, ambulances, care homes, and home-care agencies in England. This review was informed by external advisory and reference groups, which included learning disability nurses. Learning disability nurses were instrumental in providing support and challenging the design, development, and implementation of a new approach to quality inspection and monitoring of these services. The Care Quality Commission has progressed to recruit learning disability nurses into its inspection teams, providing new and exciting opportunities for learning disability nurses for the future.

The National Institute for Health and Care Excellence (NICE) is a world-renowned organisation that provides U.K. national guidance and advice on how to improve health and social care. For the first time, NICE is in the process of developing two sets of national guidelines specifically for people with learning disabilities, and they are the following

- Challenging behaviour and learning disabilities: prevention and interventions for people with learning disabilities whose behaviour challenges (due 2015)
- Mental health problems in people with learning disability: management of mental health problems in people with learning disability (due 2016)

Such developments are significant and will affect learning disability nursing practice. It is therefore important that learning disability nurses engage with such developments, which focus on improving health and health care outcomes for people with learning disabilities.

Commissioning

Starting in April 2013 in the English NHS, *Clinical Commissioning Groups* were set up to organise the delivery of NHS services in England. The aim of Clinical Commissioning Groups is to give GPs, other primary care clinicians, local communities, and local authorities the ability to influence commissioning decisions for all patients in a specific geographical location. Clinical Commissioning Groups are required to include nurses. These groups are responsible for commissioning (or buying) elective hospital care, rehabilitation care, urgent and emergency care, community health services, and mental health and learning disability services. This provides a significant opportunity for learning disability nurses to play an important role in the way health and health care services are delivered to people with learning disabilities.

Health surveillance

Another important area of practice in primary care services for learning disability nurses is the development of registers of people with learning disabilities. This is an important role for learning disability nursing for a number of reasons. Accurate registers are useful in signposting people with learning disabilities to appropriate services (Emerson and McGrother, 2010). In addition, registers highlight the extent of the known and unknown complex health and health care needs of the population of people with learning disabilities (Emerson and McGrother, 2010). Furthermore, registers are important in delivering preventive health services for people with learning disabilities (Emerson and McGrother, 2010). Demographic ignorance has been noted to have a significant affect on the implementation of a wide range of health policies for people with learning disabilities (Mafuba, 2013). Learning disability nurses need to be actively involved in developing and maintaining accurate registers to ensure adequate levels for people with learning disabilities across all age groups.

Health action planning

Health action plans (HAPs) were introduced as a part of the *Valuing People* strategy (DoH, 2001). HAPs play an important role in facilitating the maintenance and improvement of the health and health care outcomes for people with learning disabilities. The introduction of HAPs in the United Kingdom and health action planning was an important development in attempts to improve the health and healthcare outcomes for people with learning disabilities. Being the only group of professionals that exclusively specialises in working with and supporting people with learning disabilities, learning disability nurses need to engage with health action planning at both the individual and strategic levels. Learning disability nurses need to lead in translating such, and similar, policy initiatives and expectations into actual new roles. This will not only validate and enhance the value of the profession, but is likely to positively impact the implementation of wider health policies and strategies for people with learning disabilities.

Health facilitation

The importance of the 'health facilitation' role of learning disability nurses has been described in recent studies (Marshall and Moore, 2003). Although *Valuing People* (DoH, 2001) identified health facilitation, there has been a persistent lack of clarity regarding professional responsibility for this approach to meeting the health care needs of people with learning disabilities. A U.K.-wide study of community learning disability nursing roles by Mafuba (2013) has noted the extent and variation of the expected involvement of community learning disability nurses with health facilitation, despite increasing acceptance of the high regard of their health facilitation role among other professionals within primary and acute health care settings. This development has enhanced the health facilitation role of learning disability nurses among their primary care colleagues. The increasing genericisation of the delivery of health care to people with learning disabilities and the shift from treatment to preventive health interventions indicate the need for learning disability nurses to focus on enhancing their health facilitation knowledge and skills to assimilate into this relatively new role. Learning disability nurses need to be aware that such change in their roles is inevitable and unavoidable. Supporting people with learning disabilities to access health services is becoming an important role for learning disability nurses.

Health liaison

Health liaison is an important role for learning disability nurses in the implementation of health policy for people with learning disabilities (Barr et al., 1999; Stewart and Todd. 2001; Powell et al., 2004). The health liaison role of learning disability nurses is increasingly being based in acute services (Brown et al., 2011). When based in acute settings, learning disability nurses in such roles need to ensure that they are prominent. In addition, learning disability nurses need to effectively liaise with other professionals, people with learning disabilities, families, carers, and other agencies to support the development of preventive health and treatment pathways for people with learning disabilities.

Non-medical prescribing

Non-medical prescribing was introduced in the United States in 1970 (Jones and Johns, 2005). In the U.K. National Health Service, non-medical prescribing is a relatively new development aimed at changing traditional professional roles and responsibilities. Non-medical prescribing was specifically introduced to enhance the care and treatment of people with medium-term and long-term health conditions such as epilepsy. Kwentoh and Reilly (2009) have observed that many nurses who were taking up prescribing responsibilities were positive about their non-medical prescribing roles. These new roles are open to learning disability nurses, and it is in the long-term prospects and relevance of the profession for such nurses to take up these roles. People with learning disabilities often have long-term conditions, such as epilepsy and diabetes, which can benefit from non-medical prescribing.

Non-medical prescribing (epilepsy)

Epilepsy specialist nurses in Northern Ireland and Gloucestershire demonstrated the benefits to people with learning disabilities of undertaking a non-medical prescribing course. The nurses recognised opportunities to provide advice to people with learning disabilities, their families, and their carers about medication changes rather than having them wait for appointments with medical practitioners. This enabled timely and effective treatment, which resulted in the reduction of risks by preventing seizures and adverse effects of medications. The nurses are able to advise people with learning disabilities, their families, and their carers about medication changes promptly, based on assessed need. As is the case with the medical consultant who reviews the client's epilepsy at outpatient clinics, the nurses will be able to recommend medication changes to the GP, enabling a person's medical record to be updated and the necessary medication to be provided for the long term. The nurses also provide expert knowledge about epilepsy in people with learning disabilities to support GPs. This reduces the risk of sudden unexpected death in epilepsy and improving the health care outcomes for people with learning disabilities. Regular appointments, partnership working, and training can lead to improved recording and medication concordance. Reasonable adjustments can be made by strengthening links with other professionals, by providing relevant data to support access to mainstream services.

Tasks

Consider and reflect upon the implications of the non-medical prescribing role for the following

- People with learning disabilities who have epilepsy and complex needs
- Families of people with learning disabilities who have epilepsy and complex needs
- Formal and informal carers of people with learning disabilities who have epilepsy and complex needs
- Learning disability nurses (individually and collectively)
- Healthcare organisations

Source: Adapted from *UK Modernising Learning Disabilities Nursing Review, Strengthening the Commitment* (Report). Edinburgh: The Scottish Government, 2012.

Learning disability nurse consultant

The absence of a clear leadership structure at local and national levels in learning disability nursing has in the past created a significant professional leadership vacuum (Gates, 2011). There is need for a clear professional leadership structure which incorporates the learning disability nurse consultant role. Learning disability nurse consultant roles need to reflect the NHS *Key Skills Framework* (DoH, 2004) in order for their health care contributions for people with learning disabilities at local and national levels to be validated. The learning disability nursing profession needs to consider how the current *UK Learning Disability Nurse Consultant Network* can provide better leadership which has the potential to enhance professional learning disability nursing leadership at local, regional, and national levels.

School nursing

Recently, school-nursing services in Brent, Ealing, and Kent, for example, have developed teams of a mixture of learning disability nurses, paediatric nurses, and health support workers. These teams work with children and young people with moderate to profound learning disabilities from 0–18 years of age. This offers a unique opportunity for learning disability nursing to develop new areas of practice. To take full advantage of these emerging roles learning disability nurses need to develop an extensive and diverse repertoire of skills, knowledge, and experience in child health, child development, post-diagnostic counseling, safeguarding, continence promotion, immunisation and vaccination, hands-on nursing and emergency care within the school environment, and transition planning, in addition to having unique knowledge and expertise of the health and health care needs of people with learning disabilities.

Criminal justice system

A review of people with learning disabilities and learning difficulties concluded that around 20% to 30% of offenders had a learning disability or difficulty that compromised their ability to cope with the criminal justice system (Loucks, 2007). The Royal College of Nursing (2009) has recognised the contribution learning disability nurses could make to people with learning disabilities in the prison system. It is vital that people with learning disabilities are recognised and have their health and health care needs assessed to receive appropriate support during their period of incarceration. Without appropriate support, people with learning disabilities are likely to be extremely vulnerable to neglect and abuse with likely consequent poorer health and health care outcomes. Learning disability nurses are increasingly being considered a valuable addition to the nursing teams working in criminal justice service settings. The establishment of a dedicated health care service to support prisoners who have a learning disability across Surrey's four prisons (Ford, 2011) demonstrates the high regard learning disability nursing is gaining in this area of practice. The service run by a local NHS service organisation was the first countywide service of its kind in England and Wales within male and female prisons. This was led by a learning disability nurse at its inception. Learning disability nurses can and do make significant contributions, by working collaboratively with prison staff and other health care professionals within prisons and in the community during rehabilitation, to ensure that people with learning disabilities are identified and assessed for additional support so that they can access appropriate health services while they are imprisoned and following discharge. In this role, learning disability nurses need be involved in training other staff within the prison, and other health care professionals who work within the system to ensure the development of appropriate knowledge and skills necessary to meeting the health and health care needs of people with learning disabilities. Another key role for learning disability nurses working in the prison service is to undertake risk assessments and risk management plans in partnership with other professionals and people with learning disabilities to facilitate rehabilitation into the community.

CONCLUSION

The challenges posed by demographic changes to the population of people with learning disabilities will necessitate changes to future roles of learning disability nurses. The health and health care needs of people with learning disabilities, and how health care is delivered, will become increasingly complex. Consequently, learning disability nurses need to understand the need for their nursing roles to extend beyond traditional professional practice and geographical boundaries.

Nationally and internationally, health care will continue to undergo seismic shifts. Consequently, learning disability nurses, like other health care professionals, will continue to be exposed to major changes in their roles in meeting the health and health care needs of people with learning disabilities, and in where they undertake those changing roles.

Learning disability nurses need to develop formal and informal collaborations at local, national, and international levels to remain relevant. Learning disability nurses in the United Kingdom and Ireland can and need to be an important force for change of their own practice, health policy, and how health care is organised and delivered to people with learning disabilities. For this potential to be fully realised, learning disability nursing needs strong leadership, appropriate pre- and post-registration education, and engagement with workforce planning at local, national, and, to an extent, international levels. This is essential in strengthening efforts to improve the health and health care of people with learning disabilities.

REFERENCES

Alaszewski, A., Gates, B., Ayer, S., Manthorpe, G., and Motherby, E. 2000. *Education for Diversity and Change: Final Report of the ENB-Funded Project on Educational Preparation for Learning Disability Nursing.* Schools of Community and Health Studies and Nursing. The University of Hull.

An Bord Altranais. 2005. *Requirements and Standards for Nurse Registration Education Programmes* (3rd ed.). Dublin: An Bord Altranais.

Aspray, T.J., Francis, R.M., Tyrer, S.P., and Quilliam, S.J. 1999. Patients with learning disability in the community. *British Medical Journal*, 318:476–477.

Atkinson, D., Boulter, P., Hebron, C., Moulster, G., Giraud-Saunders, A., and Turner, S. 2013. The Health Equalities Framework (HEF)—An outcomes framework based on the determinants of health inequalities. (Online). Available at http://www.ndti.org.uk/uploads/files/The_Health_Equality_Framework.pdf (accessed May 24, 2014).

Backer, C., Chapman, M. and Mitchell, D. 2009. Access to secondary healthcare for people with learning disabilities: A review of the literature. *Journal of Applied Research in Intellectual Disabilities*,(22)6:514–525.

Barr, O., Gilgunn, J., Kane, T., and Moore, G. 1999. Health screening for people with learning disabilities by a community learning disabilities nursing service in Northern Ireland. *Journal of Advanced Nursing*, 29(6):1482–1491.

Beange, H., McElduff, A., and Baker, W. 1995. Medical disorders of adults with mental retardation: A population study. *American Journal of Mental Retardation*, 99(6):595–604.

Bollard, M. 2002. Health promotion and learning disabilities. *Health Education*, 16(27):47–55.

Brimblecombe, N. 2004. Making my ark. *Nurse Researcher*, 12(1):78–80.

Brown, M., MacArthur, J., McKechanie, A., Hayes, M., and Fletcher, J. 2010. Equality and access to general healthcare for people with learning disabilities: Reality or rhetoric? *Journal of Research in Nursing*, 15(4):351-361.

Brown, M., MacArthur, J., McKechanie, A., Mack, S., Hayes, M., and Fletcher, J. 2011. Learning disability liaison nursing services in south-east Scotland: A mixed-methods impact and outcome study. Journal of *Intellectual Disability Research*, doi: 10.1111/j.1365-2788.2011.01511.x

Care Quality Commission. 2012. *Learning Disability Services Inspection Programme– National Overview.* Newcastle upon Tyne: CQC.

Cooper, S.A., McConnachie, A., Allan, L., Melville, C., Smiley, E., and Morrison, J. 2011. Neighbourhood deprivation, health inequalities and service access by adults with intellectual disabilities: A cross-sectional study. *Journal of Intellectual Disability Research,* 55(3):313–323.

Department of Health and Social Security. 1971. *Better Services for the Mentally Handicapped* (Cmnd 4683). London: HMSO.

DoH. 2001. *Valuing People. A New Strategy for the 21st Century.* London: TSO.

DoH. 2004. *The NHS Knowledge and Skills Framework (NHS KSF) and the Development Review Process.* London: Department of Health.

DoH. 2007a. *Tackling Health Inequalities.* London: Department of Health.

DoH. 2007b. *Good Practice Guide in Learning Disabilities Nursing.* London: Department of Health.

DoH. 2008. *Health Care for All: Independent Inquiry into Access to Health Care for People with Learning Disabilities.* London: HMSO.

Disability Rights Commission (DRC). 2006. *Equal Treatment: Closing the Gap.* Stratford Upon Avon: Disability Rights Commission.

Durvasula, S., Beange, H., and Baker, W. 2002. Mortality of people with intellectual disability in northern Sydney. *Journal of Intellectual and Developmental Disability,* 27(4):255–264.

Emerson, E. and Baines, S. 2010. *Health Inequalities & People with Learning Disabilities in the UK.* London: HMSO.

Emerson, E. and Glover, G. 2010. Health checks for people with learning disabilities 2008/9 & 2009/10. Improving Health and Lives Learning Disabilities Observatory. (Online). Available at www.phine.org.uk/uploads/doc/vid_7393_health_checks.pdf (accessed March 13, 2014).

Emerson, E., Copeland, A., and Glover, G. 2011. The uptake of health checks for adults with learning disabilities: 2008/9 to 2010/11. (Online). Available at http://www.improvinghealthandlives.org.uk/publications/972/Health_Checks_For_People_With_Learning_Disabilities_2010–11 (accessed March 13, 2014).

Faugier, J. (2004). The predictions of nursing leaders. *Nursing Times,* 100(4):20–21.

Felce, J. and Kerr, M. 2008. The impact of checking the health of adults with intellectual disabilities on primary care consultation rates, health promotion and contact with specialists. *Journal of Applied Research in Intellectual Disabilities,* 21(6):597–602.

Ford, S. 2011. New nurse-led prison health service launched in Surrey. *Nursing Times.* (Online). Available at http://www.nursingtimes.net/nursing-practice/clinical-zones/mental-health/new-nurse-led-prison-health-service-launched-in-surrey/5034866.article (accessed May 25, 2014).

Gates, B. 2011. *Learning Disability Nursing: Task and Finish Group Report for the Professional and Advisory Board for Nursing and Midwifery—Department of Health, England.* Hatfield: University of Hertfordshire.

Ham, C. 2004. *Health Policy in Britain: The Politics and Organisation of the National Health Service* (5th ed.). Basingstoke: Palgrave MacMillan.

Heslop, P., Blair, P., Fleming, P., Hoghton, M., Marriott, A., and Russ, L. 2013. *The Confidential Inquiry into Premature Deaths of People with Learning Disabilities (CIPOLD).* Bristol: Norah Fry Research Centre.

Hollins, S., Attard, M.T., von Fraunhofer, N., McGuigan, S., and Sedgwick, P. 1998. Mortality in people with learning disability: Risks, causes, and death certification findings in London. *Developmental Medicine and Child Neurology,* 40(1):50–56.

Iacono, T. and Davis, R. 2003. The experiences of people with developmental disability in emergency departments and hospital wards. *Research in Developmental Disabilities,* 24(4):247–264.

Jackson, M. 2000. The allure of history. *British Journal of Learning Disability,* 28(2):45–57.

Janicki, M.P. 2001. Toward a rationale strategy for promoting healthy ageing amongst people with intellectual disabilities. *Journal of Applied Research in Intellectual Disabilities,* 14(3):171–174.

Janicki, M.P., Davidson, P.W., Henderson, C.M., McCallion, P., Taets, J.D., Force, L.T., Sulkes, S.B, Frangenberg, E., and Ladrigan, P.M. 2002. Health characteristics and health services utilization in older adults with intellectual disability living in community residences. *Journal of Intellectual Disability Research,* 46(4):287–298.

Jones, R.G. and Kerr, M.P. 1997. A randomised control trial of an opportunistic health screening tool in primary care for people with learning disability. *Journal of Learning Disability Research,* 41(5):409–415.

Jones, A. and Jones, M. 2005. Mental health nurse prescribing: Issues for the UK. *Journal of Psychiatric and Mental Health Nursing,* 12(5):527–535.

Kerr, M. 2004. Improving the general health of people with learning disabilities. *Advances in Psychiatric Treatment,* 10:200–206.

Kwentoh, M. and Reilly, J. 2009. Non-medical prescribing: The story so far. *The Psychiatric Bulletin,* 33:4–7. doi: 10.1192/pb.bp.107.019075.

Lennox, N. and Diggins, J.N. 1999. *Management Guidelines: People with Developmental and Intellectual Disabilities.* Melbourne: Therapeutic Guidelines Ltd.

Lennox, N., Beange, H., and Edwards, N. 2000. The health needs of people with intellectual disability. *Medical Journal of Australia,* 173 (6):328–330.

Linna, S.L., Moilanen, I., Ebeling, H., Piha, J., Kumpulainen, K., Tamminen, T., and Almqvist, F. 1999. Psychiatric symptoms in children with intellectual disability. *European Child and Adolescent Psychiatry,* 8 (suppl 4):77–82.

Llewellyn, P. and Northway, R. 2007. The views and experiences of learning disability nurses concerning their advocacy education. *Nurse Education Today,* 27(8):955–963.

Llewellyn, P.J. 2005. *An investigation into the advocacy role of the learning disability nurse.* Unpublished PhD thesis, University of Glamorgan.

Loucks, N. 2007. *No One Knows: Offenders with Learning Difficulties and Learning Disabilities—A Review of Prevalence and Associated Needs.* London: Prison Reform Trust.

Mafuba, K. 2013. 'Public Health: Community Learning Disability Nurses' Perception and Experience of Their Role'. Unpublished PhD Thesis, University of West London.

Marshall, D. and Moore, G. 2003. Obesity in people with intellectual disabilities: The impact of nurse-led health screenings and health promotion activities. *Journal of Advanced Nursing,* 41(2):147–153.

McIlfatrick, S., Taggart, L., and Truesdale-Kennedy, M. 2011. Supporting women with intellectual disabilities to access breast cancer screening: A healthcare professional perspective. *European Journal of Cancer Care,* 20(3):412–420.

Melville, C.A., Finlayson, J., Cooper, S.A., Allan, L., Robinson, N., Burns, E., Martin, G., and Morrison J. 2005. Enhancing primary healthcare services for adults with intellectual disabilities. *Journal of Intellectual Disability Research,* 49(3):190–198.

Melville, C.A., Cooper S.A., Morrison I.J., Finlayson J., Allan, L., Robinson N., Burns E., and Martin, G. 2006. The outcomes of an intervention study to reduce the barriers experienced by people with intellectual disabilities accessing primary healthcare services. *Journal of Intellectual Disability Research,* 50(1):11–17.

Mencap. 2004. *Treat Me Right! Better Health for People with Learning Disabilities.* London: Mencap.

Mencap. 2007. *Death by Indifference. Following Up the Treat Me Right Report.* London: Mencap.

Mencap. 2012. *Death by Indifference: 74 Deaths and Counting.* London: Mencap.

Messent, P.R., Cooke, C.B., and Long, J. 1999. What choice: A consideration of the level of opportunity for people with mild and moderate learning disabilities to lead a physically active healthy lifestyle. *British Journal of Learning Disabilities,* 27(2):73–77.

Michael, J. 2008. *Healthcare for All: Report of the Independent Inquiry into Access to Healthcare for People with Learning Disabilities.* London: Department of Health.

NHS Health Scotland. 2004. *Health Needs Assessment Report: People with Learning Disability in Scotland.* Glasgow: NHS Health Scotland.

NMC. 2010. *Standards for Pre-Registration Nurse Education.* London: Nursing and Midwifery Council.

Nocon, A., Sayce, L., and Nadirshaw, Z. 2008. Health inequalities experienced by people with learning disabilities: Problems and possibilities in primary care. *Learning Disability Review,* 13(1):28–36.

O'Toole, L.J. 2004. The theory–practice issue in policy implementation research. *Public Administration,* 82(2):309–329.

Parahoo, K., Barr, O., and McCaughan, E. 2000. Research utilization and attitudes towards research among learning disability nurses in Northern Ireland. *Journal of Advanced Nursing,* 29(1):607-613.

Pawar, D.G. and Akuffo, E.O. 2008. Comparative survey of comorbidities in people with learning disability with and without epilepsy. *The Psychiatrist,* 32:224–226.

Phillips A., Morrison J., and Davis R.W. 2004. General practitioners' educational needs in intellectual disability health. *Journal of Intellectual Disability Research,* 48(2):142–149.

Powell, H., Murray, G., and McKenzie, K. 2004. Staff perceptions of community learning disability nurses' role. *Nursing Times,* 100(19):40–42.

Powrie, E. 2003. Primary healthcare provision for adults with a learning disability. *Journal of Advanced Nursing,* 42(4):413–423.

Public Health Nursing Division. 2014. *Strengthening the Commitment: One Year On—Progress Report on the UK Modernising Learning Disabilities Nursing.* London: Department of Health.

Royal College of Nursing. 2004. *Promoting Excellence in Care Through Research and Development: An RCN Position Statement.* London: RCN.

Royal College of Nursing. 2009. *Health and Nursing Care in the Criminal Justice Services.* London: RCN.

Ryan, R. and Sunada, K. 1997. Medical evaluations of persons with mental retardation referred for psychiatric assessment. *General Hospital Psychiatry,* 19(4):274–280.

Scheepers, M., Kerr, M.O., Hara, D., Bainbridge, D., Cooper, S.A., Davis, R., Fujiura, G., Heller, T., Holland, A., Krahn, G., Lennox N., Meany, J., and Wehmeyer, M. 2005. Reducing health disparity in people with intellectual disabilities: A report from Health Issues Special Interest Research Group of the International Association for the Scientific Study of Intellectual Disabilities. *Journal of Policy and Practice in Intellectual Disabilities,* 2(3-4):249–255.

Scottish Executive. 2000. *The Same as You.* Edinburgh: Scottish Executive.

Stewart, D. and Todd, M. 2001. Role and contribution of nurses for learning disabilities: A local study in a county of Oxford-Anglia region. *British Journal of Learning Disabilities,* 29(4):145–150.

Straetmans, J.M.J.A.A., van Schrojenstein Lantman-de Valk, H.M.J., Schellevis, F.G., and Dinant, G.J. 2007. Health problems of people with intellectual disabilities: The impact for general practice. *British Journal of General Practice,* 57(534):64–66.

The National Development Team. 2013. The Health Equalities Framework. (Online). Available at http://www.ndti.org.uk/uploads/files/The_Health_Equality_Framework.pdf (accessed May 24, 2014).

The Scottish Government. 2000. The same as you. (Online). Available at http://www.scotland.gov.uk/Resource/Doc/1095/0001661.pdf (accessed May 24, 2014).

Thomas, G. and Kerr, M.P. 2011. Longitudinal follow-up of weight change in the context of a community-based health promotion programme for adults with intellectual disability. *Journal of Applied Research in Intellectual Disabilities,* 24(4):381–387.

Thornton, C. 1996. A focus group inquiry into the perceptions of primary healthcare teams and the provision of healthcare for adults with learning disability living in the community. *Journal of Advanced Nursing,* 23(6):1168–1176.

Torr J., and Davis R. (2007). Ageing and mental health problems in people with intellectual disability. *Current Opinion in Psychiatry,* 20(5):467-471.

UK Learning Disability Consultant Nurse Network (2006). Shaping the future: A vision for learning disability nursing. (Online). Available at http://www.rcn.org.uk/__data/assets/pdf_file/0009/354384/Shaping_the_Future_Vision_document_July_2006.pdf (accessed May 23, 2014).

UK Modernising Learning Disabilities Nursing Review. 2012. *Strengthening the Commitment* (Report). Edinburgh: The Scottish Government.

van Schrojenstein Lantman-de Valk, H.M.J., Metsemakers J.F.M., Haveman, M.J., and Crebolder, H.F.J.M. 2000. Health problems in people with intellectual disability in general practice: A comparative study. *Family Practice,* 17(5):405–407.

Webb, O.J. and Rogers, L. 1999. Health screening for people with intellectual disability: The New Zealand experience. *Journal of Intellectual Disability Research,* 43(6):497–503.

Wood, R. and Douglas, M. 2007. Cervical screening for women with learning disability: Current practice and attitudes within primary care in Edinburgh. *British Journal of Learning Disabilities,* 35(2):84–92.

FURTHER READING

Atkinson, D., Boulter, P., Hebron, C., Moulster, G., Giraud-Saunders, A. and Turner, S. 2013. *The Health Equalities Framework (HEF)-An Outcomes Framework Based on the Determinants of Health Inequalities.* http://www.ndti.org.uk/uploads/files/The_Health_Equality_Framework.pdf

Strengthening the Commitment. 2013. https://www.gov.uk/government/uploads/system/uploads/attachment_data/file/304762/Strengthening_the_commitment_one_year_on.pdf

USEFUL RESOURCES

An Bord Altranais: http://www.nursingboard.ie/en/reqs_stds_reg.aspx

Learning Disability Observatory (Public Health England): http://www.improvinghealthandlives.org.uk

NHS Careers: http://www.nhscareers.nhs.uk/explore-by-career/nursing/careers-in-nursing/learning-disabilities-nursing/

Nursing and Midwifery Council: http://standards.nmc-uk.org/Pages/Welcome.aspx

Skills for Health: http://www.skillsforhealth.org.uk/workforce-transformation/role-redesign-service/

The Health Equalities Framework: http://www.ndti.org.uk/uploads/files/The_Health_Equality_Framework.pdf

The Knowledge Network: http://www.knowledge.scot.nhs.uk/home/portals-and-topics/learning-disabilities-portal.aspx

NMC competencies for entry to the register

Learning disability nursing

Domain 1: Professional values

Field standard for competence

Learning disabilities nurses must promote the individuality, independence, rights, choice, and social inclusion of people with learning disabilities and highlight their strengths and abilities at all times while encouraging others do the same. They must facilitate the active participation of families and carers.

Competencies

1.1 Learning disabilities nurses must understand and apply current legislation to all service users, paying special attention to the protection of vulnerable people, including those with complex needs arising from ageing, cognitive impairment, and long-term conditions, and those approaching the end of life.

2.1 Learning disabilities nurses must always promote the autonomy, rights, and choices of people with learning disabilities and support and involve their families and carers, ensuring that each person's rights are upheld according to policy and the law.

3.1 Learning disabilities nurses must use their knowledge and skills to exercise professional advocacy, and recognise when it is appropriate to refer to independent advocacy services to safeguard dignity and human rights.

4.1 Learning disabilities nurses must recognise that people with learning disabilities are full and equal citizens, and must promote their health and well being by focusing on and developing their strengths and abilities.

Domain 2: Communication and interpersonal skills

Field standard for competence

Learning disabilities nurses must use complex communication and interpersonal skills and strategies to work with people of all ages who have learning disabilities and help them to express themselves. Such nurses must also be able to communicate and negotiate effectively with other professionals, services, and agencies, and ensure that people with learning disabilities, their families, and their carers are fully involved in decision making.

(continued)

Competencies

1.1 Learning disabilities nurses must use the full range of person-centred alternative and augmentative communication strategies and skills to build partnerships and therapeutic relationships with people with learning disabilities.

2.1 Learning disabilities nurses must be able to make all relevant information accessible to and understandable by people with learning disabilities, including adaptation of format, presentation, and delivery.

3.1 Learning disabilities nurses must use a structured approach to assess, communicate with, interpret, and respond therapeutically to people with learning disabilities who have complex physical and psychological health needs, or those in behavioural distress.

4.1 Learning disabilities nurses must recognise and respond therapeutically to the complex behaviour that people with learning disabilities may use as a means to communicate.

Domain 3: Nursing practice and decision making

Field standard for competence

Learning disabilities nurses must have an enhanced knowledge of the health and developmental needs of all people with learning disabilities and the factors that might influence them. Such nurses must aim to improve and maintain their health and independence through skilled direct and indirect nursing care. They must also be able to provide direct care to meet the essential and complex physical and mental health needs of people with learning disabilities.

Competencies

1.1 Learning disabilities nurses must be able to recognise and respond to the needs of all people who come into their care, including babies, children and young people, pregnant and postnatal women, people with mental health problems, people with physical health problems and disabilities, older people, and people with long-term problems such as cognitive impairment.

3.1 Learning disabilities nurses must use a structured, person-centred approach to assess, interpret, and respond therapeutically to people with learning disabilities, and their often complex pre-existing physical and psychological health needs. Such nurses must work in partnership with service users, carers, and other professionals, services, and agencies to agree on and implement individual care plans and ensure continuity of care.

5.1 Learning disabilities nurses must lead the development, implementation, and review of individual plans for all people with learning disabilities to promote their optimum health and well being and facilitate their equal access to all health, social care, and specialist services.

8.1 Learning disabilities nurses must work in partnership with people with learning disabilities and their families and carers to facilitate choice and maximise self-care and self-management and coordinate the transition between different services and agencies.

Domain 4: Leadership, management and team working

Field standard for competence

Learning disabilities nurses must exercise collaborative management, delegation and supervision skills to create, manage and support therapeutic environments for people with learning disabilities.

Competencies

1.1 Learning disabilities nurses must take the lead in ensuring that people with learning disabilities receive support that creatively addresses their physical, social, economic, psychological, spiritual, and other needs when assessing, planning, and delivering care.

1.2 Learning disabilities nurses must provide direction through leadership and education to ensure that their unique contribution is recognised in service design and provision.

2.1 Learning disabilities nurses must use data and research findings about the health of people with learning disabilities to help improve people's experiences and care outcomes and shape of future services.

6.1 Learning disabilities nurses must use leadership, influencing, and decision-making skills to engage effectively with a range of agencies and professionals. Such nurses must also be able, when necessary, to represent the health needs and protect the rights of people with learning disabilities and challenge negative stereotypes.

6.2 Learning disabilities nurses must work closely with stakeholders to enable people with learning disabilities to exercise choice and challenge discrimination.

B An Bord Altranais' competencies for entry to the register*

Domain 1. Professional/ethical practice	Indicators
1.1. Practices in accordance with legislation affecting nursing practice.	1. Integrates accurate and comprehensive knowledge of ethical principles, the Code of Professional Conduct, and within the scope of professional nursing practice in the delivery of nursing practice. 2. Fulfills the duty of care in the course of nursing practice. 3. Implements the philosophies, policies, protocols, and clinical guidelines of the health care institution. 4. Responds appropriately to instances of unsafe or unprofessional practice. 5. Integrates knowledge of the rights of clients and groups in the health care setting. 6. Serves as an advocate for the rights of clients or groups. 7. Ensures confidentiality with respect to records and interactions. 8. Practices in a way that acknowledges the differences in beliefs and cultural practices of individuals, groups, or communities.
1.2. Practices within the limits of own competence and takes measures to develop own competence.	1. Determines own scope of practice utilising the principles for determining scope of practice in the Scope of Nursing and Midwifery Practice Framework document. 2. Recognises own abilities and level of professional competence. 3. Accepts responsibility and accountability for consequences of own actions or omissions. 4. Consults with supervisors if allocated nursing assignments are beyond competence. 5. Clarifies unclear or inappropriate instructions. 6. Formulates decisions about care within the scope of professional nursing practice utilising the Decision-Making Framework in the Scope of Nursing and Midwifery Practice Framework document.

* An Bord Altranais. 2005. *Requirements and Standards for Nurse Registration Education Programmes* (3rd ed.). Dublin: An Bord Altranis.

Domain 2. Holistic approaches to care and the integration of knowledge	Indicators
2.1. Conducts a systematic holistic assessment of client needs based on nursing theory and evidence-based practice.	1. Uses an appropriate assessment framework safely and accurately. 2. Analyses data accurately and comprehensively, leading to appropriate identification of findings. 3. Incorporates relevant research findings into nursing practice. 4. Promotes research designed to improve nursing practice.
2.2. Plans care in consultation with the client taking into consideration the therapeutic regimes of all members of the health care team.	1. Establishes priorities for resolution of identified health needs. 2. Identifies expected outcomes, including a time frame for achievement. 3. Identifies criteria for the evaluation of the expected outcomes. 4. Plans for discharge and follow-up care.
2.3. Implements planned nursing care/interventions to achieve the identified outcomes.	1. Delivers nursing care in accordance with the plan that is accurate, safe, comprehensive, and effective. 2. Creates and maintains a physical, psychosocial, and spiritual environment that promotes safety, security, and optimal health. 3. Provides for the comfort needs of individuals. 4. Acts to enhance the dignity and integrity of individuals, clients, groups, or communities.
2.4. Evaluates client progress toward expected outcomes and reviews plans in accordance with evaluation data and in consultation with the client.	1. Assesses the effectiveness of nursing care in achieving the planned outcomes. 2. Determines further outcomes and nursing interventions in accordance with evaluation data and consultation with the client.
Domain 3. Interpersonal relationships	Indicators
3.1. Establishes and maintains caring therapeutic interpersonal relationships with individuals, clients, groups, or communities.	1. Reflects on the usefulness of personal communication techniques. 2. Conducts nursing care, ensuring that clients receive and understand relevant and current information about health care. 3. Assists clients, groups, or communities to communicate needs and to make informed decisions.
3.2. Collaborates with all members of the health care team and documents relevant information.	1. Participates with all health care personnel in a collaborative effort directed toward decision making about clients. 2. Establishes and maintains accurate, clear, and current client records within a legal and ethical framework.

Domain 4. Organisation and management of care	Indicators
4.1. Effectively manages the nursing care of clients, groups, or communities.	1. Contributes to the overall goal or mission of the health care institution. 2. Demonstrates the ability to work as a team member. 3. Determines priorities for care based on need, acuity, and optimal time for intervention. 4. Selects and utilises resources effectively and efficiently. 5. Utilises methods to demonstrate quality assurance and quality management.
4.2. Delegates to other nurses activities commensurate with their competence and within their scope of professional practice.	1. When delegating a particular role or function, takes account of the principles outlined in the Scope of Nursing and Midwifery Practice Framework.
4.3. Facilitates the coordination of care.	1. Works with all team members to ensure that client care is appropriate, effective, and consistent.
Domain 5. Personal and professional development	Indicators
5.1. Acts to enhance the personal and professional development of self and others.	1. Demonstrates a commitment to life-long learning. 2. Contributes to the learning experiences of colleagues through support, supervision, and teaching. 3. Educates clients, groups, or communities to maintain and promote health.

Index